7 STEPS TO GET OFF SUGAR AND CARBOHYDRATES

HEALTHY EATING FOR HEALTHY LIVING WITH A LOW-CARBOHYDRATE, ANTI-INFLAMMATORY DIET

SUSAN NEAL RN, MBA, MHS

CHRISTIAN INDIE
PUBLISHING

Editor: Janis Whipple

Cover Design: Angie Alaya

ISBN: 978-0-997-76366-9

Printed in the United States of America

I would like to dedicate this book to my sister, Kim. I am proud of you for getting off sugar and refined carbohydrates. Thank you for allowing me to share your story so that others may benefit from it. May God bless you.

CONTENTS

DISCLAIMER

Medical Disclaimer: This book offers health and nutritional information, which is for educational purposes only. The information provided in this book is designed to help individuals make informed decisions about their health; it is intended to supplement, not replace, the professional medical advice, diagnosis, or treatment of health conditions from a trained medical professional. Please consult your physician or healthcare provider before beginning or changing any health or eating habits to make sure that it is appropriate for you. If you have any concerns or questions about your health, you should always ask a physician or other healthcare provider. Please do not disregard, avoid, or delay obtaining medical or health-related advice from your healthcare professional because of something you may have read in this book. The author and publisher assumes no responsibility for any injury that may result from changing your health or eating habits.

Disclaimer and Terms of Use: Every effort has been made to ensure the information in this book is accurate and complete. However, the author and publisher do not warrant the accuracy or completeness of the material, text, and graphics contained in this book. The author and publisher do not hold any responsibility for

A FREE GIFT FOR YOU

I am excited you decided to take this journey of health and wellness. To help you succeed, I included ten appendices chock-full of plans, strategies, and summarized information. To receive a printable version of the appendices please go to SusanUNeal.com/appendix.

I created the Healthy Living Blog to provide you with helpful articles, menus, recipes, and lifestyle tips. You can subscribe to it at SusanUNeal.com/Healthy-Living-Blog.

In addition, feel free to join my closed Facebook group: 7 Steps to Get Off Sugar, Carbs, and Gluten and let me know how you are doing. In this group, I am available to answer all of your questions. I have another Facebook page, Healthy Living Series, to keep you up to date with relevant information about maintaining a healthy lifestyle at Facebook.com/HealthyLivingSeries/.

The two additional books contained in the Healthy Living Series include *Christian Study for 7 Steps to Get Off Sugar and Carbohydrates* and *Healthy Living Journal.* The mega book, *Healthy Living Series: 3 Books in 1* includes all three of the books.

If you need additional support making this lifestyle change, purchase my course, 7 Steps to Reclaim Your Health and Optimal Weight (https://susanuneal.com/courses/7-steps-to-get-off-sugar-and-carbs-course). In this course I walk you through all the material covered in my Healthy Living Series. I help you change your eating habits once and for all.

INTRODUCTION

Chronic diseases are an epidemic today, and many of them can be prevented or reversed. Excess weight and health issues may be keeping you from having a life of abundance now and in the future. Weight problems lead to other issues—lack of energy, trouble buying clothes, stress from diets, difficulty moving or keeping up with family members, physical ailments and pain, financial burdens from health-care visits and medications. Not to mention the emotional and spiritual struggles, such as self-consciousness about your appearance and how this affects the activities you choose to be involved in, or feeling you missed out on years of being who God created you to be.

If you relate to any of these struggles, would you like to improve the way you feel and look while increasing your energy level and clarity of mind? How about losing weight naturally without going on a fad diet or buying prepared meals and supplements? You can achieve these results through simply changing the types of food you eat.

As a registered nurse (RN) with a master of health science, I research and study healthy eating lifestyles to determine which foods are best for the human body. Knowing what foods to eat and avoid is essential to prevent food-related illnesses. I also understand the addictive nature of sugar and wheat and what it does to our bodies. When we consume sugar or wheat, dopamine releases in the brain, which drives us to eat more. Therefore, these products are biochemically addictive, and we must understand this so we can make the changes necessary for our health.

If anyone was addicted to sugar, it was my sister. She loved sweets. Doughnuts in the morning, soft drinks throughout the day, bread, pasta, chocolate, and candy—you get the picture. She has been overweight since she was a child. She suffered from joint pain and irritable bowel syndrome. She never knew when a specific food might set her off and she would need to be close to a bathroom for a whole day.

Being physically ill is only one aspect of how food addictions affect people. Not fitting into clothes and feeling unattractive can undermine a person's self-esteem. Then their pocketbooks are gouged, as they need to buy new clothes because the old ones don't fit. Does this sound familiar? Do you crave carbs too? When my sister was forty-nine, she asked me to help her get off sugar and carbohydrates. From my experience, this is difficult to do, so I created a seven-step plan for her to follow:

7 Steps to Get Off Sugar and Carbohydrates

1. **Decide** to improve your health through proper nutrition.
2. **Acquire** a support system and knowledge to help make a lifestyle change.
3. **Clean out** the pantry and refrigerator by removing unhealthy foods and clean out your emotions.
4. **Purchase** healthy foods plus an anti-Candida cleanse.
5. **Plan** for the start date to begin changing your eating habits.
6. **Prepare** and eat foods differently than you did before.
7. **Improve** your health through continuing this new lifestyle, never turning back to your old eating habits.

My sister not only took the seven-step plan to heart but she allowed me to share her story with you, in the hopes it will encourage you to try the plan yourself. The first time my sister tried this plan she was successful with getting off wheat because she'd tested positive for gluten sensitivity, and when she eliminated wheat her irritable bowel symptoms disappeared. This lifestyle change was easier for her because a physical pain disappeared. However, she continued to eat sugary foods, not recognizing their affect on her health. Finally, one year later, she had another health crisis, and successfully implemented the full plan.

One week after getting off sugars and refined carbohydrates, my sister's energy and rosacea skin condition improved. By the second week, her joints no longer ached, and the craving for sugar subsided. Two months later, she'd lost ten pounds and felt energized. After that, she lost five pounds per month until she got to her ideal weight and her rosacea disappeared.

If you choose to embark on this seven-step plan, you will radically improve your health and energy by merely removing sugars and refined carbohydrates. However, this plan is not a diet, where once you complete the seven steps, you're done. This is a *lifestyle change*. Typically, diets are unsuccessful because after people lose their desired weight, they go back to old eating habits, which caused them to gain weight in the first place, and find themselves facing the same challenges again and again.

The seven steps provided here are designed to incorporate your entire self—mind, body, and spirit—in making this lifestyle change so you can experience a new future, instead of another yo-yo diet that sends you back to square one. The specific instructions regarding these seven steps are provided in the next seven chapters. Each chapter begins with the following diagram, with the phase reviewed in that chapter in bold.

Decide—>Acquire—>Clean Out—>Purchase—>Plan—>Prepare—>Improve

I am excited you chose to join me on this path to wellness. God gave you a glorious body that is programmed to heal itself, if we provide it with the proper nutrition he intended. I applaud you for having the courage to take on the challenge to reclaim your body and life. I pray that God will help you and walk beside you during this journey to health.

If you have an emotional connection with food, please consider using the *Christian Study Guide for 7 Steps to Get Off Sugar and Carbohydrates*. Whether you do this study by yourself or with a group, it will help you go more in-depth to resolve an emotional issue once and for all. Please join my closed Facebook group: 7 Steps to Get Off Sugar and Carbohydrates and share with me how you are doing.

STEP 1: DECIDE TO IMPROVE YOUR HEALTH

Decide—>Acquire—>Clean Out—>Purchase—>Plan—>Prepare—>Improve

If you are motivated to start making progress toward health and even weight loss, you can't skip this first step. While you may want to get right to a food list or recipes, you can't create a new lifestyle of eating and nutrition without deciding to do what is necessary to make that change. To decide is to make a definitive choice. Make a decision to commit to implementing all seven steps. Your health is worth it.

One reason it is difficult for many to stick to decisions about food is that their bodies betray their mental commitment. That's why this book will explain how addictions affect us physically, so we can be prepared with the mental ammunition needed to stay strong. Sweets and refined carbohydrates are addictive and harmful to the human body. This book provides step-by-step instructions on how to stop the cravings and unwanted symptoms associated with eating a diet loaded with carbs. We will explore the possibility of a food addiction and candida infection of the gut. You will gain an understanding of the types of food to avoid and why. Once you have the knowledge you need to make the right decision for your health, you'll be better equipped to make the next step, and the next, until you've changed your lifestyle. With your lifestyle change, you will live the abundant life Jesus wants you to experience, not a life filled with disease and unwanted, unhealthy symptoms.

THE TROUBLE WITH SUGAR AND CARBS

One of the worst carbohydrate culprits is wheat because a polypeptide in wheat crosses the blood-brain barrier, which separates the bloodstream from the brain, and binds to the brain's morphine receptors.[1] Opiate drugs (morphine, codeine, heroin, cocaine) bind to these same receptors. Unbeknownst to us, when we eat a bagel for breakfast, we consume our crack for the day.

Take the time now to watch this five-minute Ted-Ed video, "How Does Sugar Affect the Brain?" by the neuroscientist Nicole Avena, Ph.D. Go to https://www.sciencealert.com/watch-this-is-how-sugar-affects-your-brain.[2] This video explains how we get hooked on foods with a high sugar content.

As you learned from the video, sugar causes the release of dopamine in the brain, which is part of our bodies' feel-good reward system. We enjoy the feeling of dopamine, so we keep eating carbs. Sugary foods include a food item with greater than ten grams of sugar per serving. Refined carbohydrates include rice, wheat, instant mashed potatoes, instant oatmeal, cereals, potato chips, crackers, etc. At some point, an overconsumption of sugar and refined carbohydrates rewires the brain's neural pathways and causes a person to become addicted. The brain's hijacking triggers binge eating despite its consequences of weight gain and health problems. Therefore, getting off sugar is more complex than it may seem. It is no longer about willpower and self-discipline but a *biochemical addiction*. However, we can untangle the brain's rewiring to reset it back to normal, but we need to implement all the steps outlined in this book.

We live in a culture of entitlement—where we feel we deserve to satisfy ourselves to our heart's content. Countless varieties of delicious, unhealthy foods are available to us at a whim. Even the commercials on TV entice us to indulge. It is amazing that everyone in our culture has not fallen into the *food addiction trap*. Entitlement leads to indulging, which leads to addiction. It is a slippery slope once you take your first bite of that addictive food. Down the slope you fall as you consume the whole package—which you did not intend to do. If you are addicted, you can't rely on moderation. You need to understand what is causing you to consume foods in a manner you do not want to. The average American ingests up to a staggering 150 pounds of sugar each year.[3] We eat foodlike substances full of sugar and wheat, packaged in colorful, enticing boxes and bags. These so-called foods are frequently inexpensive, as well as quick and easy to prepare. We fill that immediate craving without thinking of its long-term consequences.

However, the actual cost of a steady diet of super-processed, prepackaged foods will eventually show up in chronically poor health, increased medical costs, and use of pharmaceuticals. Doctors treat the symptoms of these chronic diseases with drugs, but they usually do not address the underlying cause. Nutritious foods prevent and even reverse conditions better than expensive medications.

Over 100 million Americans suffer from chronic, painful, expensive, and often debilitating diseases. One of the dominant causes of chronic diseases in the United States is the poor quality of food consumed. When we eat processed foodstuff, we do not provide our bodies with the nutrient-filled foods God created for humans to eat.

Food industries entice consumers to eat more of their products not to improve people's health but to improve the corporations' pocketbooks. These industries put sugar in products to lure us to buy more because they understand its addictive quality. During our seven steps, you will learn about the types of food to avoid to improve your health. You'll be educated to fight back against the food industries' tactics.

NOURISH YOUR AMAZING BODY

I am intrigued with improving the functioning of the human body. Our bodies work best when we supply them with the proper nutrition God intended. God programmed our bodies to heal themselves—like the natural healing of a cut or sprained ankle.

God gave us glorious bodies that can repair themselves of many ailments if we nourish them well. In turn, *when we are healthy, we can serve God better.* Unfortunately, when tired, foggy brained, or downright ill, we focus on ourselves instead of serving him. If you want to improve the way you feel, *make the decision* to stop eating sugar and refined carbohydrates. This is the first step of the seven-step plan.

If you choose to adopt this lifestyle, you will lose weight, but more importantly, you will improve your health. You won't starve yourself either. Recently, a friend on a cruise told me, "You eat as much as I do. How do you stay slender?" I replied, "The types of food I eat make the difference."

Many times, we do not make positive changes to improve our health until we experience a crisis. For my sister, it was rosacea. While on vacation, she got a rash all over her face. She FaceTimed me and I could see the raised, rough areas of skin. The red bumps came to a head as unsightly pustules. In her high-pitched, stressed voice she asked what I thought it might be. I didn't know, but I suggested she consult her dermatologist as soon as she returned from vacation.

The doctor wasn't sure if it was psoriasis or rosacea. He gave her two creams for her face and an antibiotic to ingest. The creams and antibiotics helped the rash go away, but as soon as she quit taking them, the outbreak came right back. A month later, her dermatologist confirmed the diagnosis of rosacea, which has no cure. Either she stayed on the medications for the rest of her life, or the rosacea reappeared.

She decided to do some research (*acquired* knowledge—step 2) of her own. She discovered sugary foods exacerbate rosacea. When she evaluated what she ate, she realized that sweets and refined carbohydrates made up a large part of her diet. However, she did not like the red, bumpy rash on her face, so she decided to make a change (*decide*—step 1). Throughout this book, we will learn about the steps she took to make a lifestyle change to heal herself of rosacea. If you choose to change your eating habits, your body may heal itself of an ailment too.

MY HEALTH CRISIS

I combated a health crisis at the age of forty-nine. In November that year, I had a crown placed on a tooth. Little did I know how that would mark the beginning of losing my good health. Ultimately, over the next nine months, this tooth abscessed and poisoned my body, resulting in ten different medical diagnoses.

One month after the crown, I began having two menstrual cycles every month. The double periods continued, and eventually, fifteen months later, I had surgery to remove two uterine polyps.

Two months later, I experienced depression and craved chocolate. Do you crave chocolate? Where I used to eat a couple of candy bars per year, now I binged on Ghirardelli chocolate every evening.

In March, I was diagnosed with an ovarian cyst, and two months later, adrenal fatigue. Although exhausted, I had difficulty sleeping. By this point, I should have known something was wrong with my body. Nevertheless, I didn't realize the severity of my physical problems even though as a Christian yoga instructor I taught my clients to be in tune with their bodies.

My doctor prescribed three different adrenal vitamins five times a day for my adrenal fatigue. That's fifteen vitamin pills per day! The physician also prescribed progesterone cream for the ovarian cyst and hormonal imbalance, as I was experiencing perimenopause. That summer I was so exhausted that I could not attend my aunt's funeral because I had no stamina to fly across the country. Even my husband and children did not understand how depleted I felt.

In July I saw flashes of light in my left eye when I quickly turned my head to the left. Two months later I was diagnosed with a hole in my retina. Retinal tears can lead to blindness if the retina becomes detached.

In August, I began experiencing visual migraines even though I had never suffered from headaches. That month I went to my dentist for a cleaning and told my hygienist I felt a bump above one of my teeth. She informed me that was not a good sign, and the dentist discovered the tooth I had crowned in November had abscessed and drained its putrid fluid into my gastrointestinal system. I still didn't realize that the affects of my abscessed tooth likely caused all the other symptoms.

I had an emergency root canal along with ten days of antibiotics and two weeks of steroids. Afterward, I was so fatigued I could not put away the groceries after shopping. No one understood how depleted my system was because on the outside I looked fine, but on the inside, I was a train wreck.

In September my doctor found I was anemic and low in vitamin D, so he told me to take iron and vitamin D supplements. He also referred me to an optometrist for the flashes of light in my eye. The optometrist performed emergency laser surgery to prevent a detached retina. When I turn my head sharply to the left, I still have a flash of light, and I will never regain that part of my vision.

In the fall, my health further declined. I felt utterly drained and sick all the time, and I could have easily stayed in bed. However, my family needed me. My doctors were unable to do much for me except recommend vitamin D, iron supplements, adrenal vitamins, and progesterone cream. So I began alternative health-care therapies such as massage, acupuncture, and colonic irrigation.

Through a colonic irrigation, the therapist found a candida infection in my colon. I had never heard of this type of infection before despite being an RN since candidiasis (candida infection from a Candida fungus) of the gut is not taught in mainstream medicine. Even my internal medicine doctor didn't know how to rid me of this yeast infection in my intestine.

A candida infection in your colon is similar to a vaginal yeast infection. Women are prone to getting vaginal yeast infections when they take antibiotics because the drug kills off beneficial flora in a person's body. Well, I had just consumed antibiotics and a steroid.

I turned fifty that August and lost my health. For fifty years, I took my good health for granted. Now I realized it was precious. Ultimately, what occurred in my body was a poisoning from an abscessed tooth resulting in ten different medical diagnoses in the following order:

1. Bimonthly periods caused by uterine polyps
2. Depression
3. Ovarian cyst
4. Adrenal fatigue
5. Hormonal imbalance
6. Retinal tear
7. Visual migraine
8. Anemia
9. Low vitamin D level
10. Candidiasis infection of my colon

My colonic therapist gave me the book *The Body Ecology Diet* by Donna Gates so I could educate myself. The information in this book confirmed I had an overgrowth of Candida in my gastrointestinal system. I followed the steps outlined in *The Body Ecology Diet* to get rid of the infection.

Candida feeds off of carbohydrates. Therefore, a physical component of my craving for sugar and carbs was an overgrowth of this harmful microorganism. Having candidiasis is like having a monster take control of your appetite. However, I fought this culprit and restored my gut flora. The gut flora consists of beneficial microorganisms (also known as probiotics) that strengthen the immune system and help defend against unfriendly bacteria and pathogens that cause disease.[4]

For the following eight months, I struggled to regain my health. To eradicate the Candida, I continued the regimen from the book and stopped eating fruit, rice, flour, sugar, and desserts. I lost a lot of weight. During this time, I took one step forward and two steps back, then three steps forward and one step back. It was a slow process, but after eight months of being on the strict anti-Candida diet, I finally regained my health.

I felt healed. The diet required great self-control, but I was determined to succeed because I desperately wanted my health back. Ultimately I beat the candida infection in my colon and restored my adrenal glands. God gave us glorious bodies that will heal themselves if we give them the right building blocks.

If you want to determine if you have a candida overgrowth in your gut, take the Candida Quiz at CandiQuiz.com.

MAKE A DECISION ABOUT YOUR HEALTH

Do you want your health back too? You may be experiencing a health crisis and need to make a change. Are you overweight or experiencing problematic symptoms such as depression, moodiness, low energy, achy joints, diabetes, hypertension, or other health problems? Do you crave unhealthy foods? Do you need guidance regarding how to improve your health and lose weight? If you want to make a change, this book will walk you through the process to regain your health through a lifestyle change so you can feel energetic again and begin to live the purposeful and fulfilled life God intended for you.

The first step to getting off sugar and carbohydrates is to decide—decide to make necessary modifications. No one can make this decision for you; it is your choice. However, the next steps will help you maintain your commitment to this life-saving decision. Several other critical components to the process of getting off sugar and carbs include acquiring the right information, obtaining a support system, and praying and asking God to give you the willpower to overcome.

If you accepted Christ as your Savior, you have the Holy Spirit inside you, as 1 Corinthians 6:19–20 states, "Don't you realize that your body is the temple of the Holy Spirit, who lives in you and was given to you by God? You do not belong to yourself, for God bought you with a high price. So you must honor God with your body." When you make healthy eating choices, you take care of the temple God gave you. You only have one body, and it needs to last a lifetime.

Gluttony, which is overeating, is a sin, as implied in Proverbs 23:1–3, "When you sit to dine with a ruler, note well what is before you, and put a knife to your throat if you are given to gluttony. Do not crave his delicacies, for that food is deceptive" (NIV), and Proverbs 23:20–21, "Do not join those who drink too much wine or gorge themselves on meat, for drunkards and gluttons become poor, and drowsiness clothes them in rags" (NIV).

Proverbs 23:1–3 is quite grave when it states, "put a knife to your throat." The truth is, if you overeat like a king, your lifespan shortens. Many chronic diseases such as diabetes and hypertension can be improved, or even cured, by changing eating habits and losing weight. For example, my aunt stopped taking blood pressure medication when she lost ten pounds, because her high blood pressure went away.

The delicacies and deceptive foods mentioned in Proverbs 23:3 are similar to the super-rich and processed foods so accessible today. Neither is nutritious for the body. A person feels awful after consuming them. These delicacies remind me of the desserts I ate on the cruise. During my cruise, I ate like a queen with three-course meals. I tried to eat more fruits and vegetables and lean meats, but I couldn't resist the desserts. After I returned home, it took a month to get my usual energy level back. Being clothed in drowsiness (Proverbs 23:21) accurately describes how people feel after consuming a heavy meal. Sleepiness descends upon them.

Overindulging to our heart's content leads to slavery over the item our flesh desires. This slavery becomes more restrictive than following healthy guidelines. Eating healthy foods gives us the boundaries we need.

FOOD ADDICTION

In our society, the overabundance of delicacies is hard to resist. At first, it seems fun to eat whatever we desire. However, that momentary pleasure is fleeting. It is unhealthy to overeat, and when that becomes a habit, eventually we become addicted to food and can't stop eating. Therefore, we binge.

Regrettably, people become addicted to sugar and carbs. In fact, their brain's circuitry goes haywire when they come into contact with these addictive foods, and their mind assigns supreme value to that food. Magnetic resonance imaging (MRI) of the brain found that addicts' neural circuitry kicks into high gear when the brain lusts for the product of addiction.[5]

Therefore, from a physical perspective, we can become addicted to sugar, wheat, and refined carbohydrates through a biochemical addiction in the brain, or through the cravings caused by Candida, or both. However, we are more than physical beings; we are spiritual as well. The struggle to get off carbs may not be only a physical battle but a spiritual one too. One of the ways we can fight food addiction is through scripture. Appendix 1 includes Bible verses to recite to tap into God's power and strength. If you are addicted to sugar and carbohydrates, like my sister, you will need God's superpower. Paul tells us in Philippians 4:13, "For I can do everything through Christ, who gives me strength."

DIET AFFECTS BRAIN HEALTH

Once you've decided to make this lifestyle change, the dietary changes outlined in step 4 may benefit not only yourself but your family members as well. A diet high in sugar is linked to dementia and Alzheimer's. Scientific studies revealed a low-glycemic, low-carbohydrate diet helps prevent and improve these prevalent, devastating diseases. If you would like more information on how to prevent these diseases, check out my pamphlet "How to Prevent, Improve, and Reverse Alzheimer's and Dementia" go to SusanUNeal.com/ALZ. This pamphlet lists twenty-four interventions to fight these diseases of the brain.

To prevent Alzheimer's and dementia, start interventions early before symptoms begin. If you contract one of these diseases, can someone in your family take care of you? I understand this situation, as my ninety-year-old mother has vascular dementia (from a stroke) and my father-in-law died of Alzheimer's disease.

Brain Testing

Take an online cognitive test to determine the health of your brain. Amazingly, the foods we eat affect our brain function. Access a free online cognitive test, the Self-Administered Gerocognitive Exam (SAGE), at ElderGuru.com. Click on Sage Alzheimer's Exam on the right lower panel.

Cognitive Assessment Results

Write down the results from your cognitive assessments here.

_____

MAKE YOUR COMMITMENT

Now that you have decided to take this seven-step plan to improving your health and your future, the following actions will help you stay accountable to your commitment and give you a baseline to measure against once you have made progress on your journey to wholeness.

Contract

Take the first step to get off sugar and carbohydrates by deciding to make a lifestyle change. Begin by writing a contract between you and God on the lines below. Include the measurable goals you would like to achieve. Ask God to help you and place your success in his loving hands.

_____

. . .

Baseline Assessment

Now that you have decided to conquer sugar and carbs, you'll need to take a few measurements before moving on. First, before changing your eating habits, obtain a baseline of your current condition. Weigh yourself and measure your waistline.

Date to implement changes:

Baseline measurement date:

Weight:

Waistline:

Symptom Checklist

Put a check by the following unhealthy symptoms you experience.

_____ Fatigue

_____ Anxiety

_____ Insomnia

_____ Irritability

_____ Depression

_____ Mood swings

_____ Poor memory

_____ Food allergies

_____ Foggy brained

_____ Decreased sex drive

_____ Hormonal imbalance

_____ Chronic fatigue, fibromyalgia

_____ Vaginal yeast infections, urinary tract infections

_____ Craving sweets and refined carbohydrates or alcohol

_____ Digestive issues (bloating, constipation, diarrhea) or disorders

_____ Skin and nail infections such as toenail fungus, athlete's foot, and ringworm

Dietary Assessment

Record the foods you ate last week. Recalling these foods will test your memory as well as help you realize the kind of foods you typically consume. How well does your memory recall? Do wheat and sugar comprise a large part of your diet?

_____

_____

_____

_____

. . .

After six months of changing your eating habits, you will objectively measure your cognitive abilities by retaking the online cognitive test, recheck your weight and waistline measurements, and note whether any unhealthy symptoms subsided. A reassessment survey is provided at the end of step 7.

TAKING STEP 1: DECIDE

Making the decision to commit to a lifestyle change, particularly if you struggle with food addiction is crucial. While it may be difficult to commit, once you have, you can look back on your contract with God when things get tough. Remember, no matter if and when you make a mistake, you can get back on track. Each chapter will end with a list of action steps to help you accomplish that step. In step 1, complete the following action steps:

1. If you haven't already, watch the Ted-Ed video, "How Does Sugar Affect the Brain?" by the neuroscientist Nicole Avena, Ph.D. Go to ScienceAlert.com/watch-this-is-how-sugar-affects-your-brain.
2. Check labels to make sure you don't consume sugary foods with greater than ten grams of sugar per serving.
3. Write and sign your contract between you and God.
4. Complete your assessments.

7 Steps to Get Off Sugar and Carbohydrates:
  STEP 1: Decide to improve your health through proper nutrition.

STEP 2: ACQUIRE A SUPPORT SYSTEM AND KNOWLEDGE

Decide—>**Acquire**—>Clean Out—>Purchase—>Plan—>Prepare—
>Improve

A decision to change one's lifestyle can't be maintained without support. The next step in the journey is to acquire that support—to gain the knowledge to make necessary changes and create a system for encouragement and accountability. We are comprised of a body, mind, and spirit, so all the components of our well-being must be addressed to successfully make the changes needed to improve our health. You will learn about food addiction and Candida (physical), which foods are beneficial versus harmful (intellectual), the benefit of obtaining a support system (emotional), and memorizing Bible verses (spiritual).

ACQUIRE KNOWLEDGE

Gaining knowledge regarding unhealthy versus healthy foods is crucial to making this lifestyle change. You cannot keep your new commitment without understanding how and why to take the next steps. Resources in this chapter will educate and equip you for this journey. Making a lifestyle change to improve your health will be challenging, including physical (biochemical), emotional, and spiritual trials. In step 2, you acquire strategies to address these challenges.

Understanding Food Addiction

We need to understand that sugar and wheat are addictive. Addiction is a compulsive repetition of an activity despite life-damaging consequences. Food addiction is a biochemical disorder that cannot be controlled by willpower alone. If you have not considered the possibility of having a food addiction, do not feel shame over the terminology. Your body has fallen prey to the accumulative effects of sugar and wheat that are ingrained in so many of our culture's food habits. The surgeon general's 2016 report indicated that addiction is a chronic brain disease, not a moral failing.[1]

Two hallmarks of addiction include persistent desire and repeated unsuccessful attempts to stop. Being addicted to food is like having an alien inside of you who takes control of your body and eats a bunch of unhealthy food. You can't stop it. Sugar and wheat hijack your body. You can't halt the craving or binges no matter what diet or method you try. Your own willpower is never enough. Understanding that food addiction is not a lack of self-control, but a rewiring of the brain, helps you to be more compassionate with yourself.

How does this addiction happen? Foods containing sugar and wheat cause the release of an excess amount of dopamine in the brain. Dopamine, a feel-good neurohormone, releases when we eat foods high in sugar, take opiate drugs, smoke cigarettes, drink alcohol, cuddle with our kids, pet a dog, or enjoy sex.[2] A dopamine rush can rewire the brain to desire more of whatever causes its release. Therefore, when a food addict sees sugary foods, dopamine releases and causes the person's focus to narrow.[3] She can think only about eating that food item to experience the euphoria it brings.

Scientists found that the part of the brain that restrains behavior (self-control) was abnormally quiet in rats with an addiction. Unfortunately, when we struggle with the desire for unhealthy foods, the part of the brain that inhibits addictive behavior becomes silent, and we lose the ability to have self-control.[4] Sugar and refined carbohydrates take over and restructure the brain.

In 2017, scientists conducted trials of a new therapy for addicts called transcranial magnetic stimulation (TMS), which treated depression and migraines for years. TMS runs an electric current through a wand that alters the electrical activity in the brain to activate the drug-damaged neural pathways that restrain behavior. So far the therapy is successful.[5] If studies continue to be successful, this could be a life-changing option for people addicted to a variety of substances.

In addition to being addictive, sugar and refined carbohydrates cause disease. Chronic ailments such as diabetes, high blood pressure, and obesity are related to the consumption of too much of the wrong types of food. Therefore, gaining knowledge is essential to changing one's eating habits.

Determining whether you are a food addict will help you understand yourself and enable you to effectively overcome this addiction. Use these online quizzes to determine if you are addicted to food: FoodAddicts.org/am-i-a-food-addict or OA.org/newcomers/how-do-i-start/are-you-a-compulsive-overeater/.

If you have an emotional connection with food, please consider using the *Christian Study Guide for 7 Steps to Get Off Sugar and Carbohydrates.* Whether you do this study by yourself or with a group, it will help you go more in-depth to resolve an emotional issue once and for all.

In my course, 7 Steps to Reclaim Your Health and Optimal Weight (https://susanuneal.com/courses/7-steps-to-get-off-sugar-and-carbs-course), I help you figure out and resolve the root cause of your inappropriate eating habit. One solved, taming your appetite is much easier. I show you how to change your eating habits once and for all.

If you are a food addict, I recommend you join a Christian-based weight-loss program or a twelve-step food addiction program along with a corresponding support group. Appendix 2 provides a resource list for these groups. Some Christian programs include:

First Place 4 Health (FirstPlace4Health.com) offers a biblical approach to weight loss through a series of Bible studies. Online groups are available, or you can check to see if one exists in your area.

Take Back Your Temple (TakeBackYourTemple.com) is a Christian online weight loss program whose motto is "Your body for God's glory. We help you take back your house so you can fulfill your God-given purpose."

The Eden Diet: A Biblical and Merciful Anti-Dieting Plan for Weight Loss (TheEdenDiet.com), a Christian weight-loss program with online support groups.

Thin Within: A Non-Diet Grace Based Approach (ThinWithin.org) is a Christian weight management program that includes online classes and groups.

Barb Raveling Christian weight loss products (Barb Raveling.com). include, a podcast—Taste for Truth: Christian Weight Loss, an app—I Deserve a Donut: and Other Lies That Make You Eat, and a couple of books—*Taste for Truth: A 30 Day Weight Loss Bible Study* and *I Deserve a Donut: And Other Lies that Make You Eat.*

Grace Filled Plate (GraceFilledPlate.com) is a website with an excellent blog which includes having a healthy mindset, recipes, nutrition, and faith.

Victory Steps for Women: Christian Weight Loss & Spiritual Wellness (VictorySteps.net/christian-weight-loss-program.html), a faith-based health and wellness coaching program, helps women overcome emotional eating, binge eating, and compulsive overeating behaviors.

Weight Loss, God's Way (CathyMorenzie.com/challenge/) is a Christian-based weight loss program that offers a free twenty-one-day challenge.

Three different online food addiction programs include:
OA.org/ (OA is Overeater's Anonymous)
FoodAddicts.org/

FoodAddictsanonymous.org/

Joining an online support group is another way to share the ups and downs of this journey. Connecting with like-minded individuals who are persevering through the same trials as you helps divide the load. Through these support groups, you can exchange acquired knowledge about your shared journey. In addition, sometimes we need to vent and express our disappointment or success with another person who understands. Life sharing nourishes the emotional side of our well-being.

Understanding Candida

Candida is the second potential physical component to a compulsion to overeat refined carbohydrates. If you crave sugar, alcohol, and processed foods, you might have an imbalance in the flora of your gut. An imbalance means the beneficial microorganisms (probiotics) have been killed off by antibiotics, steroids, unhealthy processed foods, and chemicals in foods. The destruction of these beneficial microbes allows the harmful microbe Candida to multiply quickly, taking over your digestive tract. Candida Albicans, a type of yeast common in the gut, can grow roots into the lining of your gastrointestinal (GI) system. The fungal overgrowth creates openings in the bowel walls, which is known as a leaky gut. These holes allow harmful microorganisms to enter the bloodstream. Our bodies don't recognize these particles, so our immune system creates antibodies which cause food allergies and autoimmune diseases to develop.[6] An overgrowth of Candida also causes your abdomen to become distended.

When Candida spreads out of control, it acts like a parasite sucking the life and energy out of you. Candida feeds on carbs, which is why you crave them. It is like a monster growing inside of you, craving sugar, and it is hard to fight its never-ending appetite.

I had an overgrowth of Candida in my colon, so I know how hard it is to fight this culprit. Yet I wanted my health back, so I struggled to restore my health through an anti-Candida cleanse, which I will discuss in step 4. It took eight months on a rigorous non-Candida diet to regain my health, but with determination, by the power of the Holy Spirit, I succeeded.

Below is a list of symptoms that might arise from an overgrowth of Candida. This survey is the same list you completed in step 1. Check off the ones that apply to you now. The more symptoms you experience, the more likely you are to have a candida infection.

_____ Fatigue

_____ Anxiety

_____ Insomnia

_____ Irritability

_____ Depression

_____ Mood swings

_____ Poor memory

_____ Food allergies

_____ Foggy brained

_____ Decreased sex drive

_____ Hormonal imbalance

_____ Chronic fatigue, fibromyalgia

_____ Vaginal yeast infections, urinary tract infections

_____ Craving sweets and refined carbohydrates or alcohol

_____ Digestive issues (bloating, constipation, diarrhea) or disorders

_____ Skin and nail infections such as toenail fungus, athlete's foot, and ringworm

All of the symptoms listed above are indicative of a Candida infection in your gut. If you previously took an antibiotic, you might have an imbalance of the flora in your GI tract because antibiotics kill off the beneficial microorganisms, which allows the yeast to multiply rapidly. The more times in your life that you have taken antibiotics, without replenishing your gut with probiotics that contain greater than ten strains of microorganisms for several weeks, the more likely you have candidiasis.

A simple spit test can determine if you have an overgrowth of

Candida. First thing in the morning, before you drink anything or brush your teeth, spit into a glass of water. In one to three minutes, check the cup to see if any strings hang from the spit—strings are a positive sign of Candida. The spit will resemble a jellyfish. If the water becomes cloudy or the saliva sinks to the bottom, this is also a positive sign. Healthy saliva floats on the top of the water with no strings hanging down.

There are two websites that provide a detailed explanation of the spit test. The first is NationalCandidaCenter.com. Click on the Tests tab at the top. From the menu that appears, click on Self-Test 2 - My Body Fluids.The second website is CandidaSupport.org/re-sources/saliva-test/. These two websites also include written Candida tests you can complete for further assessment.

Candida will take over your life if left untreated. If you exhibit many of the numerous symptoms listed above, you need to restore the balance of microorganisms in your gastrointestinal system. An excellent resource to help you learn more about restoring your intestinal flora is *The Body Ecology Diet* by Donna Gates. Check out her website BodyEcology.com/. Her follow-up book, *The Body Ecology Guide to Growing Younger*, is another excellent resource.

Harmful Versus Beneficial Foods

Realizing a slice of bread will raise your blood-sugar level higher than sugar should motivate you not to eat bread. Begin to learn which foods are damaging versus beneficial—the ones God gave us to eat, not the food industry's offerings.

Today, grocery stores and restaurants make non-gluten food choices readily available. Why has gluten sensitivity skyrocketed in the US? Fifty years ago, sensitivity to gluten was rare. I believe it is because the human body cannot proficiently digest the gluten in wheat the way it is hybridized now.

For centuries, people flourished by consuming bread. Nevertheless, the problem with wheat is that it is not the same today as it was one hundred years ago. Norman Borlaug received the Nobel Peace

Prize in 1970 in recognition of his contributions to world peace through increasing the food supply through hybridization—crossbreeding of different varieties—of wheat.[7]

He crossbred various types of wheat to create a high-yield dwarf wheat. No longer do tall amber waves of grain grow in the Midwest. Instead, wheat is now only a couple of feet tall, drought resistant, and prolific. *Unfortunately, the gluten changed so much that it can induce gluten sensitivity.*[8] Therefore, do not consume any wheat products. No waffles, pancakes, muffins, cake, piecrust, pizza, pretzels, bread, pasta —the list goes on and on.

Since gluten in the hybridized wheat is difficult to digest, some individuals become sensitive or intolerant to the gluten.[9] These individuals experience digestive problems when they consume foods with gluten (wheat, rye, and barley). When my sister consumes gluten, she needs to be close to a bathroom for the next twenty-four hours. Her gluten sensitivity blood test (tTG-IgA and IgG) confirmed her sensitivity to gluten.

However, gluten sensitivity tests are not always accurate. Another member of my family who is gluten sensitive had the same test with negative results. My doctor confirmed the high incidence of false-negative gluten-sensitivity test results. Instead, he recommended an individual remove wheat and gluten from their diet for a month to determine how sensitive the body might be to these foods.

If you want to find out if you are gluten sensitive, either take the Gluten Quiz at GlutenIntoleranceQuiz.com, or fast from gluten for a whole month. This length of time is necessary because the gluten molecule is so large it may take weeks before the body can eliminate it. As you reintroduce gluten back into your diet, note any adverse side effects such as gas, bloating, diarrhea, smelly feces, constipation, abdominal pain, nausea, vomiting, foggy mind, headache, joint pain, depression, nasal congestion, skin problems, fatigue, and autoimmune diseases. If you experience any of these symptoms, gluten from wheat is food you should not consume.

If a person's body does not recognize gluten as food, their immune system attacks the gluten and, unfortunately, their body at the same time. The intestinal lining becomes damaged, resulting in holes in the intestinal wall (called leaky gut). Those holes allow food to enter the bloodstream.[10] In turn, a person may become allergic to other types of food as well. It is not surprising that gluten sensitivity is often paired with an autoimmune condition because the body accidentally starts harming its own cells as it attacks the broken-down food particles in the bloodstream.

Gluten is in wheat, barley, and rye. Yet breads made of barley and rye are uncommon. Therefore, I believe the gluten culprit comes from the hybridization of wheat. Remember, a polypeptide from wheat passes through the blood-brain barrier and goes to the opiate receptors in the brain. This likely contributes to a rise of autoimmune diseases in the US.

In other words, if you get an autoimmune disease, it could have been caused by a gluten sensitivity you didn't know you had. This sensitivity could have caused your immune system to get confused and attack a part of your body. Therefore, I recommend anyone with an autoimmune disease not eat wheat.

Most Americans have no idea wheat has been bred to the point the body thinks of it as a foreign substance. This is from hybridization. But what if the body doesn't recognize genetically modified food? Again, a person's immune system might attack the foreign substance and its own body at the same time. Consequently, you should avoid any GMO foods. The only way to do so is to purchase organic foods.

The United States is one of the few industrialized nations in the world that does not label GMO food products. Finally, in July 2016 a bill passed that requires GMO food labeling within two years. The food industries fought the GMO labeling for years to avoid decreased sales or the need to change the composition of their ingredients.

Unfortunately, food manufacturers picked up on the gluten-free trend and created all sorts of unhealthy, nongluten products. Substituting wheat with gluten-free processed foods is not a healthy alternative, since they often contain rice flour, which raises blood-sugar levels.

High blood-sugar levels cause a person's pancreas to release insulin. Increased insulin causes the body to store belly fat.[11] Do you have belly fat? What you eat plays a huge role in gaining fat around the middle. High blood-sugar levels from the wrong foods lead to insulin resistance, type-2 diabetes, and dementia. In fact, dementia is referred to as type-3 diabetes—which is on the rise from consuming too much sugar and processed foods. That is why I asked you to complete the online cognitive assessment in step 1.

Delicious unhealthy foods are conveniently available to us. But just because we have access to them and the freedom to eat them doesn't mean we should. If we understand which products are harmful, we can avoid them. You may have had no idea that wheat was harmful until reading this book. However, gaining accurate knowledge about food is not always easy because of the amount of either false or conflicting information available. Be discerning as you acquire food knowledge and ensure it is from a reputable source.

If you can't or don't want to eliminate bread from your diet, make homemade gluten-free bread to avoid wheat. My sister uses the recipe Kim's Gluten Free, Dairy Free, Whole Grain Bread at GFReal-Food.com (see the last recipe in appendix 4). You could also obtain a freshly ground flour made from a nonhybridized whole-wheat berry (not just part of the berry). Einkorn wheat, a variety of nonhybridized wheat, might be available from a local provider that stone grinds the whole kernel into whole-grain einkorn flour. I found such a supplier at a local farmer's market in Pensacola, Florida. Her business is Our Daily Bread, and the Facebook page is Facebook.com/ourdailybread-bakerypensacola/. I purchase freshly ground whole grain einkorn flour from her.

To slowly wean my family off of processed white flour, I started by making pancakes, waffles, muffins, and other baked goods with 1/2 einkorn and 1/2 white flour. Surprisingly, they acclimated well to this half-and-half mixture. Then I increased the einkorn flour to 3/4 with 1/4 white flour—I got some negative feedback about this, but they got used to it (my family preferred the 50/50 combination).

My baked goods were denser but still delicious. If I made recipes with 100 percent einkorn flour, my family would not eat much of it.

So I had to settle for using 3/4 einkorn flour. With a family, making this lifestyle change can be tough, as it is hard to please everyone. Providing healthy alternatives your family will eat can be challenging.

I explained to my family that I needed to make these dietary changes to get my health back. I wanted to feel energetic again, and they desired this too—since they benefited when I felt well. (When Mama ain't happy, ain't nobody happy.) Their understanding helped them go along with my dietary changes as much as their taste buds could tolerate.

For me, I could not eat baked goods with any white flour. My gut had been too damaged when I was ill. If I eat these delicious baked products, I wake up feeling tired and foggy brained. After being weaned off unhealthy foods, I can tell when one food item affects me negatively.

With time, you should become more aware of how different foods affect how you feel. This correlation will become apparent as you keep a record of what you eat and how it makes you feel in your journal (appendix 3; we will discuss journaling later in this chapter). After a while, a pattern may emerge. If I eat something that raises my blood-sugar level, I do not feel good the next day. How do you feel the day after consuming food with high sugar content?

Roundup Ready Crops

These crops are genetically engineered to be resistant to the carcinogen glyphosate, which is the primary ingredient in the herbicide Roundup.[12] Farmers who produce Roundup Ready crops are free to spray Roundup on their fields throughout the growing season, as the plants are resistant to this herbicide. In the United States most of the nation's corn, wheat, oats, soy, and sugar beets are Roundup Ready crops.[13] Can you imagine what this carcinogen may do to the beneficial bacteria in your gut or to your overall health? Therefore, you should only eat these foods if they are organic. Organic foods are not GMO or Roundup Ready crops.

· · ·

Unhealthy Food Combinations

A friend told me she experienced painful heartburn after eating salmon, brussel sprouts, and a baked potato. She didn't know why she felt so terrible since these were healthy foods. She didn't understand what happens during digestion with different food combinations.

I explained how some food combinations cause indigestion. Combining a protein with a baked potato may cause heartburn. Conversely, eating a protein with vegetables does not cause indigestion, nor does eating a baked potato with vegetables. It's the protein/potato combination that doesn't digest well together.[14]

Also, eating fruit with your meal is not a suitable combination because fruit digests quickly, but other foods, such as proteins, do not. Therefore, eat fruit alone and wait twenty to thirty minutes before eating anything else. *The Body Ecology Diet* by Donna Gates includes a great section about food combinations and which ones cause indigestion.

Food Triggers

Another critical component to the physical nature of food addiction is understanding food triggers. Triggers cause us to get right back on the merry-go-round of desire, binging, and withdrawal. Identify your food triggers—the aroma of freshly baked cookies, a dessert table at a restaurant, a food commercial, or even an emotion. Choose to get off that merry-go-round by recognizing what stimuli set you off and avoid them. Turn the channel or pick up something to read. Call your accountability partner or recite a Bible verse. Seek help from an online support group.

Unfortunately, if you are a food addict you have to consider yourself as a recovering addict who has quit your drug—wheat and sugar. Therefore, you cannot consume these products ever again, or you will go right back to being addicted to them and having the undesirable symptoms that accompany their consumption. Yet you can live a full life without consuming these delicious but detrimental products.

ACQUIRE A SUPPORT SYSTEM

Obtaining a support system helps address the emotional aspect of this transformation. As Ecclesiastes 4:12 tells us, "Though one may be overpowered, two can defend themselves. A cord of three strands is not quickly broken" (NIV). I recommend that in addition to online or live support groups, you ask someone to be your accountability and prayer partner.

It is validating when someone understands how we feel. Perhaps no one in your family understands your struggle, so it is helpful to reach out to others. Also, family can sometimes enable our bad habits because they don't really understand, or they're in the same boat, but because you're so close you give each other permission to stay on the bad habit pathway. Having a friend for accountability who you can call when temptation arises is a crucial key to your success. It is powerful when a friend speaks the truth in love. Pray with your friend. The security of knowing someone prays for you is comforting.

At times all of us eat unhealthy foods. When this happens, we may experience guilt and depression. Having someone to pray for us during these challenges is essential to our spiritual victory. In fact, calling a friend when we feel temptation can redirect our thought process from the food. You could ask your friend to pray with you or you could meet at a coffee shop to get away from the temptation. Be open and express what's causing a challenge for you.

My sister shared the challenges she faced while she changed her eating habits. She got hungry in the afternoons, and finding a healthy snack remained difficult. I gave her suggestions and prayed with her. She decided to move her family's dinner time earlier so she could satisfy her hunger. Sharing trials with a friend helps diffuse the burden. I prayed for her and with her many times during her transitory journey.

The following scripture confirms we should share trials and confess our sins to one another: "Confess your sins to each other and pray for each other so that you may be healed. The earnest prayer of a righteous person has great power and produces wonderful results"

(James 5:16). Bringing our struggles out of the closet, and sharing them with someone we trust is valuable. Prayers are powerful, especially from someone who loves and understands us for who we truly are—including the good, the bad, and the ugly.

For additional support, please join my closed Facebook group, 7 Steps to Get Off Sugar and Carbohydrates, and share with me how you are doing.

Journal

Record your path to recovery in a journal. Writing down your actual food choices each day, as well as your thoughts, feelings, struggles, and victories, has a powerful effect. Journaling will create personal accountability. The more you journal, the more easily you'll recognize when you are eating out of emotion or for the wrong reasons. You will see what helped you battle the struggles previously. Journaling will provide clarity of your thoughts, feelings, and desires.

To help you with journaling, I created the *Healthy Living Journal*. It is full of charts and each day you'll record water and food intake, exercise, energy level, and corresponding moods. Recording your daily food consumption provides an opportunity to learn how food affects your health. When you discover negative health patterns you can change. Devotions and educational snippets are provided on a daily basis too.

If you want to create your own journal, the following information should be included in the journal (see appendix 3). Write the following items in your journal:

1. The time you eat.
2. Why you want to eat. Are you hungry, bored, angry? Is it just "time to eat" or are you with others who are having a meal?
3. If you feel a strong emotion related to this consumption of food, record the emotion.

4. Food you ate and drank, including quantity.
5. How you feel after you ate? Are you satisfied or stuffed?
6. Energy level and clarity of mind after you ate.
7. When waking up in the morning, how do you feel? See if there is a pattern of eating high-sugar-content foods and feeling sluggish the next morning.
8. What are you grateful for today?
9. Prayer requests to God.
10. Exercise—type of activity and length of time.
11. Number of glasses of water you drank and when. Did you drink on an empty stomach?
12. Every time you binge, record: what you ate, why you ate it, what triggered you to eat it, and what you might do the next time you are tempted.

As you write this information, recognize any patterns between your emotions and food consumption. Do you eat because you were hungry? If not, why? Did at least three hours lapse between meals? It takes three to four hours before food digests and your stomach empties.

You can journal on paper or electronically, on your phone or computer. The My Fitness Pal phone app is an excellent resource to track food, calories, and activity level.

If you recognize that you have a dysfunctional relationship with food, when did this dysfunction begin? The more extended the period, the longer it will take to reset your body and mind. Changing your eating habits is not an overnight process. But step-by-step you can reprogram your body, mind, and spirit. Creating a support system and journaling are vital components to your success.

Scripture
Another essential component of this lifestyle change is tapping

into God's power through reciting Bible verses. God's Word offers guidance to every area of life, including our health and our emotions. Since emotions trigger negative food habits, learn to use this weapon as you need it. Appendix 1 includes a list of scriptures categorized by the emotion a person experiences. Speak these verses out loud and with authority, believing in their power. The spoken Word of God is a double-edged sword that defeats the enemy.

Advantages of memorizing scripture include reducing stress, resisting temptation, hearing God speak, and receiving comforting reassurance of God's steadfast love. There are several steps to learning Bible verses.[15] First, you need motivation. Without God-given inspiration, memorization is difficult. So pray and ask God for the desire. For years, I thought I couldn't learn verses because they were too challenging to remember. However, with prayer and God's help, the Holy Spirit empowered me to memorize numerous scriptures.

Next, which scriptures should you memorize? Sometimes while doing a Bible study or reading the Bible, the Holy Spirit led me to learn a specific verse. A verse may be important personally. For example, as I was raising young children, verses on how to discipline children were relevant for me to memorize at the time. What are you currently going through? Seek the verses that apply to your current life situation and challenge. Many of these are listed in appendix 3, but you will find others as you search the Bible.

The second step to memorizing scripture is to write the Bible verse on an index card in the following manner: Write the verse name and number at the top and bottom of the card. Then, break the verse up into short segments that are easy to memorize. For example:

Philippians 4:13
For I can do everything
through Christ,
who gives me strength.
Philippians 4:13

This simple and effective method makes it easy to learn one line of the verse at a time. Continue to do this until the entire verse is memorized. For me, it was harder to remember the verse name and number than the verse itself. Therefore, I wrote the verse name and number at the top and the bottom of the card.

Review the Bible verse on a weekly basis to remember it. I studied the scripture cards while I worked out at the gym. My husband thought this was a creative way to exercise my body, mind, and spirit through the Word of God. This weekly repetition kept the verses at the forefront of my mind.

Bring the scripture cards with you on a walk, tape one to the bathroom mirror, or keep them in your purse to review. Be creative! Storing God's Word in your heart is like storing up treasure, as indicated in Proverbs 2:6, "For the Lord grants wisdom! His every word is a treasure of knowledge and understanding" (TLB).

If you memorize scripture, you can unsheathe the sword of the Spirit and slash the enemy when he tempts. Hiding God's Word in your heart is vital to your spiritual success on this journey to change.

Prayer

To make the lifestyle changes necessary to improve our health we need to access our heavenly father through prayer. When Jesus was in the garden of Gethsemane sweating blood, he was on his knees praying to his father. We need to follow Jesus's example. God wants to communicate with us, and that's another way we receive his power to face our struggles. Jesus's brother told us in James 5:16, "The earnest prayer of a righteous man has great power and wonderful results" (TLB).

An essential component of the arsenal God gave us is prayer, as Paul indicated in Ephesians 6:18, "And pray in the Spirit on all occasions with all kinds of prayers and requests" (NIV). Prayer helps break down the resistance you may experience as you make these changes.

During prayer, ask God to give you a willing spirit to surrender to him, and replace your desire for food with the desire to please and serve him. Also, incorporate Bible verses into your prayers. For example, "Lord, one may be overpowered, but two can defend themselves (Ecclesiastes 3:12), so please help me to find the perfect prayer partner."

God loves you, and he wants you to succeed. Use his powerful weapons—Bible verses and prayer.

Other Resources

Neurologist David Perlmutter MD wrote the book *Grain Brain: The Surprising Truth About Wheat, Carbs, and Sugar—Your Brain's Silent Killers*. He recommends taking a probiotic that contains at least ten billion active cultures from at least ten different strains of beneficial bacteria to help fight the overgrowth of Candida and balance your gut flora. As this book's subtitle (*Your Brain's Silent Killers*) indicates— wheat, sugar, and carbs harm the human brain.

The Daniel Plan by Rick Warren, recommends you stop eating sugar, wheat, and milk products for one week. Then reintroduce one of those foods at a time back into your diet to determine any adverse effects.

If you have a food addiction or emotional connection with food, please consider using the *Christian Study Guide for 7 Steps to Get Off Sugar and Carbohydrates.*

I also found *Eat Right 4 Your Type* by Dr. Peter D'Adamo to be helpful in figuring out the foods to avoid to eliminate digestive issues. This book bases food choices on a person's blood type. It recommended that those with my AB blood type not eat sunflower or sesame seeds. Normally I added those seeds to my homemade granola. Yet I often belched after I ate the granola. When I eliminated those seeds from the recipe, my indigestion ceased.

It is vital to notice how your body reacts to certain foods. If you experience digestive problems, keep track of what you ate before the symptom—in your journal. Note whether the food was consistently wheat or dairy. These two products are the usual offenders.

Dr. William Davis, the author of *Wheat Belly*, states, "Whole wheat bread increases blood-sugar as much as or more than sugar." As a cardiologist, he placed his overweight, diabetic-prone patients on a low-glycemic, whole-foods diet that excluded wheat for three months.[16] Results included:

- diabetics became nondiabetic
- acid reflux disappeared
- irritable bowel syndrome went away
- rheumatoid arthritis pain decreased
- asthma symptoms improved or resolved completely
- rashes disappeared
- energy increased
- lost weight
- experienced clearer thinking and greater focus

If you have cancer, diabetes, or a life-threatening disease I recommend trying the Hallelujah Diet at MyHDiet.com/what-is-the-hallelujah-diet/. This biblically based diet does not condone eating meat, only the types of food God gave us in the garden of Eden from Genesis 1:29.

Recipes

We need wholesome recipes that do not include wheat, sugar, white rice, or processed foods. Appendix 4 includes my favorite recipes.

The Daniel Plan: 40 Days to a Healthier Life by Rick Warren, Daniel Amen MD, and Mark Hyman MD includes meal plans with precisely what to eat for each meal as well some recipes. *The Daniel Plan Cookbook* is chock-full of healthy recipes.

Grain Brain book by David Perlmutter MD also contains beneficial recipes.

The Body Ecology Diet by Donna Gates contains tasty, nutritious recipes. Her cookbook *Living Cookbook: Deliciously Healing Foods for a Happier, Healthier World* contains delicious recipes.

Pinterest posts thousands of recipes, but not all may be good for you. You can check out the recipes I selected at Pinterest.com/SusanUNeal/.

TAKING STEP 2: ACQUIRE

Are you interested in learning more about how to become a healthier person? You are well on your way. These are the suggested action steps from this chapter:

1. Take the food addiction test.
2. Join a Christian weight loss or food addiction program.
3. Conduct the Candida spit test.
4. Either take the Gluten Quiz at GlutenIntoleranceQuiz.com, or eliminate wheat for one month, then reintroduce it into to your diet to see if you experience any ill effects.
5. Choose an accountability/prayer partner.
6. Join my closed Facebook group, 7 Steps to Get Off Sugar and Carbohydrates, at Facebook.com/groups/184355458927013/ to gain additional support.
7. Purchase the *Healthy Living Journal* or create your own journal and start recording the items listed in appendix 3.
8. Choose a scripture verse to fight temptation and write it on an index card.

7 Steps to Get Off Sugar and Carbohydrates:
　　STEP 1. Decide to improve your health through proper nutrition.
　　STEP 2. Acquire a support system and knowledge to help make a lifestyle change.

3

STEP 3: CLEAN OUT THE PANTRY AND REFRIGERATOR

Decide—>Acquire—>**Clean Out**—>Purchase—>Plan—>Prepare—>Improve

Now that you decided to change your eating habits and acquired information about damaging foods, it is time to *clean out* the pantry and refrigerator. It is necessary to remove unhealthy foods, so you are not tempted to eat them. You may need to call on your support system for the willpower and accountability to take this step.

Why do you have to remove everything unhealthy? Remember, triggers, such as a package of cookies, can cause a relapse. Just looking at the bag releases dopamine and an overwhelming desire to consume that unhealthy food.[1] Therefore, you must get these items out of the house. If a family member wants to eat foods that may tempt you, they should keep these packages hidden in their room and out of the pantry. Ask them to honor your goals and help you in this way.

Remember, think of foods as being dead or alive. *Food from a bag sitting on the shelf for months is dead and does not give your body any of the nutrients it needs to be healthy.* A fresh piece of fruit contains essential vitamins, minerals, and fiber that a body needs.

Fiber in fruit and vegetables fills your stomach and tells your body you are full. When the fiber is removed from processed foods, it takes a larger quantity of food to become full. Also, the fiber in fruit slows digestion, which reduces the effects of sugar in raising your blood-sugar levels. As you eliminate processed foods from you diet you should consume more whole, organic fruits, vegetables, whole grains (oats, brown rice, quinoa, barley), beans, fish, and meat. (We will discuss the right foods to purchase in step 4.) Your body will thank you for nourishing it properly and respond by healing.

When I was sick, it was essential to nourish myself with healthy foods so my body could create new, properly functioning cells. I wanted to get well, so I began to evaluate everything I ate.

Today, I look at any food and assess whether or not it is good for me. If a person primarily eats dead food, how does the body get the proper nutrients it needs? If a cell within the human body replicates incorrectly, it is called cancer. How can your body replace old cells with healthy new ones if you don't give it the essential vitamins and minerals it requires?

We need to consume foods similar to what God gave us in the garden of Eden. For example, green beans sautéed in olive oil is healthier than a green bean casserole with mushroom soup and processed onion rings. The casserole is not as healthy for your body as the sautéed green beans.

Check labels and try not to eat foods with more than five ingredients or 10 grams of sugar per serving. The American Heart Association recommends you limit your calories from sugar to no more than half of your total calories, which is a lot. For most women in the US that should be no more than 24 grams of sugar or 100 calories per day. For men it is 36 grams of sugar or 150 calories from sugar per day.

If you can't pronounce an ingredient, your body probably won't recognize it as food either. Begin to simplify the foods you consume. For example, eat two hard-boiled eggs for breakfast, a whole avocado for lunch, and an apple for a snack. Ask yourself, "Did the food I am about to eat exist in the garden of Eden?" Food doesn't have to be complicated.

It wasn't complicated for Adam and Eve. They picked a piece of fruit or a vegetable and ate it. It doesn't have to be difficult for us either. Instead of making an elaborate meal, eat fresh, raw vegetables, which cost less and are better for you than processed, sugar-laden products.

Farmer's markets are great venues to find fresh, local produce. It is best to eat locally grown fruit and vegetables. Buy a potato and bake it with the following toppings: olive oil, broccoli, scallions, and sea salt with kelp. The baked potato is better for you than a bag of potato chips. *Eat foods closer to the form they were in when they came out of the garden.*

FOODS TO ELIMINATE

Understanding what foods are beneficial versus which are harmful is really confusing today, especially since the food industry entices us through great marketing and by adding addictive ingredients. In step 2, we acquired knowledge about food addiction, Candida, and the importance of an accountability and prayer partner. Step 3 will continue this education by providing you with a list of unhealthy foods and the reasons why they do not nourish the human body. It is far better to eat foods as close to their value at harvest—the way God made them—rather than processed foods.

Wheat

As discussed in step 2, I do not recommend eating any foods containing wheat because today's wheat is hybridized, and therefore, is not the same healthy grain that nourished humans for centuries. The gluten in today's dwarf, drought-resistance wheat is extremely difficult for a person to digest.[2] I believe this new form of wheat created in the 1950s caused the high level of gluten sensitivity we see today.

White Flour

Eliminate wheat because it is addictive and the human body has difficulty digesting the gluten. White flour is one of the most prevalent wheat products used today, and it is far removed from the grain it once was. A wheat berry consists of three layers: bran, germ, and endosperm. White flour contains one part of the wheat kernel—the endosperm, which is mostly starch. The other two parts of the wheat contain the *fiber* and *nutrients*, and these *are not included in white flour*. The flour has also been chemically bleached, consequently, the grain no longer resembles the wholesome food God intended.

Before 1870, wheat was stone-ground, and the whole grain was mashed (all three parts of the kernel). The invention of the steel roller revolutionized grain milling. With this device, the components of the wheat berry could be separated. Removing the bran (fiber) and germ (nutrients) significantly extended the shelf life of the processed flour. Stone-ground flour contained natural oils from the wheat and became rancid after sitting for a time on the shelf.

This limited shelf life is similar to nuts and oil. Have you ever eaten a rancid nut or smelled rancid oil? The capacity of food to become spoiled is a good thing because the foul smell and taste lets you know the value of the food is gone. However, the food industries prefer products with a longer shelf life so their products won't go bad and can be sold for a longer period of time.

Unfortunately, after the bran and germ components of the wheat berry were removed from the wheat, Americans started having diseases caused by deficiencies in B vitamins because the wheat germ, which contained the grain's nutrients, was removed from flour. Therefore, in the 1940s, vitamin enrichment of bread began.

Processed foods, like white flour, with their extended shelf life, do not go bad anymore because the natural nutrients were removed. Consequently, such foods don't benefit the human body. In fact, if we eat processed foods that do not contain nutrients, we deprive ourselves of essential vitamins and minerals. A lack of nutrients leads to malnutrition. Does it make sense to add manufactured vitamins to replace the natural nutrients stripped from the food in order to have nutritional value? God already placed the nutrients in the foods. Unfortunately, food industries take those nutrients out to extend the product's shelf life, which benefits the companies' bottom line but is detrimental to our health. No wonder our bodies are unhealthy.

Recently, a friend offered me an almond-flavored, sweet cracker. I looked at it and wondered how long ago was it created? It probably sat in a box on a shelf for months, and now it could continue to stay in my pantry indefinitely. I ate a few bites and tossed it. Afterward I experienced indigestion for several hours as my body protested the foodlike substance, which was not nourishing but damaging. Shelf life means no life.

Products made from white flour contain no nutritional value. Yet humans consume wheat products made from processed white flour all the time. Our bodies do not recognize them as food. Maybe that is why many Americans experience chronic diseases.

Sugar

Sugar-sweetened drinks raise blood-sugar levels and predispose a person to diabetes, a chronic health problem in the US. Heightened blood-sugar levels cause the release of insulin. In turn, blood-sugar levels plummet, and you feel wiped out—devoid of energy. The body releases adrenaline to counteract the low blood sugar, and this causes anxiety and even panic attacks. Could that be why the incidence of anxiety disorders has increased in our society? Blood sugar fluctuations also cause a person to be more irritable and short-tempered.

Watch the excellent documentary *The Sugar Film* about what happens to a person's body after consuming 40 grams (average sugar consumption) of sugar every day for two months. This film claims 80 percent of items in the grocery store has some form of sugar added to it.

Sugar makes our blood sugar fluctuate, and causes us to become addicted to it, which causes the harmful cycle of insulin and adrenaline release. Dr. Avena's research (in the Ted-Ed talk on sugar from step 1) revealed rats binged on sugar when it was offered. She said highly processed foods, such as refined flour, may be as problematic as sugar. Her study found that pizza, chips, and chocolate were some of the most addictive foods for the human body.[3]

Wheat and sugar comprise a large part of the American diet. At church, I sat next to a mom with a twelve-month-old baby. When she got fussy, her mother pulled out a plastic bag with toast and gave some to the child. A little later, the toothless toddler held up a graham cracker she wanted to share with me. When I left, I noticed sugar-sweetened cereal all over the floor.

All of these sugary wheat products were like crack cocaine to the child's brain, since wheat goes to the same opiate brain receptors. On a Positron Emission Tomography Scan (PET) of the human brain, the same area of the brain lit up when an obese person ingested sugar and an addict received cocaine. (To see the imaging results go to Mic.-com/articles/88015/what-happens-to-your-brain-on-sugar-explained-by-science#.huzqY8vAf.)[4] As a result, many Americans become addicted to sugar and carbohydrates, especially when we begin consuming them from a young age.

Corn Syrup

Avoid high-fructose corn syrup (HFCS), an inexpensive alternative to sugar. In the late 1970s, corn syrup was introduced into the American food system to keep manufacturing costs down and that is when obesity rates began to rise. In fact, on a graph, the increased use of HFCS mirrors the rapid increase in obesity in the US. A friend of mine who is a rheumatologist believes HFCS is a major contributor to disease in this country because after its introduction, chronic diseases began rising.

. . .

White Rice

The processing of white rice resembles wheat's story; it is processed and raises blood-sugar levels. To extend its storage life, the husk, bran, and germ are removed from the rice during the milling process, which eliminates most of the grain's nutrients. Therefore, rice is enriched just like wheat products.

Taking the beneficial nutrients out of food and enriching them is not how God intended for us to consume our vitamins and minerals. God created whole grains for our body to assimilate all the nutrients and fiber. Fiber is necessary to keep the bowels moving smoothly. It is difficult to consume the recommended daily allowance of 25–30 grams of fiber by eating processed foods such as white rice. Consuming brown and wild rice are perfectly fine because they contain the whole grain of the rice including the fiber and nutrients.

Corn

Most of the corn in the United States has been genetically modified (GMO) for resistance to insects or herbicides. Genetic engineering enables the addition of insecticidal or herbicidal proteins into the seed. Corn with herbicidal proteins allows the plant to tolerate glyphosate, which is the carcinogenic chemical in Roundup.[5]

Farmers are allowed to spray as much insecticide on GMO corn as they deem necessary. As a result, we consume corn saturated with a carcinogen. Does that sound healthy? *Do not eat corn unless it is organic!* In fact, if you see the brown spot at the tip of a cornhusk, maybe even with a little worm, that corn is not GMO and is suitable to eat. Corn that bugs like is the type of corn humans consumed for centuries.

I use to enjoy eating corn tortilla chips with salsa and guacamole. Unfortunately, the next day I always woke up with a parched mouth from excessive salt and a headache from chemicals in the corn chips. The same thing happens when I eat popcorn at a movie theater. I began thinking of corn products as loaded with a carcinogen, so I changed my mind-set and do not eat them.

. . .

Milk Products

Humans are the only mammals on earth that consume milk after the age of two. Plus, we don't even drink human milk but dairy from a cow. God made cow's milk to nurture a calf so that it can grow to be the size of a cow. Get the hint? If you stop consuming dairy products, you will naturally lose weight.

Milk, similar to wheat and rice, is denatured of its nutritional value to extend its shelf life. I remember when a milkman brought fresh milk to our front door. Food industries heat raw milk to high temperatures (pasteurization), which destroys all microorganisms and most nutrients, and they add vitamin D to it. The raw milk contained enzymes that helped with digestion. Today, lactose intolerance is high.

Consume almond, cashew, or coconut milk products instead of dairy. Don't consume soy milk or soy products unless they are organic because most of the soy crops in the United States are Roundup Ready crops. I eat coconut milk ice cream and kefir. Both are delicious, and I can't tell the difference between the cow or coconut milk products. Kefir is a fermented product that contains natural gut-friendly probiotics.

Artificial Sweeteners

Do not use artificial sweeteners. People who frequently consume sugar substitutes may be at an increased risk of excessive weight gain, type-2 diabetes, and cardiovascular disease. The sugar substitute causes a person to crave sweets. The following link is an informative *Time* magazine article about weight gain associated with the consumption of artificial sweeteners: Time.com/4859012/artificial-sweeteners-weight-loss/.[6]

One of the biggest culprits containing artificial sweeteners is diet soda. Unfortunately, many people think they are being healthy by substituting diet drinks for sugary drinks, but research indicates that artificial sweeteners in diet soda make you crave sugar and increase abdominal fat. Here is the link to a corresponding article: Medical-

Daily.com/4-dangerous-effects-artificial-sweeteners-your-health-247543.[7]

Processed Meats

The World Health Organization classified processed meats (hot dogs, ham, bacon, sausage, and some deli meats) as a group 1 carcinogen.[8] Processed meats are right up there with tobacco, asbestos, and plutonium! Most people have no idea that when they feed their child a hot dog, it is comparable to giving them a cigarette.

Different types of meat processing include salting, fermenting, curing, and smoking. Avoid purchasing any prepackaged lunch meats. Instead, bake a chicken or turkey breast and cut it up to use as lunch meat. If you buy meats at a deli, make sure the attendant cuts slices from a hunk of meat that came from an animal versus the meat being shredded and formed into a mold. For example, you could buy a natural chicken breast or thigh, but often chicken parts are processed together into a molded premade, unnatural patty, which is unhealthy.

Vegetable Oils

Most vegetable oils contain omega 6 fatty acids, which promote inflammation in the human body. Therefore, lower your consumption of omega 6 foods and increase your ingestion of omega 3 foods (which are nourishing for the brain) like avocado, nuts, and fish. Olive oil contains both omega 3 and 6 fats and is high in antioxidants, therefore, it is the preferred oil to consume.

Another beneficial oil, coconut oil, resists oxidation at high heat. Therefore, use coconut oil for high-heat cooking such as frying. Coconut oil also reduces triglycerides, LDL, and total cholesterol levels.

Processed Foods

Processed foods are the foods contained in boxes and bags in the aisles of the grocery store. These foods are far from their harvested form. *Removal of their nutrients and fiber increase their shelf life. Unfortunately, they decrease the life of the person who consumes them.* Consider them dead foods that do not benefit the body but instead harm it. *Therefore, try not to eat any processed foods out of a box or bag.* This includes cereals, chips, crackers, granola bars, cookies, etc.

However, we cannot eat perfectly all the time. We may want to eat chips or crackers with a healthy dip, or we might be a guest for dinner at someone's home. Therefore, try to eat nourishing foods at least 80 percent of the time, but the rest of the time, if you choose to eat a processed food, make sure it is organic and non-GMO.

Eat to live a healthy, bountiful life. Evaluate every single thing you eat. Is it alive or is it dead? Remember, shelf life means no life.

Peanuts

Contrary to popular belief, peanuts are not a nut but a type of a vegetable called a legume (i.e., pea or bean). They grow in the ground and don't come from a tree. I also do not recommend consuming peanut butter because it is hard to digest and many people are allergic to it.

There is a peanut field right behind my house. The peanuts are dug up and left on the ground to dry for a couple of weeks. During that time, they get soaked from rain, and I can only imagine how much mold may grow on them in the humid Florida weather. Almond or cashew nuts and butter are better choices.

Two weeks after my sister got off sugar and refined carbohydrates, she ate some peanuts. Afterward she experienced a stomachache. She had eaten peanuts all her life and never noticed the harmful effects. After she weaned herself off sugar and wheat, she was more aware of the effects different foods had on her body. With time you will become more aware of this as well.

Margarine

Margarine most likely contains trans-fat, which increases the risk of heart disease, and free radicals, which contribute to numerous health problems including cancer. Instead use organic butter, olive oil, and coconut oil.

Canned Goods

Bisphenol (BPA) is an industrial chemical used to make some plastics. Canned foods are lined with BPA to prevent erosion of the can. An ongoing debate ensues between scientific studies and the Federal Drug Administration (FDA) regarding whether the level of BPA found in canned foods is safe for humans. Nonetheless, when we eat canned foods, we are exposed to this chemical. In fact, scientific studies found BPA in the urine of study participants who consumed canned food within the past twenty-four hours.[10] The FDA banned the use of certain BPA-based materials used in infant bottles, sippy cups, and infant formula packaging.[11] Therefore, try not to eat canned goods. Instead, purchase fresh vegetables, fruits, and dried beans. Foods preserved in glass (such as spaghetti sauce), not cans, is a better option.

Microwavable Foods

Many food products are microwaveable—from popcorn to frozen dinners. However, when you microwave your food or beverages the microwave alters the food, decreases hemoglobin, and raises bad cholesterol. Read further evidence in this article: Mercola.com/article/microwave/hazards2.htm.[12] Therefore, I recommend reheating leftovers in a toaster oven and limiting your use of the microwave. It takes three minutes to warm up leftovers in a toaster oven.

For popcorn, simple cook organic, non-GMO kernels in a stovetop pan with a lid. Add a little olive or coconut oil and in three minutes the kernels pop. This is about the same amount of time it takes to pop microwave popcorn. I top my popcorn with half organic butter and half olive oil, along with kelp and dulse seaweed sprinkles and sea salt.

CLEAN OUT THE PANTRY

Step 3 includes cleaning out the pantry and refrigerator. The most enlightening resource for this cleanout is a fifteen-minute video by Dr. Daniel Amen who coauthored *The Daniel Plan*. Watch "What's in Your Pantry" on YouTube.com.[13]

Remove the following unhealthy items from your pantry:

- Wheat—anything that contains wheat
- Sugar-sweetened drinks—like soda, fruit juice, Gatorade (Flavored waters with no calories are okay to keep and finish, but after they are gone it is best to drink water. If you need to, add a slice of lemon and stevia to your water.)
- Sugar—white sugar, high-fructose corn syrup—remove any item with greater than 10 grams of sugar per serving. Unfortunately, sugar does not have a recommended daily allowance.
- Rice—white rice (brown and wild rice are fine)
- Corn—all non-organic corn products such as tortilla chips and popcorn (Organic corn products are fine to consume.)
- Artificial sweeteners—saccharin, aspartame or Equal/NutraSweet, sucralose or Splenda (It is okay to keep honey, maple syrup, agave, stevia, xylitol, coconut sugar, monk fruit sugar.)
- Oils—eliminate all oils except olive oil (use when cooking at low temperatures) and coconut oil (use when cooking at high temperatures)
- Any processed food in a box or bag such as chips, crackers, cookies, and cereal unless it is organic and you choose to make this an exception

- Foods that contain partially hydrogenated vegetable oil, high-fructose corn syrup, or monosodium glutamate (MSG). Food labels disguise MSG through the following names: flavors; flavoring; enzymes; hydrolyzed, autolyzed yeast; barley malt; hydrolyzed vegetable protein; maltodextrin; natural seasonings; and glutamate.

CLEAN OUT THE REFRIGERATOR

Let's move on to cleaning out the refrigerator. Remove the following unhealthy items from your refrigerator.

- Wheat products
- Processed meats such as ham, bacon, sausage, hot dogs, and lunch meat
- Soft drinks and fruit juices—they are loaded with sugar
- Check the ingredients of condiments. If one contains high-fructose corn syrup, throw it out. Health-food stores carry better condiment substitutes, such as organic mayonnaise.
- Margarine—organic butter is a healthier choice
- All milk products except plain Greek yogurt, which contains probiotics

CLEAN OUR YOUR FREEZER

Let's open up that freezer and see what is inside. Throw out the following unhealthy products:

- Wheat products
- Dairy products (Replace your dairy products, such as ice cream, with coconut, almond, or cashew milk items.)
- Packaged frozen meals (while convenient, even the "healthy" brands of frozen foods are processed)

CLEAN OUT YOUR EMOTIONS

Food and emotions are intrinsically tied together for most of us, so we need to do an emotional check when we begin to clean out the foods that have previously brought us comfort.

Interestingly, original sin began with eating. It was probably a sweet fruit, like a fig. In Genesis 3:4–7 we read, "'You will not certainly die,' the serpent said to the woman. 'For God knows that when you eat from it your eyes will be opened, and you will be like God, knowing good and evil.' When the woman saw that the fruit of the tree was good for food and pleasing to the eye, and also desirable for gaining wisdom, she took some and ate it. She also gave some to her husband, who was with her, and he ate it. Then the eyes of both of them were opened, and they realized they were naked; so they sewed fig leaves together and made coverings for themselves" (NIV).

God gave us food to nourish our bodies. Yet food can be used for the wrong reasons. We may eat because we are sad, bored, stressed out, depressed, or happy. As we engage in emotional eating, we turn to food, instead of to God, to appease ourselves. If we feel abandoned, food can be our friend. We can swallow our angry feelings with food, instead of feeling the emotions we don't want to deal with. Food can provide an emotional escape from negative feelings.

To help you go more in-depth into the root cause of a dysfunctional relationship with food, I wrote *Christian Study Guide for 7 Steps to Get Off Sugar and Carbohydrates*. It goes into the issues of childhood wounds, abuse, and generational bondage. Getting to the root cause is vital to resolving the food issue once and for all.

In your journal (appendix 3 or *Healthy Living Journal*) document why you eat. Is it because of hunger or to relieve stress? Do you have a deep emotional wound that needs healing? If you do, journal and talk to God about it. Is there someone you need to forgive? Maybe you have a big hole in your heart that you are filling with food. God is our ultimate healer, take your wounds to him and ask him to heal you. Forgive as Jesus instructed us to do.

Sometimes we engage in mindless eating, where we munch on

something without being hungry. When a person is bored, she may look in the refrigerator or pantry but can't find anything appealing. If this happens to you, food is not what you need. First, drink two glasses of water, as you may be thirsty and don't realize it. Next, your soul may be longing for a connection with God, so spend time with him. Journal your thoughts.

Are you eating because of a negative emotion you do not want to deal with? Don't escape from negative feelings through undesirable eating. Instead, recognize dysfunctional eating behaviors and confront tough issues in your life. Bring those problems to God and be honest with him about what you experience. Each time you recognize emotional eating, clean out your emotions with God. Then you can disengage the connection between eating and feelings.

Your value to God is not determined by what you weigh. Your body is the temple of the Holy Spirit. Do not try to overcome inappropriate eating on your own, instead call on the power of the Holy Spirit to empower you to change. With God's help, you can overcome and succeed. Opening up to your accountability partner and support group is also instrumental in attaining success over emotional eating, as they can remind you of God's power in your life and can pray with you to reconnect with God when you are fighting the spiritual battle around food and emotions.

Stress also causes us to turn to food. We live in a fast-paced world where we eat on the run. We no longer have traditional meals prepared from scratch at home. Unfortunately, food industries are cooking our food for us today.

Determine the stressors (things that cause you stress) in your life, and list them in your journal. Can you do something about the stressors? Evaluate each one and brainstorm on how to minimize them. Pray to God and ask him to enlighten you and help you. Ask your accountability partner or support group for help and prayer in dealing with your stressors

How do you cope with stress? Do you tend to deal with it through undesirable eating habits? If so, recognize this and choose to do something about your stress level. Can you eliminate a stressor in your life? Some stress-relieving activities include praying with your prayer partner, enjoying a massage, journaling, and calling a friend.

Do you exercise? Exercising, a positive coping strategy for dealing with stress, burns off adrenaline and improves sleep. Do you engage in relaxation techniques such as Christian yoga or meditation? Yoga and meditation calm the mind and body. I created several Christian yoga products including DVDs, books, and card decks available at: ChristianYoga.com.

Stress tends to make people crave carbohydrates, sugary comfort foods, and junk food. These types of processed foods give you a sugar rush, but then your blood sugar crashes, and you feel rotten. The feelings from the blood-sugar fluctuation cause even more anxiety.

Plan Ahead to Avoid Emotional and Stress Eating

To develop an effective plan, document in your journal what you eat and why. A list of items to record in your journal is provided in appendix 3. Record any negative emotions you experience and determine if you eat because of your feelings. Connect the dots between your eating habits and emotions. If you discover you are engaging in emotional eating, you need to substitute it with another behavior. Also record in your journal the stressors in your life and when you are feeling stressed, so you can replace unhealthy food choices with positive behaviors.

When you recognize you are about to emotionally eat or eat out of stress, set the timer for ten minutes and spend that time with God. Express your emotions and ask him to transform your mind. Recite Bible verses out loud. After the timer rings, if you still want to eat, go on a walk, call your accountability partner, or put in a Christian yoga DVD. Break the cycle of the emotions you feel and your conditioned response to eating. A list of Food Addiction Battle Strategies is provided in appendix 10.

TAKING STEP 3: CLEAN OUT

Now that you've made it to step 3, you should feel more confident about incorporating new food choices into your healthier lifestyle. Make sure you take the following action steps:

1. Schedule a date to clean out your pantry, refrigerator, and freezer.

Date to clean out:Date accomplished:

Pantry _____

Refrigerator _____

Freezer _____

2. Cleaning out your emotions entails several steps. Do you have your journal yet? You can purchase the *Healthy Living Journal* at Susan-UNeal.com/Shop. Are you journaling what you eat and determining why you are eating? Please see the list of items you should be recording in appendix 3. Be sure to journal your thoughts and emotions too.

3. List the things in your life which cause you stress.

_____

_____

4. Think about ways that you can reduce or eliminate these stressors. List those ideas:

_____

_____

5. List some activities you would like to do to decrease your stress:

. . .

----

7 Steps to Get Off Sugar and Carbohydrates:

Step 1. Decide to improve your health through proper nutrition.- substitute positive behaviors for

Step 2. Acquire a support system and knowledge to help make a lifestyle change.

Step 3. Clean out your pantry and refrigerator by removing unhealthy foods and clean out your emotions.

STEP 4: PURCHASE HEALTHY FOODS AND AN ANTI-CANDIDA CLEANSE

Decide—>Acquire—>Clean Out—>**Purchase**—>Plan—>Prepare—>Improve

You decided (step 1) to make a lifestyle change and improve your health. Acquiring knowledge (step 2) about changing your eating habits and identifying your support system takes time but will help you keep your commitment to this decision. Cleaning out (step 3) the pantry and refrigerator was a chore, but not as difficult as cleaning out your emotions. Now it is time to *purchase* (step 4) groceries based on the healthy eating guidelines specified in this chapter.

When I told my sister that a low-glycemic diet meant she could no longer eat wheat, rice, or anything with sugar, she asked, "What *can* I eat?"

I told her, "You can eat vegetables, beans, meat, nuts, seeds, and low-sugar fruit."

To her (and probably you), this was a total change in her diet, since she ate primarily high glycemic foods. This change in eating habits felt radical and seemed limiting to her, but God gave us an incredible variety of food to enjoy and sustain our bodies, including a vast selection of different vegetables and fruits.

HEALTHY FOODS TO PURCHASE

In step 2 we reviewed a long list of resources so you can continue to educate yourself about making this lifestyle change. However, I believe our most significant resource is the Bible, so let's check out what God told us to eat. "Then God said, 'Look! I have given you every seed-bearing plant throughout the earth and all the fruit trees for your food'" (Genesis 1:29). We know what a fruit tree is, but what exactly is a seed-bearing plant? It produces seeds that can be planted again, such as grains and vegetables.

Fruits are so sweet and delicious they can be called God's candy. Instead of eating a dish of ice cream, eat a juicy strawberry, tangy green apple, or crunchy pomegranate. Fruits are not just juicy and sweet but also provide the body with the fiber, vitamins, and minerals our bodies need to be healthy. God is an artist who created different sizes, shapes, and vibrant colors of fruit.

God also created over a hundred different vegetables because the human body needs various types of nutrients essential for proper growth and performance. For example, spinach contains vitamins A and K, whereas broccoli is full of vitamin E. God gave us a variety to choose from to ensure we get the proper amounts of fiber, vitamins, and minerals.

Grains provide carbohydrates the body uses for fuel or energy. Similar to gas in a car. God offered us an assortment of grains to choose from: amaranth, barley, buckwheat, millet, oats, quinoa, rice, rye, wheat, and wild rice. Two grains I do not recommend are white rice and wheat, because of the way they are processed today, with the nutrients stripped away; all others are beneficial.

Nuts are excellent sources of protein, similar to meat. Again, God created numerous varieties to choose from including almond, brazil, cashew, chestnut, hazelnut, macadamia, pecan, pistachio, pine, and walnut. Be sure to buy raw nuts because they contain more nutrition in their natural, raw form, not roasted, salted, or sugar coated. Instead, taste the natural flavor of almonds, pecans, and walnuts. God gave us nuts to eat, and they are full of omega 3 oils, which are essential for brain function.

As previously explained, peanuts are not a nut but a type of vegetable called a legume (i.e., pea or bean). They grow in the ground and don't come from a tree. I do not recommend consuming products made with peanuts because it is hard to digest and many people are allergic to it. Other legumes (beans, lentils, and peas) may be difficult for some people to digest, but generally don't cause allergic reactions.

God gave us chia, flax, hemp, poppy, pumpkin, sesame, and sunflower seeds. Seeds are full of trace minerals the human body needs but in small amounts. Since God made us, he knows what our bodies require, and he provides it for us in different ways.

Fruits and vegetables are seasonal, which means each season (spring, summer, fall, winter) different crops are harvested. In the south, strawberries ripen in early spring. Okra and peas grow best in the summer. Pumpkins mature in the fall. Citrus fruit is picked in the winter when our bodies require more vitamin C to prevent colds. God supplies a selection of fruit and vegetables each season, and we should eat the ones that ripen in that season. Not only will we get the nutrients we need for that season but we won't tire of eating the same type of food all year long.

Sometimes we get into the habit of eating the same sort of food over and over again, but it is healthier to eat an assortment to get a variety of nutrients. We can choose from a vast number of fruits, vegetables, grains, nuts, and seeds, and each is unique in its flavor and amount of nutrients. God knew what he was doing when he created these nutrient-rich foods for us to consume. They not only provide what our body needs but they are delicious to enjoy as well. God wants us to enjoy all of his creation.

Yet God never put food in a box or bag and had them sit on the shelf for months. He didn't label them with an expiration date. He gave humans a vast selection of food since their bodies need a broad range of nutrients to function correctly. *By eating different foods from each food category (vegetable, fruit, grain, nut, seed), you take proper care of your body.* God did not give us vitamin pills either. Instead he created fresh food right from the plant or tree and loaded them with vitamins and minerals so our bodies will function at their highest potential.

After the flood, God introduced meat into the human diet. As God directed Noah in Genesis 9:2–3, "'All wild animals and birds and fish will be afraid of you,' God told him; 'for I have placed them in your power, and they are yours to use for food, in addition to grain and vegetables'" (TLB). After humans began consuming meat, their life-span significantly shortened. I am not saying we shouldn't eat meat. However, there are healthy protein alternatives to meat such as nuts and beans.

When you purchase meat, make sure it is organic, grass fed, or free range with no hormones or antibiotics. I think the antibiotics we consume from our meat also harm our gut flora.

We do not need to consume meat at every meal. From a blood analysis, my sister discovered she had an excess amount of protein. Too much protein in a person's diet causes the body to extract calcium from the bones and send it into the bloodstream to balance its pH.[1] This calcium leaching weakens a person's bones and is a factor in osteoporosis. In fact, incidences of osteoporosis in third-world countries with a low-protein diet are lower than industrialized nations.[2]

One summer I bought a new fruit and vegetable every week at the grocery store. It was an excellent experience for our children and me as I got out of the rut of cooking the same meals over and over, and we found different foods we liked such as red cabbage, star fruit, and bok choy.

HEALTHY EATING GUIDELINES

The following healthy eating guidelines are my secret to maintaining optimal weight and brain health. This is a low-carbohydrate, low-glycemic, anti-inflammatory eating plan, which is the type of diet recommended for improving memory and cognition and preventing and reversing type-2 diabetes. A summary of Healthy Eating Guidelines is included in appendix 5.

A low-glycemic diet does not raise blood sugar or insulin levels. Foods high in carbohydrates cause a release of glucose into the bloodstream and a corresponding rise in insulin. Avoid the following high-carbohydrate foods: cakes, crackers, sugary cereals and drinks, flours, bread products, jellies/jams, and refined potato products. These types of foods are addictive.

Low-carbohydrate, anti-inflammatory dietary guidelines include:

- About 50 percent of food items are fresh organic vegetables.
- Eat one fresh, raw serving of low-glycemic fruit per day. Low-glycemic fruits include green apples, berries, cherries, pears, plums, and grapefruit.
- Do not always eat cooked foods. Eat a couple of servings of raw vegetables every day. Have a salad for lunch with either nuts or meat. When eating out, order a salad or coleslaw as sides, since both are raw.
- Another 25 percent of your daily food intake should come from an animal or vegetable protein such as beans, nuts, and lean meats. Fish is exceptionally nutritious. Try to eat it once a week.
- A variety of different nuts and seeds are excellent sources of protein, minerals, and essential fatty acids.
- Avoid sugar, flour, rice, pasta, and bread. Instead, eat more fruits, vegetables, and low-glycemic grains such as quinoa and pearled barley.
- Do not eat sugary cereals. Instead, eat oatmeal, fruit, or

granola. Be careful, as the sugar content of granola may be high. My favorite granola recipe appears in appendix 4.

- Try not to eat anything containing more than 10 grams of sugar in one serving.
- Eat nontraditional grains such as quinoa, amaranth, pearled barley, wild rice, and organic oats.
- Eat cultured foods such as kimchi, sauerkraut, and cultured plain Greek yogurt since they contain natural probiotics. Add one to two tablespoons of these foods to a meal twice a week or eat the yogurt as a snack. Personally, I take a probiotic capsule every day.
- Replace undesirable ingredients with whole foods. *The Daniel Plan Cookbook* by Rick Warren provides a chart titled Foods and Ingredients to Avoid and suggests replacements.[3] A few recommendations from this book include:
- Replace sugary snacks with nuts, nut butter, dark chocolate, and plain Greek yogurt with berries.
- Replace condiments and sauces containing MSG or high-fructose corn syrup with spices, vinegar, and herbs.
- Replace table salt with kosher or sea salt.
- Replace fried foods with baked foods.

My additional healthy eating tips include:

- Make homemade granola from organic oats (recipe in appendix 4). For breakfast, I add fresh berries to a bowl of granola.
- Buy or whip up a flavorful dip like hummus or guacamole to eat with a platter of fresh vegetables (not chips or pita bread).
- Substitute beans for meat for some meals.
- Squeeze a slice of lemon and add a couple drops of liquid stevia into a glass of water. It is like drinking lemonade.
- Boil eggs and keep them in the refrigerator for a snack.

- Chew your food thoroughly because this is where digestion begins.

Please try not to be overwhelmed by all of this information. Guide your eating with the 80/20 percent rule. *If you eat healthy 80 percent of the time and not so healthy 20 percent of the time, this will probably be an improvement.*

I don't eat perfectly, but I try. With God's help, I attempt not to eat more than 10 grams of sugar at one sitting. If I mess up, the next day I get to start new, as indicated in Lamentations 3:22–23, "Because of the LORD's great love we are not consumed, for his compassions never fail. They are new every morning; great is your faithfulness" (NIV).

Each morning as I wake up, my body tells me how well I ate the previous day. If I did not experience any blood sugar fluctuations, I have a clear mind and abundant energy. The incredible sensation of how God created our bodies to feel motivates me to continue to eat well every day. I am more productive when I eat healthy foods.

While shopping at a grocery store, shop along the edges of the store in the dairy, meat, and produce sections. Stay away from the center of the store where processed foods experience an extended shelf life. Remember, *a long shelf life means the nutritional value of the food has been removed.* Otherwise, the food becomes rancid at some point. If a food spoils, it is beneficial, but if it does not spoil, it contains no nutrients.

HEALTHY SUBSTITUTIONS TO PURCHASE

Many unhealthy food choices can be replaced with healthy alternatives that are whole, unprocessed, and natural. In addition to the replacements mentioned above from Rick Warren's book *The Daniel Plan Cookbook*, the following sections offer a number of options to replace the unhealthy foods you eliminated in step 3 with healthy, flavorful foods as God intended.

. . .

Sugar Substitutes

Substitute sugar with a natural sweetener, stevia, which is an herb. Purchase stevia in a health food store because popular stevia products at the grocery store are too refined. Another option is local honey. However, honey raises blood sugar levels. I use a powder form of stevia for baking. Also, I found a natural sweetener with zero calories that rates zero on the glycemic index—Lakanto Monkfruit Sweetener (Lakanto.com/); which is made from monk fruit.

In the following list I rank the best natural sugar substitutes based on their glycemic index:

stevia-0

monk fruit sweetener-0

xylitol-12

agave-15

coconut sugar-35

honey-50

maple syrup-54

Try out these different sweeteners. Choose a natural, low-glycemic sweetener that you can live with and use it sparingly.

Pasta Substitutes

My sister wanted to know what she would use for pasta in her new lifestyle. I told her to buy spaghetti squash, use shirataki noodles, or spiralize zucchini. Spaghetti squash can sit on a counter for a couple of weeks, just like a box of spaghetti, and it is simple to cook. Cut it in half, scrape the seeds out of the center, and put it, cut side up, on a baking sheet with 1/4 inch of water in the pan. Bake at 350° for 30–40 minutes. When done, scrape the inside with a fork for a low-glycemic "spaghetti." The squash absorbs any flavor you put on it, such as shrimp scampi or spaghetti sauce. This vegetable also tastes great as a side dish with olive oil and seasonings.

To spiralize zucchini, purchase a spiralizer. Push the zucchini through the device and out comes your zucchini noodles. For shirataki noodles, cook them as directed on the package and add your sauce. Again, zucchini and shirataki noodles absorb the flavor of the sauce added to them.

Meat Substitutes

Fish, nuts, and beans are excellent sources of protein, which are healthier for you than meat. Every week, prepare a few meals with one of these meat substitutes as the primary protein source. Serve fish one night, beans another, and nuts on your salad for a third.

Nuts also contain omega-3 fatty acids. Pecans grow in the south, walnuts in the Carolinas, macadamia nuts in Hawaii. What types of nuts grow in your area? I recommend that during the nut-harvesting season in your area you purchase a lot of nuts. Every year, I freeze at least twelve pint jars of pecans. I use one every month. This is an excellent way to obtain local, fresh nuts at an economical price.

Beans are another great substitute for meat. I recommend cooking one meal a week with beans as the main source of protein. Appendix 4 contains a lot of flavorful recipes that include beans. Dried beans are better for you than canned. Soak beans overnight and throw out the water. The water contains the beans' gas-causing substance. If you need to, take a digestive enzyme from the health food store to prevent flatulence.

Try to substitute fish for meat. Fresh wild-caught salmon is available in upper-end grocery stores from July–October. I try to serve this twice a month during this time. Plan on preparing fish once a week. Leftover fish is not as palatable as fresh, so I included a delicious fish stew recipe in appendix 4.

Another alternative to meat is whole grain quinoa, which contains five grams of protein in one serving (1/2 cup cooked). I sauté fresh vegetables and combine them with quinoa for a satisfying meal that takes only twenty minutes to prepare. Countless vegetable combinations can be created: sautéed scallions, mushrooms, and spinach along with sunflower and pumpkin seeds; sautéed onion, bell peppers, and kale with a fresh avocado on top; sautéed bok choy, snow peas, and carrots with cashews and sesame seeds.

Dairy Substitutes

It is best not to consume milk products. However, several healthy dairy substitutes include almond, cashew, and coconut milk. Personally, I enjoy the flavor of toasted coconut almond blend, which combines both of these milks. If you like soy milk, be sure to purchase organic soy products as soy is one of the Roundup Ready crops I discussed in step 2.

WATER

Most people do not nourish and cleanse their bodies with an adequate amount of water on a daily basis. The human body is comprised of 75 percent water, and we can't survive for more than a few days without it. Some people think drinking tea, juice, soda, or other drinks will hydrate their body, but they don't. In fact, caffeinated beverages are a diuretic, which causes you to urinate more frequently and lose fluid. Drink an average of eight glasses of water per day.

However, your water requirements depend upon your size. Various sources recommend: "Drink half your weight in ounces every day." Using this formula, a 130-pound person should drink eight glasses of water. (130/2 = 65 ounces; 65/8 ounces (1 cup) = 8 glasses.)

Scheduling when to drink water throughout the day can be tricky because it is best to drink on an empty stomach. Therefore, drink two glasses of water early in the morning before breakfast. Drink two more glasses before lunch. In the afternoon, when you desire an afternoon snack, drink two glasses of water, which will help curb your appetite. Consume your last two glasses before dinner. Yes, you will go to the bathroom more often; don't think of it as a burden but as a process whereby toxins expel from your body. Don't drink any beverage after dinner to prevent getting up during the night to go to the bathroom.

If you do not consume an adequate amount of water, your body suffers the consequences. Some common symptoms of dehydration include constipation, fatigue, dry skin and mouth, bladder and kidney problems, and high blood pressure since the blood is thicker. Our blood is 90 percent water.

My mother and aunt did not like water. They preferred sweet tea and coffee. My aunt contracted bladder cancer and my mother experienced frequent urinary tract infections (UTI). Water helps cleanse the body of toxins. If we don't drink enough water to flush the toxins out of our kidneys and bladder, the toxins accumulate in these organs and cause infection and disease.

Consider these additional tips for your water intake each day:

- Do not drink with meals because the fluid dilutes digestive enzymes, which secrete to break down the food. Instead, drink between meals, usually three hours after a meal, which gives time for food digestion. You may drink up to ten minutes before you eat.
- Drink an average of eight glasses of water every day or the recommended amount for your weight. Other than coffee or tea, water should be the only beverage consumed. Do not count coffee and tea toward the number of glasses of water.
- If you feel hungry, drink water. Scientists reported that two 8-ounce glasses of water is an effective weight loss strategy because many times when a person feels hungry, they are actually thirsty.[4] So drink water and see if that fills you up before eating. You may be pleasantly surprised.

The *Healthy Living Journal* contains a Water Tracker Chart for you to keep track of how much water your drink on a daily basis.

FOODS THAT CAUSE INFLAMMATION

Some medical literature claims inflammation is the root of chronic disease. Where do you think inflammation comes from? It generates from what we put into our bodies and most likely from the food we ingest.

We eat many foods that are far from the product that they were when it was harvested. The human body does not recognize some of these so-called foods as beneficial and so it reacts negatively and causes inflammation. Inflammation causes a wide-range of negative effects across many systems in the body. It is important to identify what food is causing a negative effect in you. A week after my sister stopped eating wheat, her joint pain went away. This is an example of the positive effects that occur when you eliminate inflammatory foods.

Limit milk products because they cause mucus formation and inflammation. In fact, dairy is recognized as one of the top five inflammatory foods.[5] If you are lactose intolerant, like me, do not eat or drink milk products. However, if you choose to ingest dairy, take a lactaid tablet to help with digestion.

Sugar and wheat are two other major inflammation-causing foods. I taught The Daniel Plan by Rick Warren, which recommends you stop eating sugar, wheat, and milk products for one week. Then you reintroduce one of those foods at a time to determine any adverse effects. Every time I reintroduced dairy products, I experienced additional phlegm and postnasal drip. I realized milk products caused inflammation in my system, yet I had consumed them for fifty years. It is vital for you to figure out what may be causing an inflammatory response in your body too. When you track the foods you eat and your bodies response to them you determine which foods cause inflammation in your body.

Our food today contains all sorts of chemicals and additives. Conversely, a vegetable or piece of fruit does not contain artificial additives except for the pesticides and herbicides sprayed on them. I do not want to consume any glyphosate (carcinogen) residue contained in Roundup Ready crops such as oats, wheat, soy, corn, or sugar beets. Consequently, I buy organic and I recommend you do too.

If you choose to purchase nonorganic fruits and vegetables, understand that the thinner the skin, the deeper the pesticide and herbicide penetrate the fruit. For example, strawberries soak up the chemicals, but bananas have a thicker skin and therefore do not.

I met a woman at a conference who suffered from inflammation so severely she experienced swelling throughout her whole body, including her fingers. As we reviewed the three primary food culprits —sugar, wheat, and dairy—she told me it couldn't be dairy because she loved cheese and ate it her whole life. I explained to her that a high consumption of cheese might be causing an inflammatory response in her body, but she wouldn't find out until she stopped eating it for at least a week and observed her symptoms when she reintroduced it.

If you think there may be a specific food causing you problematic symptoms in your body, eliminate it for at least a week. When you reintroduce it, be sure to record in your journal what symptoms you experience. If you would like me to coach you during this process, I offer healthy and wellness coaching services at SusanUNeal.com/Health-Coaching.

GUT HEALTH

You may have an imbalance in the flora of your gut if you crave sugar, alcohol, wheat, and processed foods. If your gut is not healthy, you are not healthy. An excellent resource that will explain what occurs when you develop an intestinal imbalance is *The Body Ecology Diet* by Donna Gates.[6] Check out her website Bodyecology.com.

After taking antibiotics and steroids due to an abscessed tooth, I suffered from candidiasis (an overgrowth of yeast) in my gut. A person's abdomen becomes distended when they have an overgrowth of yeast. Is your stomach distended? Candidiasis is like a parasite growing inside of you, and you don't even know it. The Candida begins to grow roots into the lining of your GI tract and makes you crave carbs because that is what it eats. Stopping this parasite's cravings and killing the Candida is tough, but I did and you can too!

To kill the overgrowth of yeast, I stopped eating specific foods for eight months. These foods included: sugar, fruit, wheat, and rice. I had to limit my alcohol consumption to vodka because it is distilled not fermented, therefore, it does not contain a grain like wheat. Most, if not all, alcoholics have candidiasis.

I was successful in killing the yeast in my colon, but I still cannot eat foods with high sugar content or the Candida starts to grow again. I can tell it is growing when I start to crave carbohydrates and feel tired.

During the eight months of my strict anti-Candida diet, I also took large doses of probiotics (up to 100 billion units/day). Probiotics for colon and vaginal health helped target those problem areas. Today, I still take probiotics but not such a large dose. The *Grain Brain* author, Dr. David Perlmutter, recommends taking a probiotic that contains at least ten billion active cultures from at least ten different strains including Lactobacillus acidophilus and Bifidobacteruim.[7] Therefore, I change the brand of my probiotic every time I purchase a new one, so I can get a wide-range of beneficial microorganisms.

To determine if you have a candida overgrowth in your gut, take the Candida Quiz at CandiQuiz.com.

FIBER

Be sure you get enough fiber. Most of us do not consume the recommended 25–30 grams of fiber per day. You should have a bowel movement (BM) at least once a day. Meat slows digestion. As you increase the fruits and vegetables in your diet, having a daily BM will not be a problem.

We need something like a broom to sweep out the inside of our colons and remove the buildup of fecal matter. Our natural broom is raw fruits and vegetables. Every spring when my garden produces its first crop, my number of BMs increase as fresh vegetables sweep my colon. Eating fresh fruits and vegetables is a natural method to cleanse a colon. You may notice an increase in your BMs as you increase your consumption of vegetables instead of processed foods. If you experience constipation, supplement with oxygenated magnesium, ground flaxseed, or other natural fiber supplements from a health food store.

WEEKLY MENU PLANNING

Planning my weekly menu takes about an hour, and I usually do this on Sunday afternoons. If the weather is nice, I sit by the pool and get my vitamin D naturally from the sun. Twenty minutes of sun without sunscreen is beneficial and won't cause sun damage. I use one recipe book and something to write on, or I use the notes app on my smartphone.

Create two lists—a grocery list and a menu for the breakfast, lunch, snack, and dinner for the week. Post the menu on the refrigerator. Next, hit the grocery store or local farmer's market. Your family will appreciate your planning and food preparation, and being prepared will keep you from making unhealthy impulsive choices when you grocery shop.

Be sure to purchase an anti-Candida cleanse from a health food store or online. An attendant at the health food store can tell you the best cleanse that they carry. Food addiction and Candida overgrowth are the most likely reasons a person craves sugary foods and refined carbohydrates.

JOURNAL

During each step of this lifestyle change, continue to journal. Have you purchased the *Healthy Living Journal* or created your own journal yet? The journal's purpose is to record what you eat, drink, and exercise, as well as the emotional and spiritual implications you have with food. See appendix 3 for specific documentation suggestions.

Keep track in your journal of the number of glasses of water you consume per day. Also write down how frequently you exercise a week. This tracking is important for your physical health, yet one of the most valuable components of your journal is what takes place in your mind. When you choose to binge, what have you told yourself? Write it down. Just as it is important to determine the nutritional content of food, it is vital to figure out the strongholds you have in your mind. Understanding yourself and what your inner voice tells you about food is instrumental to determine the root cause of dysfunctional food habits.

Jesus told us in John 10:10, "The thief's purpose is to steal, kill and destroy. My purpose is to give life in all its fullness" (TLB). Are you living life to its fullness? Is your health or weight impeding you from embracing a healthy, bountiful life? Remember to evaluate every single thing you purchase to eat. Is it dead or is it alive?

TAKING STEP 4: PURCHASE

This step helps you purchase the right foods and plan for buying and eating the right foods to continue on this healthy journey. Make sure you take the following action steps:

1. Become familiar with the healthy eating guidelines provided in step 4 and appendix 5. Print out a printable version of this appendix at SusanUNeal.com/appendix.
2. Determine what alternatives you will use for sugar, pasta, dairy, and to some extend meat.
3. Plan your menu for the week and a corresponding grocery list.
4. Purchase healthy, organic fruits, vegetables, whole grains, nuts, seeds, fish, and meats.
5. Take the Candida Quiz at CandiQuiz.com.
6. Buy and implement an anti-Candida cleanse.
7. If you haven't done so already, purchase the *Healthy Living Journal* or create your own journal.

7 Steps to Get Off Sugar and Carbohydrates:

Step 1. Decide to improve your health through proper nutrition.

Step 2. Acquire a support system and knowledge to help make a lifestyle change.

Step 3. Clean out your pantry and refrigerator by removing unhealthy foods and clean out your emotions.

Step 4. Purchase healthy foods and an anti-Candida cleanse.

5

STEP 5: PLAN FOR THE START DATE

Decide—>Acquire—>Clean Out—>Purchase—>**Plan**—>Prepare—>Improve

We need both a physical and spiritual *plan* for getting off sugar and carbohydrates. We are complex beings with a body, mind, spirit, and soul. From step 2, we understand the biochemical component of addiction to wheat and sugar. However, the spiritual component remains—that these products may be a stronghold we turn to instead of God to meet our needs. A seven-day plan of how to wean our physical bodies off of these highly addictive products and a detailed five-step spiritual plan for resisting temptation is examined in step 5.

Once you have eliminated unhealthy foods (step 3) and purchased good, nutritious foods (step 4), begin changing your eating habits by following the seven-day outline below. If you work, I recommend starting this program on a Wednesday so you can rest on the weekend. The first few days will be difficult (similar to a drug addict coming off of a drug), but with the help of Christ, prayer, an accountability partner, and these guidelines you can succeed! I included scripture verses in appendix 1 for you to recite when tempted to eat unhealthy foods.

My sister followed the Seven-Day Eating Plan. She started the plan on a Wednesday. She experienced a headache on Saturday and Monday after eliminating sugar and processed foods. Fortunately, by Monday evening her bothersome symptoms associated with stopping the sugar addiction subsided. After a week of being off sugar, she felt more energetic. She also noticed her joint pain was gone and she no longer passed gas. The first week was tough, but she did it.

You can succeed too—my sister did, I did—so let's ask God to help you: "Dear heavenly Father, please be with the reader who wants to change the way she eats so she can live the abundant life you planned for her. Please give her the power and strength to succeed. For Psalm 138:3 states, 'As soon as I pray, you answer me; you encourage me by giving me strength.' Please Lord, give her strength. Through Jesus's holy name we pray. Amen."

Appendix 6 includes a summary of this Seven-Day Eating Plan.

SEVEN-DAY EATING PLAN

Day 1 (Start on Wednesday)
1. Consume Water
Drink up to two cups of coffee or tea per day, but no more. The only other beverage you should drink is filtered water. I use a filter on my refrigerator water dispenser and a water filter on a pitcher. Before breakfast drink two glasses of water, two before lunch, two midafternoon, and two more before dinner. Do not drink during meals and do not drink anything after dinner. Drink up to ten minutes before eating.

2. Take a Probiotic
Begin taking a probiotic every day. I usually buy several probiotics from a health food store with at least ten different strains of beneficial bacteria, and I take a different one each day to vary the flora in my

gastrointestinal system. I store my probiotics in the refrigerator door. After I take a probiotic, I move the bottle to a different shelf, so I can keep track of the one I took last.

3. Stop Eating High-Sugar Foods

Stop eating anything containing greater than 10 grams of sugar per serving. The American Heart Association recommends you limit your calories from sugar to no more than half of your total calories, which is a lot. For most women in the US that should be no more than 24 grams of sugar or 100 calories per day. For men it is 36 grams of sugar or 150 calories from sugar per day. Check labels for the number of grams of sugar per serving size.

Day 2

1. Eliminate Wheat

Do not eat anything containing wheat. No more bagels, toast, pancakes, biscuits, pasta, pretzels, crackers, cookies, cake, or pie. Eliminating wheat is like going off a drug. Be aware that you may experience the following symptoms for a few days: irritability, foggy brain, and fatigue. You might even feel fluish. However, within a week your symptoms will subside. After this, never eat wheat or more than 10 grams of sugar in one serving again, or your addiction will start all over again. (Ugh.)

Day 3

1. Eliminate Processed Foods

Do not eat processed foods from boxes and bags.

2. Implement Healthy Eating Guidelines

Make 50 percent of your food fresh and raw. Follow the Healthy Eating Guidelines provided in appendix 5.

Add digestive enzymes to your meals if you're having trouble digesting food (belching, indigestion). A health-food store attendant can provide advice regarding which digestive enzyme to purchase.

. . .

Days 4 and 5 (Saturday and Sunday)

Continue to implement all the steps listed on day one through three as you proceed.

1. Rest

Focus on you. Rest, read, pray, and ask God to help you to succeed.

2. Use the Sword of the Spirit

Now is the time to fight the thief Jesus spoke of in John 10:10, for Satan wants you to fail: "The thief's purpose is to steal, kill and destroy. My purpose is to give life in all its fullness" (John 10:10 TLB).

Fight the thief with the sword of the Spirit—the Word of God. Write verses on index cards or put them on the notes app on your smartphone. Use verses that will remind you of the help God provides in any struggles you may be facing at this point, such as Philippians 4:13: "For I can do everything through Christ, who gives me strength." Every time you get the urge to go back to your old eating habits, speak the verse out loud to cut the demonic influence out of your life. Our spiritual nature needs to be addressed as well as our physical.

Day 6

1. Start the Anti-Candida Cleanse

Now let's kill the bug in your gut—Candida. Today, start the anti-Candida cleanse you purchased in step 4. If you are not ready to begin this step because you are still experiencing symptoms of withdrawal (headache, exhaustion, irritability, mental fogginess, fluish symptoms), wait a few days until you feel better. Read the instructions on the cleanse package for how to administer it. Initially, I recommend taking the cleanse every other day for the first week to minimize lethargy and headaches. You will feel awful if the dead Candida is not quickly expelled from your colon. To avoid becoming constipated, drink plenty of water. During the second week, begin taking the Candida cleanse every day as recommended.

How long should you stay on the Candida cleanse? The cleanse label provides specific instructions, though it depends on the severity of your Candida overgrowth. Through a colonic irrigation, my therapist found I had a severe Candida infection. I stayed on the cleanse until I finished the bottle—about a month. In fact, I took a second bottle as well. Currently, I go on the cleanse every time I begin having symptoms of a Candida infection (crave carbs and feel fatigued), and I usually stay on the cleanse for one week.

During this cleanse you need frequent bowel movements to eliminate the dead Candida from your colon. If you become constipated, you will get a headache. Prevent a headache by increasing the fiber in your diet through a fiber supplement (which usually comes with your Candida cleanse), water, and raw fruits and vegetables.

The first three days you are on the cleanse, you may not feel well, but after a week you will begin to feel better than you have in a long time. You are just about to get the life back Jesus wants you to experience—one that is abundant and full.

Regarding bowel movements (BM), humans should have at least one a day, if not two, when you are not on a cleanse. When my sister started the cleanse, she had four BMs in one day. She had a lot of fecal matter built up in her colon. Think of a colon like a pipe with sludge built up on the inside. A colon could have a half-inch of fecal matter sticking to it. We use Drano to clean out our drain and pipes. The cleanse is kind of like Drano for the colon. This cleanse is milder than a colonoscopy prep. My sister lost a pound that day!

Day 7

1. Get Up and Exercise

If you are still feeling the symptoms of withdrawal, be gentle with yourself by performing a simple form of exercise such as walking or yoga.

It doesn't matter what type of exercise you do just as long as you do it. Walking, jumping rope, lifting weights, or taking a group fitness class like Pilates or water aerobics are a few examples of exercise. After you begin feeling better, try to exercise for twenty minutes three times a week. I found the book *Eat Right 4 Your Type* by Dr. Peter D'Adamo informative regarding the type of activity each blood type is most inclined to enjoy. It was right on for me with yoga, swimming, bicycling, and hiking.

Record the exercise you perform in your journal that you set up in step 2. If you haven't been or aren't exercising, determine why you don't do it more. Is it because you don't have the time or you're too tired? Is there any type of exercise you enjoy? Figure out what you like to do and put it on your calendar. Ask a family member, friend, or neighbor to join you on a regular basis, so you encourage each other to keep up this beneficial habit.

If you previously consumed high-sugar products, the fluctuations in your blood sugar may have caused lethargy, especially when blood-sugar levels plummeted. As you remove these products from your diet, at first you will become even more tired, but after a week or two, your energy level will increase. At that time, you can explore additional exercise activities. Is there a type of physical endeavor you enjoyed when you were younger? Maybe it's time to try it again.

Recently, I joined a Facebook group that schedules hikes on Saturday mornings. I enjoy meeting new people and conversing as we walk in a unique setting each week. The time flies while walking with friends. Do you have someone you could walk with? Sharing workouts with another person makes it more enjoyable and adds accountability.

I love to swim because when I am under the water, it feels like a different world. If you find an activity you enjoy, it becomes a pleasure instead of a burden. Figure out what you like to do, carve out the time, and do it!

Irrefutable evidence exists that regular physical activity prevents numerous chronic diseases such as diabetes, cancer, obesity, depression, hypertension, osteoporosis, osteoarthritis, and cardiovascular disease.[1] In fact, the most physically active people are the ones with the lowest risk of contracting these chronic diseases.[2] So get out and do whatever physical activity you appreciate. What matters is that you get moving.

Two months after my sister started this lifestyle change, she joined a gym. The trainer set up her routine for the machines and weights. As she tried different group fitness classes, she found Zumba was too fast for her, but she enjoyed the pace of yoga.

I teach Christian yoga. For years I could've found an excuse to not go to the gym--it's raining, I'm tired--you get the picture. But because I taught the class I had to show up. Join an exercise class where you have accountability (you paid for the class, or you have someone to hold you accountable to attend).

The gentle Christian yoga class I teach is called Scripture Yoga™. I created two DVDs, "God's Mighty Angels" and "What the Bible Says about Prayer," and two books, *Scripture Yoga* and *Yoga for Beginners*. Seniors love my class because it improves their flexibility. I have clients who attend up into their eighties. If you desire gentle exercise, yoga may do the trick. Check out my website at ChristianYoga.com and Facebook page at Facebook.com/ScriptureYoga.

Mindfulness exercises such as yoga and meditation train a person to pay attention to cravings without reacting to them. The idea is to ride out the wave of intense desire. As a person becomes more mindful she notices why she wants to indulge. Meditation quiets the part of the brain that can lead to a loop of obsession.[3]

Day 8 and Beyond

You are well on your way to changing your lifestyle, but more than that you will change your life for the better. Your health, mood, and energy level will improve. Each week you will lose weight, and the body God gave you will heal itself of many ailments.

As your body heals some diseases can be reversed, you will be able to reduce or eliminate medications because you will no longer suffer from the maladies these medications were treating. However, before stopping any prescription medication be sure to consult with your physician.

Improvement in your vitality will allow you to experience activities you were not able to be involved in before. Overall your well-being and emotional countenance will become revitalized. You are in the process of getting your life back, the one that God wants you to enjoy to its fullest.

PLAN FOR PITFALLS

No one is perfect. You will have days when you eat sugar, wheat, or processed foods. That's okay. This happens to everyone; don't let it discourage you. Share your feelings with your accountability/prayer partner. Pray together. Share with your online group if you joined one. Write about your feelings, obstacles, and victories in your journal. Changing the way you eat will be a challenging journey, but one you can conquer.

Every morning spend time with God and plan your day. Determine your menu for the day and what temptations you might encounter. What time of the day would you most likely engage in unhealthy eating? Decide how you will fight food temptation for that specific day. Select a scripture verse and begin the day by reciting it out loud.

When you recognize temptation, remove yourself from the area containing the food, and record the trigger in your journal. Also, write down five reasons why you do not want to eat the food. Put the timer on for ten minutes and spend that time with God. Some strategies for resisting temptation include: pray, go for a walk, recite your Bible verse, call your prayer partner, drink two glasses of water, listen to praise music and start praising God, or utilize other helpful strategies that you develop (see appendix 10 for a list of Food Addiction Battle Strategies). Also, think about how far you have come in overcoming your food addiction and whether you want to experience the withdrawal symptoms again.

If you relapse, get up, brush the dust off yourself, and start again. Realize what triggered your cravings. Was it your emotions? In your journal, keep track of what you ate, why you ate it, what triggered you to eat it, and what you might do the next time you are tempted. *It is vital you record every single time you binge.* Confess your sin to God, and his mercies are new every morning (Lamentations 3:22–23). Ask him to help you do better next time.

Were you tempted by something you saw on TV? If yes, don't watch the commercials. Was it food someone else in your family ate? If yes, ask them not to eat it in front of you. Ask them to store the tempting food products somewhere else in the house. Through journaling, you can identify your triggers and learn how to avoid them.

It is a normal process for people to stay the course and fall off the wagon and binge. This cycle continues to repeat itself, but as you continue to turn to God and rely on his mighty strength, slowly but surely, you will gain control of your body, mind, and spirit.

The changes in your eating habits are a lifelong lifestyle journey so you can live the abundant life Jesus wants you to experience. Not a life filled with disease and unwanted, unhealthy symptoms.

BINDING THE STRONG MAN IN YOUR LIFE

To master addictions, I created the Five-Step Binding the Strong Man Plan. My family had a history of alcoholism, and I did not want to pass this on to my children. I enjoyed consuming alcohol. In fact, I turned to it to relieve my stress instead of God. Alcohol was my spiritual stronghold. A stronghold is something you turn to instead of God. Through using this plan, I tied up the strong man of addiction and kicked him out of my life.

This five-step plan should help a person with any addiction, including food. Before beginning this plan, let's look at God's advice in the Bible in two different translations:

How can anyone enter a strong man's house and carry off his possessions unless he first ties up the strong man? Then he can rob his house.

Matthew 12:29 (NIV)

One cannot rob Satan's kingdom without first binding Satan. Only then can his demons be cast out!

Matthew 12:29 (TLB)

I did not fully understand this verse initially, so I researched its meaning. Adam Clark's commentary states, "Men, through sin, become the very house and dwelling place of Satan (*probably to one of his demons*), having of their own accord surrendered themselves to this unjust possessor; for whoever gives up his soul to sin gives it up to the devil. It is Jesus, and Jesus alone, who can deliver from the power of this bondage. When Satan is cast out, Jesus purifies and dwells in the heart" (emphasis mine).[4] In other words, when a person surrenders to a specific sin over and over again, he or she becomes the dwelling place of an evil spirit. Theological controversy exists about whether Christians can be possessed or only oppressed.

Some examples of spirits of addiction include: alcohol, cigarettes, caffeine, drugs, food, sex, pornography, masturbation, TV, video games, shopping/buying, gambling, etc., but there are also spirits of fear, worry, greed, anxiety, depression, loneliness, unworthiness, unforgiveness, hatred/anger, etc. All of these can be strongholds in one's life.

How can you tell when a particular spirit is a strong man in your life? You can recognize it when these manifestations cause a desire so overpowering you succumb to the temptation over and over again. Even when you don't want to, you can't help it—it's like a battle raging inside you.

Paul struggled with sin as indicated in Romans 7:14-15, "The trouble is with me, for I am all too human, a slave to sin. I don't really understand myself, for I want to do what is right, but I don't do it. Instead, I do what I hate."

What drove you to eat poorly? Is it a food addiction, emotional issue with food, spiritual bondage, Candida infection, or lack of understanding about which foods negatively impact your health? Record the answer to this question in your journal.

When people yield themselves to a vice often enough, the power of the sin becomes attached to them, and they soon become driven by it. They no longer merely think a thought; the thought commands them. That is a strong man—a spirit that attaches itself to your being in a strong way. It has a stronghold in your life, and it won't let go.

Remember, "We are not fighting against people made of flesh and blood, but against persons without bodies—the evil rulers of the unseen world, those mighty satanic beings and great evil princes of darkness who rule this world; and against huge numbers of wicked spirits in the spirit world" (Ephesians 6:12 TLB). Even though the fight gets intense, with God we can overcome any temptation.

Since there is a war going on in the spiritual realm, we may be exposed to an evil spirit at some time in our lives. No one is immune from demonic harassment. If you get to the point where you can identify the strong man for who and what he is, you can do something about it. More specifically, you can bind the strong man who comes against you, as stated in Matthew 12:29.

To be quite frank, what I am addressing is whether you have an evil spirit of addiction oppressing you. Have you taken the food addiction test? Do you think the craving for refined carbohydrates is merely a Candida infection or is there a possibility of a spiritual component?

If you think your food addiction has a spiritual connection, because you feel helpless to control the way you eat, the five-step plan will help you fight domination by an evil spirit. This plan will help you take your life back! See appendix 8 for a summary of this plan.

Five-Step Binding the Strong Man Plan
1. Name what controls you.
Name the thing controlling you—food addiction, anxiety, eating disorder, depression, etc.—whatever it may be, and declare (out loud) Jesus Christ is your Lord in its place![5]

For me, it was the desire to drink alcohol. I liked the way it made me feel. I identified that this desire was a generational curse handed down from my grandfather to my father and from him to me. I wanted it to stop. I did not want to hand this curse down to my children. I recognized alcohol became a stronghold in my life because I turned to a drink to handle my stress rather than turning to God. Turning to alcohol happened over and over again until I used the steps in this plan to tie up the strong man of alcohol addiction in my life.

Stand up to the evil spirit who brought bondage into your life by saying, "Evil spirit, you won't lord over me nor entice me through (insert your addiction) anymore. Jesus is my Lord!" A person obtains spiritual power and authority through Christ. Declare that the spiritual powers of darkness will not have lordship over your life. They will not rule you, govern your behavior, capture your thought life, nor lead you into temptation and sin because "the one who is in you is greater than the one who is in the world" (1 John 4:4 NIV).

"For when Satan, strong and fully armed, guards his palace, it is safe—until someone stronger and better armed attacks and overcomes him and strips him of his weapons and carries off his belongings."

Luke 11:21–22 (TLB)

Get ready, for *you are capable of evicting the addiction strong man in your life*. If you accepted Jesus as your Lord and Savior (see appendix 7 to find out how), the Holy Spirit lives within you and the Spirit is stronger than Satan. Day after day, declare out loud that Jesus reigns as the Lord of your life—not your addiction.

What food problems have been with you since childhood? My sister was hooked on candy and sugary foods since a child. For me, it was the generational bondage of alcoholism. Take some time with God and record in your journal what instances from your past resulted in the way you eat today.

. . .

2. Submit yourself completely to God.

"Submit yourself to God, resist the devil and he will flee from you."
James 4:7 (NIV)

There is a secret to resisting the devil—you must first submit yourself
to God. How in the world do you do that? In my experience, you no
longer do your will but God's will by submitting your life to him. For
me, it was not without a fight.

I finally recognized the Holy Spirit's desires within me after I read
The Purpose Driven Life. The Spirit's wishes felt like my conscience.
After this recognition, God began nudging me to grow with simple
requests like spending more time with him.

At first after I struggled with wanting my way, not Gods, but I
recognized what was going on, and repented. Now when I recognize
the Holy Spirit's leading in my life, I try to obey. I am not perfect,
therefore, I repent when I realize I did not submit my will to God, and
I ask him to help me do better the next time.

If you are a food addict, after binging, ask God to forgive you and
help you not to binge the next time. Record your experience in your
journal. Once you ask for forgiveness, God chooses not to remember
your sins, as indicated in Hebrews 8:12: "And I will be merciful to
them in their wrongdoings, and I will remember their sins no more"
(TLB). Don't fret over a stumble. Get up and try again using this Five-
Step Binding the Strong Man Plan.

3. Use the name of Jesus.

Jesus told his disciples, "Look, I have given you authority over all
the power of the enemy" (Luke 10:19). If you are a disciple of Jesus
(see appendix 7 to find out how) you can accept the authority he
gave you.

In the book of Acts, the apostles healed and worked miracles in the name of Jesus. Use Jesus's name as Peter did in Acts 3:6: "in the name of Jesus Christ of Nazareth, walk" (TLB). Using the name of Jesus is key to binding the strong man because then you operate under Jesus's authority.

Picture a person tied in ropes. That's the way a spiritual strong man afflicts his victim. However, if you declare Jesus is Lord over your life, not the strong man (addiction), and use Jesus's name, you are under his authority. Then the ropes, tied around you by the evil spirit, break. Eventually, the spiritual ropes loosen and fall off. Next, comes the moment to take action by tying the strong man through binding him with the Word of God.

4. Use the Word of God.

"For when Satan, strong and fully armed, guards his palace, it is safe—until someone stronger and better armed attacks and overcomes him and strips him of his weapons and carries off his belongings."

Luke 11:21–22 TLB

The Holy Spirit inside of you is stronger than Satan and his demons. By using the name of Jesus, you are not only under his authority but you can speak with his authority. You are much better armed than Satan. Now is the time to stand up to him, strip him of his weapons, and kick him out of your life through the Word of God!

Say to the strong man, "In the name of Jesus, you won't oppress me anymore. I bind your power in the name of Jesus and by the Word of God."

Search the Bible for a verse that is the opposite of your addiction. A list of verses is provided in appendix 1. Here are two examples:

. . .

No discipline is enjoyable while it is happening—it's painful! But afterward there will be a peaceful harvest of right living for those who are trained in this way.

Hebrews 12:11

Dear friends, I warn you as "temporary residents and foreigners" to keep away from worldly desires that wage war against your very souls.

1 Peter 2:11

I used Ephesians 5:18: "Don't drink too much wine, for many evils lie along that path be filled instead with the Holy Spirit and controlled by him." Use the specific scripture you chose to bind the strong man every time he tempts you. Write this verse on an index card and memorize it.

While at a party, I implemented this plan to fight Satan and I won. There was a band, catered food, and an open bar. Oh my! How I wanted a drink, but didn't want one at the same time. The spiritual battle was on. Who would win? I had three fundamental factors on my side:

1. I had sworn God was the Lord of my life—I was not going to turn to alcohol but to God.

2. I submitted my will to God.

3. I memorized the verse about not drinking too much wine.

The desire to consume an alcoholic beverage at the open bar came upon me again and again that evening. At that time, I had no idea an evil spirit bound me in spiritual chains that went as far back as my childhood. To fight my addiction, I recited Ephesians 5:18 to bombard the strong man over and over again.

Praise God, I did not succumb to the temptation to drink. When I left the party, I felt like I fought the devil and won! Through the power of the Holy Spirit, Jesus's authority, and the Word of God, I bound that evil spirit—the strong man.

Luke 11:22 states the strong man was stripped of his weapons and his belongings were carried off. Matthew 12:29 asserts when Satan was bound his demons could be cast out. Well, the evil spirit that gave me the desire to drink was cast out of my life. Now the urge to drink alcohol is no longer an uncontrollable temptation since the evil spirit was stripped of his weapons.

After you tie up the strong man with the Word of God—ignore him. He will try to hobble after you because he doesn't give up easily. If he did, he wouldn't be a strong man. Remember, the next time you are tempted, you're facing a critical moment. When you give him (the spirit of addiction) your attention by drinking, eating sugary foods, worrying—whatever addiction it was—you are, in effect, untying the strong man.

To help you continue ignoring the strong man, recite your opposing Bible verse and ask God for help.

5. Praise God and practice gratitude.

When you praise God and thank him for his blessings, the strong man won't hang around. Don't be satisfied with binding the strong man and walking away—punish him.

Fill your mind, heart, and body with the Spirit of God by putting the right things in your spirit. Listen to praise music; read the Bible and pray; memorize scripture; attend church, Sunday school, or a Bible study. Also, start doing more to help others. Performing acts of service and helping others fills your heart with honorable feelings and humility. Every day, write in your journal about all you can praise God for and thank him.

When you embrace a mind-set of gratitude, dopamine releases in your brain. Remember that dopamine, the feel-good neurohormone, releases when you eat sugar and wheat. Instead of getting the positive feeling from a bad habit, get it from a good one—by journaling gratefulness. If you would like to become more grateful, check out my friend's book The Gratitude Journal: A 21 Day Challenge to More Gratitude, Deeper Relationships, and Greater Joy. Next time you want to eat something unhealthy, grab your journal instead.

Beat the strong man by declaring Bible verses out loud. Stomp him into the ground by singing praises to God. I created a worship playlist on my phone, and I listen to it every morning as I get ready for work. Before long, I lift my arms in praise and worship to our almighty God. The devil can't stand to be around someone who worships the Lord.

Become God's warrior by using his mighty unseen weapons. Paul advises, "It is true that I am an ordinary, weak human being, but I don't use human plans and methods to win my battles. I use God's mighty weapons, not those made by men, to knock down the devil's strongholds" (2 Corinthians 10:3-4 TLB). Get ready to knock out and tie up the strong man of addiction in your life. (A simplified version of the Five-Step Binding the Strong Man Plan is included in appendix 8.) You are God's mighty conqueror!

To assist you with the spiritual implications regarding dysfunctional food habits I created Christain Study Guide for 7 Steps to Get Off Sugar and Carbohydrates. This in-depth study goes into more detail regarding accessing God's power, changing your mind-set, and using the armor of God.

TAKING STEP 5: IMPLEMENT THE PHYSICAL AND SPIRITUAL PLANS

Planning is crucial for maintaining this new way of eating you committed to. Take these action steps below as you plan:

1. Implement the Seven-Day Eating Plan listed in appendix 6. Go to SusanUNeal.com/appendix for a printable version of the appendices. Date you will start this plan: _____.

2. Plan for the pitfalls. Print the list of Food Addiction Battle Strategies from appendix 10, and use these strategies as you stumble.

3. Implement the Five-Step Binding the Strong Man Plan and print a copy of the plan.

4. Choose a specific verse to use when the strong man of addiction tempts you. Write the verse on an index card and memorize it.

5. Continue to record pertinent information in your journal such as: what food problems have been with your since childhood, and write about all you can praise God for and thank him.

7 Steps to Get Off Sugar and Carbohydrates:

Step 1. Decide to improve your health through proper nutrition.

Step 2. Acquire a support system and knowledge to help make a lifestyle change.

Step 3. Clean out your pantry and refrigerator by removing unhealthy foods and clean out your emotions.

Step 4. Purchase healthy foods and an anti-Candida cleanse.

Step 5. Plan for the start date to begin changing your eating habits.

Day 1: Drink eight glasses of water per day. Stop eating sugar. Take a probiotic.

Day 2: Stop eating wheat.

Day 3: Do not eat processed foods out of boxes and bags. Make 50 percent of your food be fresh and raw. Follow the Healthy Eating Guidelines provided in appendix 5.

Day 4 and 5: Focus on you. Rest, read, pray, and ask God to give you the willpower to succeed.

Day 6: Begin the anti-Candida cleanse.

Day 7: Get up and exercise.

Five-Step Plan for Binding the Strong Man of addiction in your life.

1. Name your addiction and declare (out loud) that Jesus Christ is your Lord in its place!

2. Submit yourself completely to God.

3. Bind the strong man with the name of Jesus.

4. Use the Word of God to bind the strong man (evil spirit of addiction).

5. Punish the strong man by praising God and being grateful.

6

STEP 6: PREPARE AND EAT FOODS DIFFERENTLY

Decide—>Acquire—>Clean Out—>Purchase—>Plan—>**Prepare—
>Improve**

You have decided to change your eating habits, acquired knowledge, cleaned out the pantry, purchased healthy food, and planned the physical and spiritual steps; now it's time to get to work in the kitchen. In step 6, we will *prepare* for eating in a healthier way, with a suggested weekly menu. Post your menu on the refrigerator, so you know what you planned to cook for each meal during the week. Appendix 4 is full of recipes.

Cooking from scratch is important. For example, do not buy garlic already minced in a jar. You have no idea how old it is. The nutrients from fruits and vegetables begin to break down as soon as you cut them. Instead, mince a fresh clove of garlic.

It might take longer to cook from scratch, but the food will be more nutritious and low in sugar. Also, you will save time and money with less trips to the doctor. Your health is worth it. Your family will appreciate the time you invest into preparing healthy, delicious meals.

Make the transition from eating convenience foods, such as processed foods or eating out, to cooking at home. It doesn't have to be difficult. When Adam and Eve were in the garden of Eden, they picked a fruit or vegetable and ate it. Pretend you are in God's garden that he created for you and dream up what you could prepare. Create a salad with an avocado or nuts (protein). Load a sliced green apple with almond butter. Dip fresh vegetables into a healthy dip like guacamole or hummus. Blend a fruit smoothie with kale or spinach. Bake a large sweet potato—it is very filling. Simple meals work just as well as complicated, complex dishes.

God made you in his image, and he prizes and loves you. You are worthy of the time and effort it takes to invest in yourself. Choose to put yourself higher on your list of priorities. If you do, you will do a better job of living out the life God created for you.

TIPS FOR A HEALTHIER LIFESTYLE

The following tips should assist you to successfully make healthy lifestyle changes. Simple hints like drinking plenty of water or eating only until you are full will help you be more prepared, especially when it comes to choosing healthy foods when eating out.

Only Eat Until You're Full

As you prepare to eat healthier, one positive change you can make is to notice the sensation of fullness as you eat. Some individuals may not be in touch with that feeling anymore. Focus on recognizing when you are full so you do not overeat. You may have to change some of your mealtime habits as well. Eat slowly, chew your food thoroughly, and pay attention to how the food tastes. As you learn to enjoy the taste of foods in their purest form, you'll begin to look for more ways to prepare meals with the variety of amazing foods God created for our health.

When you eat processed foods, versus meals you prepare from scratch, it takes a larger quantity of the refined product to fill your stomach because these foods do not contain the original food's fiber. Think of crushing a bag of chips versus shredding carrots and celery. The fresh vegetables will satiate your hunger with a smaller volume.

When you eat foods closer to their form at harvest, you will become full with smaller portions. The feeling of fullness stays with you for a longer period too, so you don't need to snack as much. By following this simple lifestyle change, you will eat a smaller quantity of food loaded with vitamins, minerals, fiber, and all the nutrients the human body needs—the way God intended for you to eat.

Pay attention to portion size. Think of your stomach as the size of your fist—before it is stretched out by food. Put less food on your plate than you think you will eat. Use a smaller plate. As soon as you feel full, stop eating and put the timer on for five minutes. When the timer rings, you shouldn't feel hungry anymore since it takes a little while for your brain to recognize your stomach reached its capacity. If you stop eating at the first sign you feel the sensation of fullness, in five minutes your brain receptors catch up with the feeling in your stomach.

Eating Out

Realistically, you won't be able to prepare meals at home all the time. Our lives are busy and many days we are unable to eat at home, so on occasion we will eat out. Let's first address fast food. We need to use drive-throughs when traveling or in a hurry. Most fast-food restaurants provide a selection of healthy options to choose from, such as a fresh salad with raw ingredients. However, be sure to use either no dressing or as small a portion as you can. If you use more than one fast-food package of salad dressing, you just made your positive eating choice into a negative one.

Healthy eating choices at a dine-in restaurant are a vegetable plate, fish, or chicken. First, check the menu for the ingredients in your meal choice, and make sure you ask for your food to be served in the healthiest way: no sauces and baked or gilled instead of fried. When your food arrives, the serving size may be substantial. Therefore, when served a large plate of food, before you begin eating, determine how much you will eat to prevent overeating. You might even ask for a to-go container at the beginning of your meal to store what you will not eat at this meal. It is difficult to stop unless you establish boundaries before you begin eating delicious foods.

Drink Your Daily Water Intake

If you get hungry in between meals, drink two glasses of water. Water usually curbs your appetite. Most people mistake the feeling of thirst for hunger. Our bodies desperately need water to flush out the toxins and prevent dehydration. You also will have more energy when you drink an adequate amount of water.

My sister found it challenging to incorporate drinking eight glasses of water into her daily routine, especially on an empty stomach. It is best not to drink during meals because the fluid dilutes gastric juices that break down food. She previously drank sweet tea and sodas instead of water and this increased her sugar consumption. I suggested she drink two glasses of water before breakfast, two before lunch, two midafternoon, and two before dinner (my recommendation in steps 4 and 5).

I stop drinking fluids at 6 pm, so I don't have to get up to go to the bathroom as much at night. Try not to forget about drinking all day long and then consume a lot of water after dinner. Getting up in the middle of the night to go to the bathroom disrupts sleep. Plan when you will consume your eight glasses of water during the day.

Follow the Healthy Eating Guidelines

As you prepare your weekly menu, keep in mind these Healthy Eating Guidelines from step 4 (purchase) listed below and also in appendix 5:

- Buy organic fruits, vegetables, and meats.

- About 50 percent of your food should be fresh, organic vegetables.
- Eat one fresh, raw serving of a low-glycemic fruit per day. Low-glycemic fruits include green apples, berries, cherries, pears, plums, and grapefruit.
- Do not always eat cooked foods. Eat a couple of servings of raw vegetables every day. Eat a salad for lunch with nuts, meat, or an avocado. When eating out, order a salad or coleslaw as sides since both are raw.
- Plan for 25 percent of your food to be an animal or vegetable protein such as beans, nuts, and lean meats. Fish is especially nutritious.
- A variety of different nuts and seeds are excellent sources of protein, minerals, and essential fatty acids.
- Eat nontraditional grains such as quinoa, amaranth, pearled barley, and oats.

MEAL PLANNING

To help my sister on this journey to change her eating habits I provided her with examples of healthy meals. The following daily meal categories include a list of appropriate healthy food options for your menu planning and shopping lists.

Breakfast

- oatmeal with pecans and cinnamon
- pancakes made with almond flour (A link for this recipe: Pinterest.com/SusanUNeal/breakfast/)
- quinoa with a smashed banana, almond milk, and walnuts
- scrambled eggs with hash browns
- omelet with green onions, red peppers, and mushrooms
- berries with plain Greek yogurt
- chia parfait with fruit

- homemade granola with berries and/or Greek yogurt
- hash browns with onions, peppers, and a sliced avocado on top
- mashed avocado with two fried eggs on top
- pancakes made with two eggs and one smashed banana

Lunch

- a salad or vegetable plate, if eating out
- romaine lettuce wrap sandwich with any meat or vegetable
- cucumber sandwich—cut a cucumber in half and load it with meat (not lunch meat) and veggies
- salad with fish, chicken, nuts, or avocado
- baked potato bar with olive oil, broccoli, scallions, sunflower seeds
- guacamole or hummus with sliced vegetables
- whole avocado and an heirloom tomato
- baked sweet potato with butter, cinnamon, and honey

Snack

- sliced green apple with almond or cashew butter
- berries with whipped cream made with coconut milk
- raw vegetables with hummus or guacamole
- boiled egg or deviled eggs (made with organic mayonnaise)
- carrots and celery sticks
- berries with slivered almonds
- nuts—raw almonds, pecans, pistachios, macadamia nuts, or cashews
- organic popcorn popped on the stove (not microwave popcorn)

Dinner

- chicken fajitas with guacamole, lettuce, tomato, and avocado on a coconut tortilla wrap (available at health food stores)
- spaghetti with a baked spaghetti squash for the noodles
- steak, mushrooms, green beans with slivered almonds, and a salad
- salmon, sautéed red cabbage, and wild rice
- baked or grilled chicken, quinoa, and sautéed or grilled zucchini and yellow squash
- chili made with lean meat
- fish, salad, and asparagus
- beef stew with potato, carrots, celery, bok choy, and onions
- black bean soup
- fresh field peas with sliced tomatoes, fried okra, and corn pone bread (recipe in appendix 4)
- shrimp fettuccine alfredo with shirataki noodles, and a salad
- roasted whole chicken with onions, potatoes, carrots, and bok choy
- salad with berries, nuts, and seeds

Dessert

- dark chocolate (at least 70 percent chocolate)
- dark chocolate almond cookies (recipe in appendix 4)
- chocolate nut clusters (see directions in the section Curb the Sweettooth)
- dark chocolate–covered strawberries

- one dried date to seven pecan halves (be careful, as dates are high in sugar)

MENU PLANNING

If you haven't planned your menu already, choose a pleasant spot (outside, by a fire, coffee shop), to plan your menu and corresponding grocery list. This may take up to an hour, but is well worth your time and effort. Use this book, another healthy cookbook, or an app on your phone to find recipes. I have a provided a list of recipe resources in step 2.

I list what I plan to cook for breakfast, lunch, dinner, and snack for every day of the week. As I choose a recipe, I put the corresponding ingredients that I need on my grocery list. For years, as my children were growing up, I posted on their chalkboard what the menu was for every day of the week. Everyone in the family knew what I would be serving.

I cooked on Sunday and Monday and listed leftovers (from Sunday) to be served on Tuesday. Wednesday we all ate at church, and Thursday I served leftovers from Monday. Two nights of cooking took care of four meals. To liven up a leftover, I would cook one new item (such as a vegetable) to be served with the previous meal, and this new item gave the meal new interest.

I created a standard grocery list for the store I used. For me, it was Walmart. To create this list, initially I walked through the store and either wrote or dictated into my smartphone notes app the items I normally purchased on those aisles. For example, I would start in the refrigerated section and would include eggs, butter, coconut milk, and non-dairy yogurt on the list for that aisle. Then I proceeded to the next aisle, cleaning supplies and paper products. I listed Clorox wipes, toilet paper, napkins, paper towels, paper plates, etc. At home, I typed out this list based on each grocery store aisle and the products I normally purchased. It took work to create this list, but it has stream-lined my grocery store planning for years.

Each week I printed a fresh new list and my family knew that if we ran out of an item, they circled it on the list or wrote it out. I made a rule to guide us—if it wasn't on the list it didn't get purchased. I put the responsibility on them, not all on me.

Every week I made some sort of fresh, raw salad (broccoli salad, beet salad, coleslaw, salad with lettuce) and I ate that for my lunch. For my children's lunch boxes, I tried to include one fresh fruit and vegetable. When they wanted a fruit roll-up, I explained that I was giving them something better by giving them a real piece of fruit (their choice) because it was loaded with the natural vitamins and minerals that God put into the fruit to nourish our bodies. My children learned the importance of whole God-given foods.

After you plan your menu and purchase all those groceries, it is time to start cooking healthy homemade meals. If you need help with planning your menu, join my blog at HealthLivingSeriesBlog.com where I post menus and corresponding grocery lists.

PREPARE TO COOK

As I planned my menu I also designated who would be cooking the meal. I assigned each of my children a night to assist me in the kitchen at least one time per week. Mealtime preparation can be a great opportunity for bonding.

Each morning I checked my menu posted on the refrigerator to determine if I needed to defrost any frozen items. I determined the time to serve our meal and began cooking one hour prior to that time. Most meals required some sort of chopping of vegetables, so if another family member assisted me, I had them do this job. When cooking alone, I turned on my praise music and enjoyed creating a colorful, delicious meal. I felt I was providing my family with a beautiful love offering.

I always cooked more than was needed so I would have enough food left over for future meals. If I was taking the time to prepare a healthy meal from scratch, I wanted to make sure that my efforts were fully utilized. I had everyone serve themselves, and whoever did not assist me in cooking had kitchen clean-up duty.

CURB YOUR SWEET TOOTH

Surprisingly, taste buds change when you eat natural foods. As you eliminate sugar from your diet, your pallet changes, and the healthy snacks listed below will seem sweet to you. When the craving for sugar arises, I eat one of these nutritious snacks (this list is also provided in appendix 9):

- Slice a green apple, which is low in sugar, and add almond or cashew butter to each slice. It tastes sweet; conversely, the almond butter is high in protein. Both the apple and nut butter provide fiber and fill me up.
- Melt 70-percent dark chocolate in a pan on the stove and add different types of nuts until well coated with the chocolate. Place mounds of nut clusters on wax paper. After an hour they harden. Keep in an airtight container on the counter or refrigerator for a week. Nuts contain fiber and are filling.
- Sparingly eat one date along with seven pecan halves. Dates are high in natural sugar, so you only need a smidgen to attain the sweetness. Don't eat too many dates, but instead fill up on the pecans, which are high in protein.
- I grow fruit trees in my yard, so from June through December I pick fresh blueberries, apples, grapes, pears, and oriental persimmons. I eat one serving of fruit each day either for breakfast or as an afternoon snack.
- Curb sweet cravings by adding a teaspoon of raw, unfiltered, unpasteurized apple cider vinegar in a cup of water with a couple of drops of stevia.

Learning a new skill is difficult at the beginning, but with time, your new eating habits will become routine. Recognize you can say no to the voice in your head that demands unhealthy food. Instead of giving in to this voice, put the timer on for fifteen minutes to delay food gratification. Training yourself to wait before you eat will help you gain better self-control. During that time preoccupy yourself by writing in your journal.

JOURNAL

In step 2 and appendix 3, I recommended that you purchase the *Healthy Living Journal* or write the following items in your journal any time you eat:

1. The time you eat.
2. Why you are about to eat. Are you hungry, bored, angry? Is it just "time to eat" or are you with others who are having a meal?
3. If you feel a strong emotion related to this consumption of food, record the emotion.
4. What you ate and drank, including quantity.
5. How you feel after you ate? Satisfied or stuffed?
6. After you eat, record how the food makes you feel regarding your energy level and clarity of mind.
7. When waking up in the morning, how do you feel? See if there is a pattern of eating high-sugar-content foods and feeling sluggish the next morning.
8. What are you grateful for today?
9. Prayer requests to God.
10. Exercise—type and length of time.
11. Number of glasses of water you drink and when. Did you drink on an empty stomach?
12. Every time you binge, record: what you ate, why you ate it, what triggered you to eat it, and what you might do the next time you are tempted.

As you write this information, determine if there is a pattern to your behavior as it relates to eating. Do you eat because you are hungry? If not, why do you want to eat? Do you have at least three hours in between meals? It takes three to four hours for your previous meal to digest, and your stomach to empty. Change your mind-set from immediate gratification to thinking about how this food will make you feel and whether it will nourish the temple of the Holy Spirit.

Continue to journal for the first three months as you make this lifestyle change. You may continue journaling longer if you feel it is helping you achieve your goals. However, as you improve your eating habits, you may only need to journal if and when you binge (see #12 above).

SPIRITUAL PREPARATION

You prepared the kitchen by cleaning out the pantry and refrigerator, planned the menu, purchased food, and prepared meals. However, you also need to prepare spiritually because the enemy will attack. Post the Five-Step Binding the Strong Man Plan from appendix 8 on your refrigerator or bathroom mirror and use it when tempted to overeat unhealthy foods.

To overcome a spiritual battle with food, I recommend the study *Christian Study Guide for 7 Steps to Get Off Sugar and Carbohydrates*. It goes into renewing the mind by bringing every thought captive to Jesus Christ. Whether you do this study by yourself or with a group, it will help you go more in-depth to resolve the spiritual component of a food addiction.

You are in a battle, so you need to develop a strategy. From journaling, have you identified your food triggers? Do you have a plan for how to reduce those triggers? Have you told yourself lies that justify inappropriate eating? Journal those lies. Replace those lies with the Word of God.

I challenge you to learn one new scripture verse per week. Choose the verse, write it on an index card, and memorize it. Step 2 includes tactics to help you memorize Bible verses. When you choose to learn God's Word it will affect you in positive ways you can't begin to imagine. We are supposed to store his word in our hearts so we can draw upon it when the enemy tells us lies. Store the sword of the Spirit in your mind and you can defeat Satan, and successfully achieve the goals in the contract you wrote to God in step 1.

Develop and document your battle strategies in your *Healthy Living Journal*. Some of your Food Addiction Battle Strategies (listed in appendix 10) should include:

1. Record pertinent information in your journal.
2. Find a specific Bible verse to oppose your food issue and write it on an index card. Keep it with you until you memorize it. Speak the verse out loud every time you feel the urge to eat unhealthy foods.
3. Ask a friend to be your accountability and prayer partner.
4. Join a Christian weight loss program or an online food addiction program.
5. Determine food triggers and eliminate them.
6. Implement the Five Steps to Binding the Strong Man Plan:
7. Name the thing controlling you—your food addiction, anxiety, eating disorder, depression, etc.—whatever it may be, and declare (out loud) Jesus Christ is your Lord in its place!
8. Submit yourself completely to God.
9. Bind the strong man (evil spirit of addiction) with the name of Jesus.
10. Use the Word of God to bind the strong man.
11. Punish the strong man by praising God.

Do you have an accountability/prayer partner, yet? Acquiring a support system is integral to successfully make this lifestyle change. Have you joined a Christian weight loss program or one of the online food addiction programs? A list of these programs is provided in appendix 2. If you need to, reread step 2 about how to create your support system.

When you binge, be sure to journal afterward—every single time. There is a Binge Eating Tracker chart in the *Healthy Living Journal*. Figure out what you told yourself that validated why it was okay to eat the item. Then go through the Five Steps to Binding the Strong Man Plan (appendix 8). If you journal and implement this five-step plan every time you binge, you will experience success. Retraining your mind is like disciplining a child; consistency is vital to conformity.

Don't tell yourself lies such as "a little bit of food with sugar will curb my appetite." Instead, sugar will open up the floodgate for you to binge on that sweet food item. My hairdresser asked me how I was able to not eat sugary foods or refined carbohydrates. She said she eliminates these foods for a while, but as soon as she eats one item with sugar, she starts craving it all over again. She is completely right. Therefore, do not eat anything with more than 10 grams of sugar in one serving, or 24 grams for a woman or 36 grams for a man per day. (Check out the list of natural sweet snacks to Curb the Sweet Tooth in appendix 9.)

If you tell yourself lies to break your eating rules and eat what you regret, I recommend you get the app "I Deserve a Donut and Other Lies That Make You Eat" by Barb Raveling. Some of the lies this app evaluates include:

"I'll never be skinny so I might as well eat."

"I deserve this."

"I need this."

You can't serve God to your fullest if your body doesn't function well. The Holy Spirit inside of you is holy, so you should honor the body that carries the Spirit. First Corinthians 6:19–20 states, "Don't you realize that your body is the temple of the Holy Spirit, who lives in you and was given to you by God? You do not belong to yourself, for God bought you with a high price. So you must honor God with your body." *You honor God with your body through making this lifestyle change to improve your health.*

Scripture indicates you are a priest to serve God: "To him who loves us and has freed us from our sins by his blood, and has made us to be a kingdom and priests to serve his God and Father" (Revelation 1:6 NIV). If you are overweight or develop a chronic disease, it will be hard to fulfill your privilege and responsibility to the Lord. Of course, not all diseases can be cured by proper nutrition. However, diabetes, obesity, high blood pressure, cardiovascular disease, and cancer can be affected, positively or negatively, by your diet.

Changing your eating habits for the better reminds me of accepting Christ as your Lord and Savior. Many people choose not to accept Jesus's precious gift. Will you choose to accept this lifestyle change to improve your health? The decision is yours.

You should feel great about the steps you have taken to improve your health and well-being. I am proud of you and so is God. You are well on your way to achieving your goals.

TAKING STEP 6: PREPARE

This step helps you prepare for a new way of eating not only in your menu and meal plans but in spiritual preparation for the changes you are making. Take the action steps listed below:

1. Plan your menu for the week and post it on the refrigerator.
2. Create a standardized grocery list that you can print out every week when planning your menu.
3. Go grocery shopping.
4. Prepare healthy meals from scratch using the Healthy Eating Guidelines in appendix 5. For a a printable version of the appendix go to SusanUNeal.com/appendix.
5. Pay attention to:
6. Portion control
7. Water intake
8. Eat fresh and raw items at fast-food restaurants.
9. Use techniques to curb your sweet tooth (see appendix 9).
10. Continue to record pertinent information in your journal.

Have you identified your food triggers? Do you have a plan for how to reduce those triggers? Have you told yourself lies that justify inappropriate eating? Journal those lies. Replace those lies with the Word of God.

11. Memorize one scripture verse per week. Choose the verse, write it on an index card, and memorize it.

12. Download the app "I Deserve a Donut and Other Lies That Make You Eat" by Barb Raveling.

7 Steps to Get Off Sugar and Carbohydrates:

Step 1. Decide to improve your health through proper nutrition.

Step 2. Acquire a support system and knowledge to help make a lifestyle change.

Step 3. Clean out your pantry and refrigerator by removing unhealthy foods and clean out your emotions.

Step 4. Purchase healthy foods and an anti-Candida cleanse.

Step 5. Plan for the start date to begin changing your eating habits.

Step 6. Prepare and eat foods differently than you did before.

7

STEP 7: IMPROVE YOUR HEALTH

Decide—>Acquire—>Clean   out—>Purchase—>Plan—>Prepare—
>Improve

When you take the steps outlined in this book, your health, and energy levels *improve* because you eat healthy foods that nourish your body. After a week of being off sugar, cravings for it and for carbohydrates cease. Understanding your food triggers helps you stay away from unhealthy foods. Now you need to continue this lifestyle change for the rest of your life, never turning back to your old eating habits.

Don't make your expectations too high. Remember the 80/20 rule: if you improve your eating 80 percent of the time, you will improve your diet. This lifestyle change is not an all-or-nothing situation. If you don't follow the dietary guidelines provided in this book 100 percent of the time, don't have the mind-set that you failed. Instead, give yourself grace as God does. Try to do well, but if you don't eat correctly 20 percent of the time, that's okay. It's probably better than the way you ate before.

Expect to stumble. You will not change your eating habits entirely. Don't get discouraged when you do not meet your expectations.

Making this lifestyle change is difficult, but with the help of Christ, you can succeed.

GIVE YOURSELF GRACE

Many people get into a cycle of diets. They do well for a while, but when they make a mistake, they feel terrible about themselves, as if they failed. So they return to unhealthy eating habits.

An all-or-nothing attitude is perilous. If you blow your eating guidelines, stop overeating as soon as possible and continue to follow the healthy eating standards for the rest of the day. Just because you slipped doesn't mean you should binge. As with any attempt to improve your life, when you stumble, get up and try again.

Our thought life can sabotage our success. We must change our thought process from negativity and despair to positivity and hope if we are to make the lifestyle changes necessary for a healthy future. We are far from perfect, so don't create expectations of perfection for yourself on this journey. Improvement is the correct mind-set to succeed. Replace any negativity about yourself with God's grace.

Another way to think of grace is to consider how you would advise your best friend who calls you after she binges on food. You would show her grace and help her start again. When you mess up, think about what you would tell her. Don't be so hard on yourself. Understand that at some point you will eat unhealthy foods, and you will overeat. Expect it and move on.

James Allen, a nineteenth-century self-help-movement pioneer, stated, "The greatest discovery of our generation is that human beings can alter their lives by altering their attitudes of mind. As you think, so shall you be."[1] This quote is similar to Proverbs 23:7: "For as he thinks in his heart, so *is* he" (NKJV). What do you think of yourself? Record the answer to this question in your journal. Open up your heart to God and ask him to give you an optimistic mind-set as you give yourself grace.

LET YOUR MISTAKES MOTIVATE YOU

As your diet improves, when you eat foods high in sugar or refined carbohydrates you will feel sluggish. You may not even feel like getting out of bed the next day, and you will be foggy brained. Whereas, if you eat clean, raw foods, your clarity of thought and energy improves.

Every time I slip, I pay for it the next day and that motivates me to eat healthier. I like waking up feeling energized and ready to start my day, rather than feeling groggy. That way, I can serve God to the best of my ability.

Unfortunately, as I write this chapter, I have just overindulged in ice cream (made with coconut milk), and I feel terrible. My blood sugar spiked and then plummeted. I feel drained, and I have a slight headache. I can't concentrate, and I don't feel like working on anything. Do you understand this feeling? I recognize what I did. I will eat better for the rest of today. Tomorrow is a new day, and I will feel better then.

FOOD ADDICTION REVISITED

If you did not previously take the test to determine if you are a food addict, I suggest that you do so. The first step in dealing with any addiction is to acknowledge it. Even if you don't see yourself this way, understanding your body's reaction to foods is crucial for making improvement in your eating and feeling the benefits of a healthier approach to food. Use these links to online quizzes to determine if you are addicted to food: FoodAddicts.org/am-i-a-food-addict and OA.org/newcomers/how-do-i-start/are-you-a-compulsive-overeater/. If you do discover you are a food addict, take the steps necessary to begin to overcome this (see step 1) to improve your lifestyle and food habits.

Addiction rewires the neural circuits in a person's brain. Therefore, the brain assigns a higher value to sugar and wheat than other foods. Subliminal food cues excite the brain's reward system and contribute to a relapse. People fall prey to these unseen triggers. That is why it is imperative to identify what sets off your desire and eliminate the trigger. Similarly, an alcoholic should not go into a bar. As your health improves from eating well, you cannot let down your guard. Recognizing you have a food addiction and avoiding the triggers will keep you in recovery mode and allow you to maintain this healthier lifestyle.

If you are a food addict and are not able to stop the cycle of addiction with the suggestions in this book, I strongly recommend you use the *Christian Study Guide for 7 Steps to Get Off Sugar and Carbohydrates* or join a twelve-step program along with a corresponding support group. You could also join my closed Facebook group: 7 Steps to Get Off Sugar and Carbohydrates. Appendix 2 includes a list of Christian Weight Loss and Food Addiction Programs.

BENEFITS OF HEALTHY EATING

Whether you are dealing with addiction or not, as you nourish your body with the proper nutrients God intended for you to ingest, your body will begin to heal itself of diabetes, hypertension, headaches, allergies, skin problems, joint pain—the list goes on. Complete healing will take some time, yet some unhealthy symptoms may disappear right away. Also, you will lose weight naturally without starving yourself. Your mental clarity will improve, as will the speed of your thought processes. You will love the new you!

How long will it take to stop struggling with food? To answer that question, you need to determine how long you have had a problem with food. If it is more than a decade, it may take over a year to rewire the pathways of your brain and spiritually tie up the strong man of addiction and kick him out of your life. Don't think of this as an overnight fix. It took a while to get into this condition, and it will take a while to get the healthy you back, so be patient. It took me eight months on the anti-Candida diet to kill the yeast in my colon.

THE PATH TO RECOVERY AND HEALTH

If you have a food addiction, your recovery will not be short or easy, but you can do it. "Because the one who is in you is greater than the one who is in the world" (1 John 4:4 NIV). Through the Holy Spirit inside of you, you are powerful. *God is on your side.* Use his powerful words to fight the enemy.

How do you look at food? Are you using food to comfort and meet an emotional need, or do you think of food as a necessity to keep your body functioning? Have you journaled about this? Do you turn to food to help you deal with the challenges of life? If so, food is your stronghold. A stronghold is something you put before God.

Pray and ask the Lord to help you turn to him instead of food. You need to get to the root cause of your dysfunctional food eating issue so you can heal. Turn to God first to meet your needs, not food. You will need to continue to turn to God over and over again asking for his help to free you from food addiction. Getting off sugar and carbohydrates reminds me of training a child. It takes years and a lot of repetition. But at some point, the child gets it and becomes well behaved, most of the time.

During this journey of change, learn from your mistakes. Have you ever thought, *I'll take one bite and that will satisfy my sugar craving?* If so, you understand that logic never works. You can't take only one bite, because dopamine releases in the brain and causes a physiological response that your self-control cannot manage.[2]

Even before you take the first bite, if you desire the food item, dopamine secretes in the brain. Scientists proved this through MRI imaging of the brains of addicts. Therefore, when you feel the temptation to eat refined carbohydrates, recognize it and use one of your strategies we developed in this book (see Food Addiction Battle Strategies in appendix 10). If you understand what is going on in your brain, you can more effectively fight the temptation.

If you need more guidance, I created the course, 7 Steps to Reclaim Your Health and Optimal Weight (SusanUNeal.com/courses/7-steps-to-get-off-sugar-and-carbs-course). This course will help you figure out and resolve the root cause of your inappropriate eating habits. One solved, taming your appetite is much easier. I show you how you can change your eating habits once and for all.

TURN TO GOD

The transformation from food addiction cannot come from dietary boundaries and self-control alone; it must come from God helping you. Turn to the Lord when you want to eat inappropriately. Explore your emotions with him and ask him to stabilize your feelings. Allow him to minister to your heart and mind, and your eating habits will improve. Use your journal to help you know what is triggering your temptations and ask God to help you overcome these specific triggers.

Memorize his Word so you can live by it and recite it. Turn to him when your journey gets tough. Do not count on your self-control as you have in the past; count on him. Hand over control of your eating habits to the Lord. Relinquish the outcome of your lifestyle change to God. Submit your life to him. Live in victory through total reliance on him. If you do, you will be transformed by a renewing of your mind as indicated in Romans 12:2: "Don't copy the behavior and customs of this world, but let God transform you into a new person by changing the way you think. Then you will learn to know God's will for you, which is good and pleasing and perfect." Be patient and trust God for he is faithful.

My sister feels like a new person. Her rosacea disappeared, as well as her excess weight. Her joints no longer ache. Big chores, like house cleaning, don't seem like such a difficult task for her to accomplish anymore. She feels good inside and out because the glorious body God gave her healed through providing it with proper nutrition. As you continue to nourish your body, weak-functioning cells will be replaced by new ones, and your body will work to heal itself of diseases the way the Lord intended.

As a Certified Health and Wellness Coach, I encourage and guide others to regain their health. A client told me her pediatric endocrinologist diagnosed her son as obese and prediabetic. We reviewed the types of food her family ate and developed a plan to cut out unhealthy foods. She resolved to eliminate wheat, milk, and fruit juice from her family's diet. I encouraged her to try to improve their eating habits 80 percent of the time and not worry about what they ate the other 20 percent of the time, since no one can be perfect. If you would like me to assist you on this journey to improve your health as your wellness coach go to SusanUNeal.com/Health-Coaching.

SIX-MONTH SELF-ASSESSMENT

You started this journey with a self-assessment of your physical health. Six months after you start this program, perform another assessment. At that time, record your results here and note the healthy improvements you will have experienced.

Date:

Weight:

Waistline:

Cognitive Assessment Results:

Put a check by the following unhealthy symptoms you still experience.

_____ Fatigue

_____ Foggy brained

_____ Poor memory

_____ Insomnia

_____ Irritability

_____ Mood swings

_____ Anxiety

_____ Depression

_____ Hormonal imbalance

_____ Decreased sex drive

_____ Chronic fatigue, fibromyalgia

_____ Craving sweets and refined carbohydrates or alcohol

_____ Digestive issues: bloating, constipation, diarrhea

_____ Skin and nail infections such as toenail fungus, athlete's foot, and ringworm

_____ Vaginal yeast infections, urinary tract infections

In the space below, write the types of food you ate for the past week. Recalling these foods will test your memory (which should have improved). Note the difference between the foods you just ate and those you recorded in step 1, which are the foods you ate before you began the process of making a lifestyle change.

CONTINUE THE JOURNEY

Understand this is a spiritual battle as well as a physical one. But you can break free from the control of food. God is full of grace and mercy to help you. He is not condemning but loving. Be loving of yourself while you are on this journey to a healthier you, the you God created you to be.

Hebrews 12:1–2 states, "Let us strip off every weight that slows us down, especially the sin that so easily trips us up. And let us run with endurance the race God has set before us. We do this by keeping our eyes on Jesus, the champion who initiates and perfects our faith." I pray you attain the results you desire in obtaining a body that functions well. Be sure to give your body the organic foods God created.

Dear friend, I am praying that all is well with you and that your body is as healthy as I know your soul is.

3 John 2 (TLB)

Blessings, Susan Neal

TAKING STEP 7: IMPROVE YOUR HEALTH

Congratulations on taking these seven steps to get off sugar and carbs and improve your health, life, and future! As you continue on with these lifestyle changes, remember to utilize the following actions steps:

1. Remember the 80/20 percent rule. If you improve your eating 80 percent of the time you will improve your diet and health. However, healing takes time so be patient.

2. Expect to stumble. No one is perfect, but give yourself grace, as God does, when you do mess up and eat poorly.

3. Rely on God. Turn to him and the Bible verses you memorized when you stumble.

4. Document your path to recovery in your journal. How do you look at food? Are you using food to comfort and meet an emotional need, or do you think of food as a necessity to keep your body functioning? Have you journaled about this? Do you turn to food to help

you deal with the challenges of life? If so, food is your stronghold. Learn from your mistakes as you record what occurred, and figure out why so you can prevent these mishaps in the future.

5. Hand over control of your eating habits to the Lord. Relinquish the outcome of your lifestyle change to God. Submit your life to him. Live in victory through total reliance on him.

6. Perform your self-assessment at six months into your journey. Compare this assessment to the first one you took at the beginning of this journey. Note your areas of improvement in your journal and let these victories motivate you to continue to improve and maintain your new healthy lifestyle.

7 Steps to Get Off Sugar and Carbohydrates:

Step 1. Decide to improve your health through proper nutrition.

Step 2. Acquire a support system and knowledge to help make a lifestyle change.

Step 3. Clean out your pantry and refrigerator by removing unhealthy foods and clean out your emotions.

Step 4. Purchase healthy foods and an anti-Candida cleanse.

Step 5. Plan for the start date to begin changing your eating habits.

Step 6. Prepare and eat foods differently than you did before.

Step 7. Improve your health through continuing this new lifestyle never turning back to your old eating habits.

APPENDIX 1: SCRIPTURE VERSES

When you experience temptation, negative emotions, or sinful thoughts regarding your journey to a healthy lifestyle, speak the Word of God out loud and thrust the sword of the Spirit toward the evil forces that might be influencing you. Spoken Bible verses become a double-edged sword to defeat the enemy. State these scripture verses boldly and with authority, believing in their power. This offensive weapon drives the enemy away from you. But first, repent of any sins.

These scripture verses are categorized into various topics you might face in your journey to wholeness. You may find others to add to this list. Seek to memorize as many as you can so you can mentally access them whenever you need to call upon the power of God's Word in your daily battles. To help in memorization, I suggest you write individual verses and their references on an index card to carry with you as you go.

ADDICTION

I can do anything I want to if Christ has not said no, but some of these things aren't good for me. Even if I am allowed to do them, I'll refuse to if I think they might get such a grip on me that I can't easily stop when I want to.

1 Corinthians 6:12 (TLB)

We demolish arguments and every pretension that sets itself up against the knowledge of God, and we take captive every thought to make it obedient to Christ.

2 Corinthians 10:5 (NIV)

Let us strip off every weight that slows us down, especially the sin that so easily trips us up. And let us run with endurance the race God has set before us. We do this by keeping our eyes on Jesus, the champion who initiates and perfects our faith.

Hebrews 12:1–2

Teach me to do your will, for you are my God. May your gracious Spirit lead me forward on a firm footing.

Psalm 143:10

Each time he said, "My grace is all you need. My power works best in weakness." So now I am glad to boast about my weaknesses, so that the power of Christ can work through me.

2 Corinthians 12:9

And let us not get tired of doing what is right, for after a while we will reap a harvest of blessing if we don't get discouraged and give up.

Galatians 6:9 (TLB)

Rather, clothe yourselves with the Lord Jesus Christ, and do not think about how to gratify the desires of the flesh.

Romans 13:14 (NIV)

I have been crucified with Christ and I no longer live, but Christ lives in me. The life I now live in the body, I live by faith in the Son of God, who loved me and gave himself for me.

Galatians 2:20 (NIV)

No discipline seems pleasant at the time, but painful. Later on, however, it produces a harvest of righteousness and peace for those who have been trained by it.

Hebrews 12:11 (NIV)

Therefore, I urge you, brothers and sisters, in view of God's mercy, to offer your bodies as a living sacrifice, holy and pleasing to God—this is your true and proper worship.

Romans 12:1(NIV)

"It is not by force nor by strength, but by my Spirit, says the LORD of Heaven's Armies."

Zechariah 4:6

Well then, shall we keep on sinning so that God can keep on showing us more and more kindness and forgiveness? Of course not! Should we keep on sinning when we don't have to? For sin's power over us was broken when we became Christians and were baptized to become a part of Jesus Christ; through his death the power of your sinful nature was shattered. Your old sin-loving nature was buried with him by baptism when he died; and when God the Father, with glorious power, brought him back to life again, you were given his wonderful new life to enjoy.

Romans 6:1–4 (TLB)

ANGER

And "don't sin by letting anger control you."

Ephesians 4:26

Stop being angry! Turn from your rage! Do not lose your temper—it only leads to harm.

Psalm 37:8

A gentle answer turns away wrath, but a harsh word stirs up anger.

Proverbs 15:1 (NIV)

A hot-tempered person starts fights; a cool-tempered person stops them."

Proverbs 15:18

ANXIETY AND WORRY

"So be strong and courageous! Do not be afraid and do not panic before them. For the LORD your God will personally go ahead of you. He will neither fail you nor abandon you."

Deuteronomy 31:6

"So don't worry about tomorrow, for tomorrow will bring its own worries. Today's trouble is enough for today."

Matthew 6:34

Don't worry about anything; instead, pray about everything. Tell God what you need, and thank him for all he has done. Then you will experience God's peace, which exceeds anything we can understand. His peace will guard your hearts and minds as you live in Christ Jesus.

Philippians 4:6–7

DEPRESSION / DISCOURAGEMENT / DESPAIR

The eyes of the LORD watch over those who do right; his ears are open to their cries for help. But the LORD turns his face against those who do evil; he will erase their memory from the earth. The LORD hears his people when they call to him for help. He rescues them from all their troubles.

Psalm 34:15–17

Why am I discouraged? Why is my heart so sad? I will put my hope in God! I will praise him again—my Savior and my God!

Psalm 42:5–6

He will call on me, and I will answer him; I will be with him in trouble, I will deliver him and honor him. With long life I will satisfy him and show him my salvation.

Psalm 91:15–16 (NIV)

But God, who encourages those who are discouraged, encouraged us by the arrival of Titus.

2 Corinthians 7:6

FEAR

I prayed to the LORD, and he answered me. He freed me from all my fears.

Psalm 34:4

For God has not given us a spirit of fear and timidity, but of power, love, and self-discipline.

2 Timothy 1:7

Be strong and courageous. Do not be afraid or terrified because of them, for the LORD your God goes with you; he will never leave you nor forsake you.

Deuteronomy 31:6 (NIV)

But even if you suffer for doing what is right, God will reward you for it. So don't worry or be afraid of their threats.

1 Peter 3:14

GUILT AND CONDEMNATION

But if we confess our sins to him, he is faithful and just to forgive us our sins and to cleanse us from all wickedness. If we claim we have not sinned, we are calling God a liar and showing that his word has no place in our hearts.

1 John 1:9–10

Who dares accuse us whom God has chosen for his own? No one—for God himself has given us right standing with himself. Who then will condemn us? No one—for Christ Jesus died for us and was raised to life for us, and he is sitting in the place of honor at God's right hand, pleading for us.

Romans 8:33–34

For God made Christ, who never sinned, to be the offering for our sin, so that we could be made right with God through Christ.

2 Corinthians 5:21

HATRED

"So now I am giving you a new commandment: Love each other. Just as I have loved you, you should love each other. Your love for one another will prove to the world that you are my disciples."

John 13:34–35

"But I say, love your enemies! Pray for those who persecute you! In that way, you will be acting as true children of your Father in heaven."

Matthew 5:44–45

INSECURITY

As soon as I pray, you answer me; you encourage me by giving me strength.

Psalm 138:3

Our purpose is to please God, not people. He alone examines the motives of our hearts.

1 Thessalonians 2:4

"Don't be afraid, for I am with you. Don't be discouraged, for I am your God. I will strengthen you and help you. I will hold you up with my victorious right hand."

Isaiah 41:10

For I am convinced that neither death nor life, neither angels nor demons, neither the present nor the future, nor any powers, neither height nor depth, nor anything else in all creation, will be able to separate us from the love of God that is in Christ Jesus our Lord.

Romans 8:38–39 (NIV)

JEALOUSY

I am not saying this because I am in need, for I have learned to be content whatever the circumstances.

Philippians 4:11 (NIV)

And this same God who takes care of me will supply all your needs from his glorious riches, which have been given to us in Christ Jesus.

Philippians 4:19

Yet true godliness with contentment is itself great wealth. After all, we brought nothing with us when we came into the world, and we can't take anything with us when we leave it. So if we have enough food and clothing, let us be content.

1 Timothy 6:6-8

LONELINESS

Turn to me and have mercy, for I am alone and in deep distress.

Psalm 25:16

"And be sure of this—that I am with you always, even to the end of the world."

Matthew 28:20 (TLB)

"And I will be your Father, and you will be my sons and daughters, says the LORD Almighty."

2 Corinthians 6:18

MERCY

Because of the LORD's great love we are not consumed, for his compassions never fail. They are new every morning; great is your faithfulness.

Lamentations 3:22–23 (NIV)

PRAYER

And pray in the Spirit on all occasions with all kinds of prayers and requests. With this in mind, be alert and always keep on praying for all the Lord's people.

Ephesians 6:18 (NIV)

REJECTION

"You didn't choose me. I chose you."

John 15:16

Even before he made the world, God loved us and chose us in Christ to be holy and without fault in his eyes. God decided in advance to adopt us into his own family by bringing us to himself through Jesus Christ."

Ephesians 1:4–6

But despite all this, overwhelming victory is ours through Christ who loved us enough to die for us.

Romans 8:37 (TLB)

REVENGE

Dear friends, never avenge yourselves. Leave that to God, for he has said that he will repay those who deserve it. Don't take the law into your own hands.

Romans 12:19 (TLB)

"I will take revenge; I will pay them back. In due time their feet will slip. Their day disaster will arrive, and their destiny will overtake them."

Deuteronomy 32:35

"The LORD will grant that the enemies who rise up against you will be defeated before you. They will come at you from one direction but flee from you in seven."

Deuteronomy 28:7 (NIV)

SELFISHNESS

Don't think only of yourself. Try to think of the other fellow, too, and what is best for him.

1 Corinthians 10:24 (TLB)

He died for all so that all who live—having received eternal life from him—might live no longer for themselves, to please themselves, but to spend their lives pleasing Christ who died and rose again for them.

2 Corinthians 5:15 (TLB)

SPIRITUAL WARFARE

For I can do everything God asks me to with the help of Christ who gives me the strength and power.

Philippians 4:13 (TLB)

"Look, I have given you authority over all the power of the enemy."

Luke 10:19a

"You, dear children, are from God and have overcome them, because the one who is in you is greater than the one who is in the world."

1 John 4:4 (NIV)

For though we live in the world, we do not wage war as the world does. The weapons we fight with are not the weapons of the world. On the contrary, they have divine power to demolish strongholds. We demolish arguments and every pretension that sets itself up against the knowledge of God, and we take captive every thought to make it obedient to Christ.

2 Corinthians 10:3-5 (NIV)

STRESS

Give all your worries and cares to God, for he cares about you.

1 Peter 5:7

"And besides, what's the use of worrying? What good does it do? Will it add a single day to your life? Of course not! And if worry can't even do such little things as that, what's the use of worrying over bigger things?

"And don't worry about food—what to eat and drink; don't worry at all that God will provide it for you. All mankind scratches for its daily bread, but your heavenly Father knows your needs. He will always give you all you need from day to day if you will make the Kingdom of God your primary concern."

Luke 12:25–26, 29–31 (TLB)

TEMPTATION

Submit yourselves, then, to God. Resist the devil, and he will flee from you.

James 4:7 (NIV)

There he told them, "Pray that you will not give in to temptation."

Luke 22:40

Don't do as the wicked do. Avoid their haunts—turn away, go somewhere else.

Proverbs 4:14–15 (TLB)

God is our refuge and strength, an ever-present help in trouble.

Psalm 46:1 (NIV)

For God is working in you, giving you the desire and the power to do what pleases him.

Philippians 2:13

My son, if sinful men entice you, do not give in to them. My son, do not go along with them, do not set foot on their paths."

Proverbs 1:10, 15 (NIV)

"Watch and pray so that you will not fall into temptation. The spirit is willing, but the flesh is weak."

Mark 14:38 (NIV)

Happy is the man who doesn't give in and do wrong when he is tempted, for afterwards he will get as his reward the crown of life that God has promised those who love him.

James 1:12 (TLB)

No temptation has overtaken you except what is common to mankind. And God is faithful; he will not let you be tempted beyond what you can bear. But when you are tempted, he will also provide a way out so that you can endure it.

1 Corinthians 10:13 (NIV)

UNFORGIVENESS

"But when you are praying, first forgive anyone you are holding a grudge against, so that your Father in heaven will forgive your sins, too."

Mark 11:25

Be kind and compassionate to one another, forgiving each other, just as in Christ God forgave you.

Ephesians 4:32 (NIV)

A further reason for forgiveness is to keep from being outsmarted by Satan, for we know what he is trying to do.

2 Corinthians 2:11 (TLB)

APPENDIX 2: CHRISTIAN WEIGHT LOSS AND FOOD ADDICTION PROGRAMS

First Place 4 Health (FirstPlace4Health.com) offers a biblical approach to weight loss through a series of Bible studies. Online groups are available, or you can check to see if one exists in your area.

Take Back Your Temple (TakeBackYourTemple.com) is a Christian online weight loss program whose motto is "Your body for God's glory. We help you take back your house so you can fulfill your God-given purpose."

The Eden Diet: A Biblical and Merciful Anti-Dieting Plan for Weight Loss (TheEdenDiet.com) is a Christian weight-loss program with online support groups.

Thin Within: A Non-Diet Grace Based Approach (ThinWithin.org) is a Christian weight management program that includes online classes and groups.

Barb Raveling Christian weight loss products (Barb Raveling.com) include, a podcast—Taste for Truth: Christian Weight Loss, an app—I Deserve a Donut: and Other Lies That Make You Eat, and a couple of books—*Taste for Truth: A 30 Day Weight Loss Bible Study* and *I Deserve a Donut: And Other Lies that Make You Eat.*

Grace Filled Plate (GraceFilledPlate.com) is a website with an excellent blog which includes having a healthy mindset, recipes, nutrition, and faith.

Victory Steps for Women: Christian Weight Loss & Spiritual Wellness (VictorySteps.net/christian-weight-loss-program.html) is a faith-based health and wellness coaching program, helps women overcome emotional eating, binge eating, and compulsive overeating behaviors.

Weight Loss, God's Way (CathyMorenzie.com/challenge/) is a Christian-based weight loss program that offers a free twenty-one-day challenge.

Three different online food addiction programs include:
    OA.org/ (OA is Overeater's Anonymous)
    FoodAddicts.org/
    FoodAddictsAnonymous.org/

Joining an online support group is another way to share the ups and downs of this journey. Connecting with like-minded individuals who are persevering through the same trials as you helps divide the load. Through these support groups, you can exchange acquired knowledge about your shared journey. In addition, sometimes we need to vent and express our disappointment or success with another person who understands. Life sharing nourishes the emotional side of our well-being.

APPENDIX 3: HEALTHY LIVING JOURNAL

Write the following items in your journal:

1. The time you eat.
2. Why you want to eat. Are you hungry, bored, angry? Is it just "time to eat" or are you with others who are having a meal?
3. If you feel a strong emotion related to this consumption of food, record the emotion.
4. Food you ate and drank, including quantity.
5. How you feel after you ate? Are you satisfied or stuffed?
6. Energy level and clarity of mind after you ate.
7. When waking up in the morning, how do you feel? See if there is a pattern of eating high-sugar-content foods and feeling sluggish the next morning.
8. What are you grateful for today?
9. Prayer requests to God.
10. Exercise—type of activity and length of time.
11. Number of glasses of water you drank and when. Did you drink on an empty stomach?
12. Every time you binge, record: what you ate, why you ate it,

what triggered you to eat it, and what you might do the next time you are tempted.

As you write this information, recognize any patterns between your emotions and food consumption. Did you eat because you were hungry? If no, why?

APPENDIX 4: RECIPES

The following recipes will help you keep sugar and refined carbohy-drates out of your diet and still enjoy delicious meals made with whole, natural foods. The recipes are divided into breakfast, snacks/desserts, dips, vegetables/side dishes, entrees, and bread.

BREAKFAST

Granny Sue's Granola
    8 cups organic oats
    1 cup almonds
    1 cup pecans
    1 cup walnuts
    ½ cup sunflower seeds
    $1/3$ cup sesame seeds
    1/3 cup pumpkin seeds
    ¾ cup coconut or olive oil
    ½–2/3 cup of honey
    Combine all ingredients. Pour into two large greased baking pans.
Bake at 325 degrees for 18–20 minutes; take out and stir. Cook for

another 18–20 minutes, stir and add the following ingredients: 1–2 cups of dried fruit—berries, dates, apricots, raisins, or craisins.

Cook for 10 more minutes. Store granola in two-quart mason jars. Put one on the kitchen counter and the other in the refrigerator. Makes two quarts.

Banana Pancakes

1 smashed banana (lower in sugar if green)

1 egg

½ cup almond flour

1 tablespoon coconut oil

¼ teaspoon baking soda

Combine all ingredients. Cook just like a pancake, but make the cakes small, so they are easier to flip.

Strawberry/Almond Coffee Cake

Preheat oven to 350 degrees and spray an 8X8 pan with olive oil.

2½ cups almond flour

½ teaspoon baking soda

¼ teaspoon salt

¼ cup melted coconut oil

1 tablespoon honey or maple syrup

1 teaspoon baking stevia

1 teaspoon vanilla

Combine all ingredients with a mixer.

Fold 2 cups diced strawberries into the mix.

Put in the pan and add the following topping.

Topping

½ cup almond flour

3 tablespoons softened coconut oil

1 tablespoon honey or maple syrup

1 teaspoon baking stevia

½–1 cup sliced almonds

Combine topping ingredients (except nuts) with a pastry cutter.

Add nuts and sprinkle mixture on top of the coffee cake. Bake for 25–30 minutes until a toothpick comes out clean.

Apple Quinoa Breakfast Muffins

Preheat oven to 375 degrees. Spray a muffin pan with olive oil.

1 cup cooked quinoa

½ cup applesauce

1 mashed banana (lower in sugar if green)

½ cup almond or coconut milk

1 tablespoon honey or maple syrup

2 teaspoons baking stevia

1 teaspoon vanilla

1 teaspoon cinnamon

2½ cups orgainic oats

1 chopped apple

Mix all ingredients. Pour ingredients into muffin pan. Bake for 20–25 minutes.

Chia Parfait

4 tablespoons chia seeds

1 cup almond or coconut milk

½ teaspoon cinnamon

1 teaspoon vanilla

$1/_8$ teaspoon baking stevia

1 cup of fruit of your choice (berries, banana—lower in sugar if green)

½ cup of organic oats

½ cup slivered almonds (or another nut)

Mix the first five ingredients and put in the refrigerator overnight.

In the morning layer the chia mixture with oats, nuts, and fruit in parfait glasses. Top with fresh fruit. (Makes 4 servings.)

Hash Brown Cups

Preheat oven to 350 degrees. Spray muffin pan with olive oil.

1 bag shredded hash browns

3 chopped green onions

½ teaspoon salt

¼ teaspoon pepper

2 tablespoons olive oil

Combine all ingredients. Spoon into muffin pan. Bake for 60–75 minutes. Makes 12 muffins.

Banana Quinoa Oatmeal

1 cup of quinoa cooked in 2 cups of water (about 4 cups cooked)

2 smashed slightly green bananas (lower in sugar if green)

¾ cup chopped walnuts

1 teaspoon cinnamon

1 teaspoon vanilla

1 tablespoon honey or 1 teaspoon of stevia

¾ cup almond or coconut milk

Combine ingredients on stovetop and warm.

Banana Egg Pancakes

1 smashed banana (lower in sugar if green)

2 eggs

$1/_8$ teaspoon cinnamon

Mix ingredients together and pour small-sized pancakes in a hot skillet so they flip easily. These delicious pancakes need no syrup because the banana is sweet. (Makes one serving.)

Apple Oatmeal Cups

Preheat oven to 350 degrees and spray muffin pan with olive oil.

2 cups organic oats

1 teaspoon baking soda

$1/_8$ teaspoon salt

½ teaspoon cinnamon

1 cup almond or coconut milk

1 egg

1 mashed banana (lower in sugar if green)

1 diced apple

Mix all ingredients. Pour into a muffin pan and bake for 20–25 minutes.

SNACKS/DESSERTS

Dehydrated Fruit

A food dehydrator is a terrific investment when beginning to change to a healthier style of eating. Simply cut your fruit into similar sized slices. Place on dehydrator trays and turn on for the length of time indicated by your dehydrator's instructions. If the fruit is in different sizes, the small pieces will get overdone, and the large pieces will not be completely dried. Store dried fruit in mason jars. I give specific instructions on how to dehydrate foods in my YouTube video at Youtube.com/c/SusanNealScriptureYoga.

Coconut Macaroon Cookies

3 egg whites

¼ teaspoon salt

1 teaspoon vanilla

1–2 teaspoon stevia

1 tablespoon monk fruit sugar

1½ cups unsweetened, shredded coconut

Whip the egg whites and vanilla until peaks form. Fold the rest of the ingredients into the whipped egg whites. Let mixture stand for 5 minutes. Bake for 10–15 minutes on a greased cookie sheet at 350 degrees until the macaroons are lightly brown.

Frozen Berries

Either pick or purchase your berries (organic is best). Rinse with water and drain in a colander. Place berries on an ungreased cookie sheet. Make sure the berries do not touch. Place in freezer several hours until frozen. Place frozen berries in mason jars and put in the freezer. Since the berries are frozen individually, you can take as much or as little out of the jar as you need when making your fruit smoothie. My youngest daughter loved to crunch on frozen blue-berries.

Berry Smoothie

1 cup coconut or almond milk

1 cup frozen berries

1 teaspoon coconut oil

Stevia to sweeten

1 cup ice

Protein smoothie: add ½ cup of nuts (almond, pecan, walnut) or 2 tablespoons of almond butter.

Green smoothie: add ½ cup of spinach or kale.

Dark Chocolate–Covered Nuts, Seeds, and Currants

Melt 1–2 bars of dark chocolate (at least 70 percent cocoa), which is healthy and low in sugar. Add a mixture of nuts, seeds, and currants until coated. Drop by tablespoons onto a sheet of wax paper. As the mixture cools, the nut clusters will harden.

Granny Sue's Cranberry Relish

1 large package of raspberry-cranberry Jello

Replace ¾ cup of sugar (from the Jello package's directions) with appropriate measurement of powdered stevia, monk fruit sugar, or half and half mixture.

Prepare the Jello as directed, using the sugar substitute, and place in refrigerator.

Meanwhile, chop the following ingredients by hand or in food processor:

2 cups apples

2 cups celery

2 cups lightly roasted pecans

12-oz package of cranberries

Mix these four ingredients into the Jello and refrigerate until firm.

Dark Chocolate Chip Pecan Cookies

3 cups of almond flour (could substitute 1 cup with coconut flour)

¼ teaspoon salt

1 teaspoon baking soda

¼ cup of coconut or olive oil

1 teaspoon of stevia for baking

¼ cup of maple syrup

1 egg

1 teaspoon vanilla

½ cup dark chocolate chips (more than 70 percent cocoa)

½ cup pecans, almonds, or walnuts (optional)

Combine dry ingredients. In a separate bowl, mix oil, stevia, syrup, eggs, and vanilla with a hand mixer. Slowly add dry ingredients. Mix by hand when adding chocolate chips and nuts. Bake at 375 degrees for 15 minutes.

Almond Butter

Bake almonds for 15 minutes at 325 degrees on an ungreased cookie sheet.

Let almonds cool and place them in a food processor.

Blend on high for about 7–10 minutes. Stop and stir the mixture about every minute.

If you like crunchy nut butter, take a few tablespoons of nuts out of the food processor after blending it for about 30 seconds. I set five tablespoons aside for a one-pint mixture.

Store in the refrigerator.

Almond Flour

Bake almonds for 15 minutes at 325 degrees on an ungreased cookie sheet.

Let almonds cool and place them in a food processor.

Blend on high for about 2–3 minutes until it is the consistency of uncooked grits.

Store in a pint jar in the refrigerator or freezer. Use it just like you would white flour.

Trail Mix

  2 cups almonds
  2 cups walnuts
  2 cups pecans
  1 cup sunflower seeds
  ½ cup sesame seeds
  ¾ cup raisins
  ¾ cup craisins
  Mix all ingredients together and store in the refrigerator.

Organic Popcorn

  2 tablespoons coconut oil
  ¼–$^1/_3$ cup organic popcorn kernels (1 serving)
  Cook oil and popcorn on high in a pan with a lid on the stove top.
  Toppings: ½–1 tablespoon butter, 1 tablespoon olive oil, kelp, dulse (seaweed), sea salt

DIPS

Guacamole

  5–6 smashed avocados
  ½ cup diced cherry tomatoes
  2 tablespoons cilantro
  2 tablespoons olive oil
  2 tablespoons red wine vinegar
  ½ cup chopped purple onion or scallion
  2 cloves minced garlic (use fresh garlic, not from a jar)
  1 tablespoon lime juice
  Mix all ingredients together. Leave the avocado pits in the dip for better storage.

Hummus

  1 cup sesame seeds
  1 clove of garlic
  2 tablespoons olive oil

Bake sesame seeds at 350 degrees for 20 minutes. Put roasted seeds in food processer with 1 garlic clove and 2 tablespoons of oil. This is tahini. Set aside.

4 cups dried garbanzo beans
   3 lemons juiced
   ½ cup lemon zest
   ½ teaspoon salt
   ½ teaspoon cumin

Soak garbanzo beans in water overnight. Pour out water. Cook garbanzo beans in water that is one inch over the top of the beans for 40 minutes or until tender. Cool and drain but set aside 1 cup of the water. Blend the beans and rest of ingredients in the food processor. If needed, add some of the water you set aside until the consistency of the mixture is creamy. Add the tahini and blend.

VEGETABLES/SIDE DISHES

Barb's Asian Slaw
   1 cabbage head, shredded
   4 chopped green onions
   ½ cup slivered or sliced almonds

Dressing
   ½ cup olive oil
   ¼ cup tamari or soy sauce
   1 tablespoon honey or maple syrup
   1 tablespoon baking stevia

Heat up dressing ingredients in a saucepan on the stove until thoroughly mixed.

Mix all ingredients when you are ready to serve.

Blueberry Cantaloupe Avocado Salad
   1 diced cantaloupe
   2–3 chopped avocados

1 package of blueberries
¼ cup olive oil
$^1/_8$ cup balsamic vinegar
Mix all ingredients.

Beet Salad (from Israel)

2–3 fresh, raw beets grated or shredded in food processor
3 tablespoons olive oil
2 tablespoons balsamic vinegar
¼ teaspoon salt
$^1/_3$ teaspoon cumin
Dash stevia powder or liquid
Dash pepper
Mix all ingredients together for the best raw beet salad.

Broccoli Salad

1 head broccoli, chopped
2–3 slices of fried bacon, crumbled
1 diced green onion
½ cup raisins or craisins
½–1 cup of chopped pecans
¾ cup sunflower seeds
½ cup of pomegranate

Dressing

1 cup organic mayonnaise
¼ cup baking stevia
2 teaspoons white vinegar
Mix all ingredients together. Mix dressing and fold into salad.

Rosemary Garlic Potatoes

Preheat oven to 425 degrees.
5 red new potatoes, chopped
¼ cup olive oil
2–3 cloves of minced garlic

1 tablespoon rosemary

Stir all ingredients together in a bowl. Pour onto a baking sheet and bake for 30 minutes.

Sweet and Sour Cabbage

1 tablespoon honey or maple syrup

1 teaspoon baking stevia

2 tablespoons water

1 tablespoon olive oil

¼ teaspoon caraway seeds

¼ teaspoon salt

$^1/_8$ teaspoon pepper

2 cups chopped red cabbage

1 diced apple

Cook all ingredients in a covered saucepan on the stove for 15 minutes.

Barley and Lentil Salad

1 head romaine lettuce

¾ cup cooked barley

2 cups cooked lentils

1 diced carrot

¼ chopped red onion

¼ cup olives

½ chopped cucumber

3 tablespoons olive oil

2 tablespoons fresh lemon juice

Mix all ingredients together. Add kosher salt and black pepper to taste.

ENTREES

Homemade Chicken Broth

1 tablespoon olive oil

1 chopped onion

2 chopped stalks celery

2 chopped carrots

1 whole chicken

2+ quarts of water

1 tablespoon salt

½ teaspoon pepper

1 teaspoon fresh sage

Sauté vegetables in oil. Add chicken and water and simmer for 2+ hours until the chicken falls off the bone. Keep adding water as needed. Remove the chicken carcass from the broth, place on a platter, and let it cool. Pull chicken off the carcass and put it into the broth. Pour broth mixture into pint and quart mason jars. Be sure to add meat to each jar. Leave one full inch of space from the top of the jar or it will crack when it freezes as liquids expand. Place jars in freezer for up to a year. Take out and use whenever you make a soup.

Homemade Vegetable Broth

1 tablespoon olive oil

1 chopped onion

2 chopped stalks celery

2 chopped carrots

1 head bok choy

6 cups or 1 package fresh spinach

2+ quarts of water

1 tablespoon salt

½ teaspoon pepper

1 teaspoon fresh sage

Sauté vegetables in oil. Add water and simmer for 1 hour. Keep adding water as needed. Pour broth mixture into pint and quart mason jars. Leave one full inch of space from the top of the jar or it will crack when it freezes as liquids expand. Place jars in freezer for up to a year. Take out and use whenever you make a soup.

Fish Stew

1 tablespoon olive oil

1 chopped onion or leek
2 chopped stalks celery
2 chopped carrots
1 clove minced garlic
1 tablespoon parsley
1 bay leaf
1 clove
$^1/_8$ teaspoon kelp or dulse (seaweed)
¼ teaspoon salt
Fish—leftover, cooked, diced
2–3 cups chicken or vegetable broth
Add all of ingredients and simmer on the stove for 20 minutes.

Quinoa with Vegetables

2 cups water
1 cup dried quinoa
Assorted fresh vegetables
Cook quinoa in water.
Sauté an assortment of vegetables in olive oil. Different vegetable combinations include:

- sautéed scallions, mushrooms, and spinach along with sunflower and pumpkin seeds;

- sautéed onion, bell peppers, and kale with a fresh avocado on top;

- sautéed bok choy, snow peas, and carrots with cashews and sesame seeds.

Either serve vegetables on top of quinoa or combine.

Black Bean Soup

1 pound dry black beans (soak in water overnight and drain water)
1 tablespoon olive oil

2 cups chopped onion or 1 leek

1 cup chopped carrots

4 cloves minced garlic

2 teaspoons cumin

¼ teaspoon red pepper flakes

4 cups chicken broth

4 cups water

¼ teaspoon thyme

2 chopped tomatoes or 1 (14 oz) can tomatoes

1½ teaspoon salt

Optional: add bacon or ham to flavor

Chopped green onions to garnish

Sauté vegetables in oil. Add rest of ingredients and cook on stovetop on medium-low heat for 1 hour.

Richard's Best Chicken

2 tablespoons olive oil

8 chicken thighs

6 cloves garlic

1 jar artichoke hearts, drained

¾ cup chicken broth

3 fresh squeezed oranges

1 sliced Meyer lemon

¼ cup capers

½ cup olives

In a cast-iron skillet, fry chicken on each side in oil until skin is golden and crispy. Remove from skillet. Sauté garlic and artichokes for a few minutes, add chicken (skin up). Pour in rest of ingredients and bring to a boil. Place skillet with all ingredients uncovered in a 350-degree oven for 30 minutes.

White Bean and Cabbage Soup

1 tablespoon olive oil

4 chopped carrots

4 chopped stalks of celery or 1 chopped bok choy

1 chopped onion

2 cloves minced garlic

1 chopped cabbage head

½ lb northern beans soaked in water overnight (drained)

6 cups chicken broth

3 cups water

Sauté vegetables in oil. Add rest of ingredients and cook on medium-low heat for 30 minutes.

Brooke's Chili

2 lb organic ground beef

1 diced onion

3 cloves minced garlic

6 diced tomatoes

1 jar tomato sauce

1 tablespoon salt

1 cup water

1 cup kidney beans soaked in water overnight (drained)

1 cup pinto beans soaked in water overnight (drained)

2 tablespoons chili powder

1 tablespoon cumin

1 tablespoon honey or maple syrup

1 teaspoon baking stevia

1 teaspoon pepper

In a large pot, brown the ground beef and drain the grease. Add the onion and garlic and cook until translucent. Add rest of ingredients and simmer for 1 hour.

Lentil Soup

2 tablespoons olive oil

2 chopped onions

1 chopped red pepper

1 chopped carrot

2 cloves minced garlic

½ teaspoon cumin

¾ teaspoon thyme

1 bay leaf

8 cups chicken broth

2 chopped tomatoes

½ pound dried lentils (1¼ cup)

Optional: add bacon or ham to flavor

1 teaspoon salt

¼ teaspoon pepper

Handful of spinach

Sauté vegetables in oil. Add rest of ingredients (except spinach and spices). Cover and cook on low for 2 hours. Add spinach and spices.

White Chicken Chili

1 tablespoon olive oil

1 pound of chicken strips cut into pieces

2 teaspoons cumin

½ teaspoon oregano

½ teaspoon salt

½ teaspoon pepper

1 chopped onion

1 chopped red bell pepper

4 cloves minced garlic

4 cups chicken broth

2 cups northern beans soaked in water overnight (drained)

Sauté chicken and spices in oil and remove from pan. Sauté onion and red pepper. Add rest of ingredients including chicken and cook on medium-low heat for 15 minutes.

Mixed Vegetable Soup

1 tablespoon olive oil

1 chopped leek

1 chopped bok choy

4 chopped carrots

2 cloves minced garlic

1 chopped zucchini

2 chopped tomatoes

1 cup garbanzo beans soaked in water overnight (drained)

5 chopped potatoes

8 cups broth

1 teaspoon basil

½ cup amaranth

Sauté first four ingredients, add garlic for last minute. Add rest of ingredients and simmer on the stove for 25 minutes.

Potato Soup

2 tablespoons olive oil

1 diced onion

4 minced cloves garlic

1 teaspoon thyme

1 bay leaf

4 diced red potatoes

6 cups water

1 sliced leek

3 diced celery stalks

2 teaspoons salt

¼ teaspoon pepper

Sauté onion, garlic, thyme, and bay leaf in oil until translucent. Add rest of ingredients and simmer for about 20 minutes.

BREAD

Granny Sue's Corn Pone

Preheat oven to 440 degrees and spray a cookie sheet with olive oil.

¼ teaspoon salt

1 cup oatmeal

1 cup organic cornmeal

¼ cup sesame seeds

¼ cup sunflower seeds

¼ cup pumpkin seeds

1 cup hot water

Combine all ingredients and stir.

Pour mixture onto a greased cookie sheet and shape like large oval cookies about ½ inch thick. Bake for 35 minutes.

Kim's Gluten Free, Dairy Free, Whole Grain Bread[1]

3 large eggs lightly beaten

1 teaspoon apple cider vinegar

¼ cup oil of choice (canola, olive, corn, coconut, grapeseed, etc.)

$1^1/_3$ cup milk of choice—unsweetened (rice, hemp, almond, cow) warmed to about body temperature

1 tablespoon +1 teaspoon honey

3 tablespoons brown sugar

½ cup millet, sorghum, quinoa, amaranth, or buckwheat flour (choose one)

½ cup second choice of flour: millet, sorghum, quinoa, amaranth, or buckwheat flour (choose one)

1 cup multigrain rice flour, brown rice flour, or (my favorite) teff flour

½ cup tapioca flour

½ cup cornstarch (potato starch works too)

3 teaspoons xanthan gum

1½ teaspoons salt

2¼ teaspoons dry active yeast

optional add ins:

flax seeds

sesame seeds

sunflower seeds

add in a total of about a ¼ cup

Combine first six ingredients in bread maker pan. Sift next seven ingredients and then add on top of liquid ingredients. Toss in your add ins. Make a little well in the dry ingredients and add the yeast in the hole. Start the bread maker on the gluten-free bread setting. Gluten-free bread needs less time as there is no need for additional punch downs like with wheat bread.

APPENDIX 5: HEALTHY EATING GUIDELINES

Low-carbohydrate, anti-inflammatory dietary guidelines include:

- About 50 percent of food items are fresh organic vegetables.
- Eat one fresh, raw serving of low-glycemic fruit per day. Low-glycemic fruits include green apples, berries, cherries, pears, plums, and grapefruit.
- Do not always eat cooked foods. Eat a couple of servings of raw vegetables every day. Have a salad for lunch with either nuts or meat. When eating out, order a salad or coleslaw as sides, since both are raw.
- Another 25 percent of your daily food intake should come from an animal or vegetable protein such as beans, nuts, and lean meats. Fish is exceptionally nutritious. Try to eat it once a week.
- A variety of different nuts and seeds are excellent sources of protein, minerals, and essential fatty acids.
- Avoid sugar, flour, rice, pasta, and bread. Instead, eat more fruits, vegetables, and low-glycemic grains such as quinoa and pearled barley.
- Do not eat sugary cereals. Instead, eat oatmeal, fruit, or

granola. Be careful, as the sugar content of granola may be high. My favorite granola recipe appears in appendix 4.

- Try not to eat anything containing more than 10 grams of sugar in one serving, or 24 grams for a woman or 36 grams for a man per day.
- Eat nontraditional grains such as quinoa, amaranth, pearled barley, wild rice, and oats.
- Eat cultured foods such as kimchi, sauerkraut, and cultured plain Greek yogurt since they contain natural probiotics. Add one to two tablespoons of these foods to a meal twice a week or eat the yogurt as a snack. Personally, I take a probiotic capsule every day.
- Replace undesirable ingredients with whole foods. *The Daniel Plan Cookbook* by Rick Warren provides a chart titled Foods and Ingredients to Avoid and suggests replacements. A few recommendations from this book include:
- Replace sugary snacks with nuts, nut butter, dark chocolate, and plain Greek yogurt with berries.
- Replace condiments and sauces containing MSG or high-fructose corn syrup with spices, vinegar, and herbs.
- Replace table salt with kosher or sea salt.
- Replace fried foods with baked foods.

APPENDIX 6: SEVEN-DAY
EATING PLAN

Day 1 (Start on Wednesday)

1. Consume Water

Drink up to two cups of coffee or tea per day, but no more. The only other beverage you should drink is filtered water. I use a filter on my refrigerator water dispenser and a water filter on a pitcher. Before breakfast drink two glasses of water, two before lunch, two midafternoon, and two more before dinner. Do not drink during meals and do not drink anything after dinner. Drink up to ten minutes before eating.

2. Take a Probiotic

Begin taking a probiotic every day. I usually buy several probiotics from a health food store with at least ten different strains of beneficial bacteria, and I take a different one each day to vary the flora in my gastrointestinal system. I store my probiotics in the refrigerator door. After I take a probiotic, I move the bottle to a different shelf, so I can keep track of the one I took last.

3. Stop Eating High-Sugar Foods

Stop eating anything containing greater than 10 grams of sugar per serving, or 24 grams for a woman or 36 grams for a man per day. Check labels for the number of grams of sugar per serving size.

Day 2

1. Eliminate Wheat

Do not eat anything containing wheat. No more bagels, toast, pancakes, biscuits, pasta, pretzels, crackers, cookies, cake, or pie. Eliminating wheat is like going off a drug. Be aware that you may experience the following symptoms for a few days: irritability, foggy brain, and fatigue. You might even feel fluish. However, within a week your symptoms will subside. After this, never eat wheat or more than 10 grams of sugar in one serving again, or your addiction will start all over again. (Ugh.)

Day 3

1. Eliminate Processed Foods

Do not eat processed foods from boxes and bags.

2. Implement Healthy Eating Guidelines

Make 50 percent of your food fresh and raw. Follow the Healthy Eating Guidelines provided in appendix 5.

Days 4 and 5 (Saturday and Sunday)

Continue to implement all the steps listed on day one through three as you proceed.

1. Rest

Focus on you. Rest, read, pray, and ask God to help you to succeed.

2. Use the Sword of the Spirit

Now is the time to fight the thief Jesus spoke of in John 10:10, for Satan wants you to fail: "The thief's purpose is to steal, kill and destroy. My purpose is to give life in all its fullness" (John 10:10 TLB).

Fight the thief with the sword of the Spirit—the Word of God. Write verses on index cards or put them on the notes app on your smartphone. Use verses that will remind you of the help God provides in any struggles you may be facing at this point, such as Philippians 4:13: "For I can do everything through Christ, who gives me strength." Every time you get the urge to go back to your old eating habits, speak the verse out loud to cut the demonic influence out of your life. Our spiritual nature needs to be addressed as well as our physical.

Day 6

1. Start the Anti-Candida Cleanse

Now let's kill the bug in your gut—Candida. Today, start the anti-Candida cleanse you purchased in step 4. If you are not ready to begin this step because you are still experiencing symptoms of withdrawal (headache, exhaustion, irritability, mental fogginess, fluish symptoms), wait a few days until you feel better. Read the instructions on the cleanse package for how to administer it. Initially, I recommend taking the cleanse every other day for the first week to minimize lethargy and headaches. You will feel awful if the dead Candida is not quickly expelled from your colon. To avoid becoming constipated, drink plenty of water. During the second week, begin taking the Candida cleanse every day as recommended.

Prevent a headache by increasing the fiber in your diet through a fiber supplement (which usually comes with your Candida cleanse), water, and raw fruits and vegetables. The first three days you are on the cleanse, you may not feel well, but after a week you will begin to feel better than you have in a long time. You are just about to get the life back Jesus wants you to experience—one that is abundant and full.

Day 7

1. Get Up and Exercise

If you are still feeling the symptoms of withdrawal, be gentle with yourself by performing a simple form of exercise such as walking or yoga. It doesn't matter what type of exercise you do just as long as you do it. Walking, jumping rope, lifting weights, or taking a group fitness class like Pilates or water aerobics are a few examples of exercise. After you begin feeling better, try to exercise for twenty minutes three times a week. Record the exercise you perform in the *Healthy Living Journal* or the journal that you set up in step 2.

Mindfulness exercises such as yoga and meditation train a person to pay attention to cravings without reacting to them. The idea is to ride out the wave of intense desire. As a person becomes more mindful she notices why she wants to indulge. Meditation quiets the part of the brain that can lead to a loop of obsession. Check out my website at ChristianYoga.com.

Day 8 and Beyond

You are well on your way to changing your lifestyle, but more than that you will change your life for the better. Your health, mood, and energy level will improve. Each week you will lose weight, and the body God gave you will heal itself of many ailments. As your body heals the disease processes, you will be able to reduce or eliminate medications because you will no longer suffer from the maladies these medications were treating. However, before stopping any prescription medication be sure to consult with your physician. Improvement in your vitality will allow you to experience activities you were not able to be involved in before. Overall your well-being and emotional countenance will become revitalized. You are in the process of getting your life back, the one that God wants you to enjoy to its fullest.

APPENDIX 7: HOW TO BECOME A CHRISTIAN AND DISCIPLE OF JESUS CHRIST

Accepting Jesus as your Savior

Salvation begins when we recognize our sinfulness and ask God to forgive us. We accept that Jesus Christ humbled himself in obedience to God by dying on a cross to pay for our sins. Sin is simply to miss the mark, to live our lives by our own selfish desires instead of following God's ways.

Since Jesus never sinned, he was an acceptable sacrifice to pay the debt (eternal damnation) for our sins. Once we accept Jesus' gift and ask him to come into our hearts, we are filled with the Holy Spirit. Accepting Jesus places the helmet of salvation on our heads. Our Savior's Spirit within us gives us the ability to come before God and receive his grace and mercy to help us in our times of need.

Accepting Jesus as your savior is simple. All you need to do is pray. In this prayer ask God to forgive you for your sins and tell him that you will turn away from those sins. Ask Jesus to come into your heart and lead your life. At that moment you receive the Holy Spirit.

When we accept Christ as our Savior, God adopts us as his children and loves us unconditionally like a parent. Nothing can take his love away from us. Since we are his children, we can access his power by faith and apply it to any area in our lives.

Becoming a Disciple of Jesus Christ

We become righteous when we ask God to forgive us of our sins and accept Jesus Christ as our Lord and Savior; at that moment God replaces our sin with our Savior's righteousness—since he never sinned. To maintain this right standing, we must accept God's moral standards as our values. Living our life in obedience to those values is part of becoming a disciple of Jesus Christ.

We become Jesus' disciple when we submit our lives to him and allow him to lead us. How do we let Jesus lead our lives? Through following his Word and responding to the prompting of the Holy Spirit inside of us. We should pay attention to the gentle nudging the Spirit gives us and pray throughout the day. Remain in contact with Jesus spiritually through silently talking to him and asking for his help and guidance as you need it. He wants to be a part of your life.

It is important to spend time with God, maybe through reading a devotion or a Bible verse as well as spending meditative time in God's presence. Ask him to lead you and he will. Search for him, and you will find him. Jeremiah 29:13 (NIV) "You will seek me and find me when you seek me with all your heart." So start seeking.

Through salvation, we received the Holy Spirit. Receiving God's Spirit compares to a seed which needs soil, sunlight, water, and fertilizer to grow. As the seed grows so does our faith. The following four habits can help us to stand firm in our faith:

1. Studying and memorizing scripture verses
2. Spending time with the Lord
3. Fellowship with other Christians
4. Submitting control of our lives to Jesus

These practices will make us spiritually strong and wise.

APPENDIX 8: FIVE-STEP BINDING THE STRONG MAN PLAN

1. Name what controls you.

Name the thing controlling you—food addiction, anxiety, eating disorder, depression, etc.—whatever it may be, and declare (out loud) Jesus Christ is your Lord in its place![5]

Stand up to the evil spirit who brought bondage into your life by saying, "Evil spirit, you won't lord over me nor entice me through (insert your addiction) anymore. Jesus is my Lord!" A person obtains spiritual power and authority through Christ. Declare that the spiritual powers of darkness will not have lordship over your life. They will not rule you, govern your behavior, capture your thought life, nor lead you into temptation and sin because "the one who is in you is greater than the one who is in the world" (1 John 4:4 NIV).

"For when Satan, strong and fully armed, guards his palace, it is safe—until someone stronger and better armed attacks and overcomes him and strips him of his weapons and carries off his belongings." Luke 11:21–22 (TLB)

Get ready, for *you are capable of evicting the addiction strong man in your life*. If you accepted Jesus as your Lord and Savior (see appendix 7 to find out how), the Holy Spirit lives within you and the Spirit is stronger than Satan. Day after day, declare out loud that Jesus reigns as the Lord of your life—not your addiction.

2. Submit yourself completely to God.

"Submit yourself to God, resist the devil and he will flee from you." James 4:7 (NIV)

There is a secret to resisting the devil—you must first submit yourself to God. How in the world do you do that? In my experience, you no longer do your will but God's will by submitting your life to him. For me, it was not without a fight.

If you are a food addict, after binging, ask God to forgive you and help you not to binge the next time. Record your experience in your journal. Once you ask for forgiveness, God chooses not to remember your sins, as indicated in Hebrews 8:12: "And I will be merciful to them in their wrongdoings, and I will remember their sins no more" (TLB). Don't fret over a stumble. Get up and try again using this Five-Step Binding the Strong Man Plan.

3. Use the name of Jesus.

Jesus told his disciples, "Look, I have given you authority over all the power of the enemy" (Luke 10:19). If you are a disciple of Jesus (see appendix 7 to find out how) you can accept the authority he gave you.

In the book of Acts, the apostles healed and worked miracles in the name of Jesus. Use Jesus's name as Peter did in Acts 3:6: "in the name of Jesus Christ of Nazareth, walk" (TLB). Using the name of Jesus is key to binding the strong man because then you operate under Jesus's authority.

Picture a person tied in ropes. That's the way a spiritual strong man afflicts his victim. However, if you declare Jesus is Lord over your life, not the strong man (addiction), and use Jesus's name, you are under his authority. Then the ropes, tied around you by the evil spirit, break. Eventually, the spiritual ropes loosen and fall off. Next, comes the moment to take action by tying the strong man through binding him with the Word of God.

4. Use the Word of God.

"For when Satan, strong and fully armed, guards his palace, it is safe—until someone stronger and better armed attacks and overcomes him and strips him of his weapons and carries off his belongings." Luke 11:21–22 TLB

The Holy Spirit inside of you is stronger than Satan and his demons. By using the name of Jesus, you are not only under his authority but you can speak with his authority. You are much better armed than Satan. Now is the time to stand up to him, strip him of his weapons, and kick him out of your life through the Word of God! Say to the strong man, "In the name of Jesus, you won't oppress me anymore. I bind your power in the name of Jesus and by the Word of God."

Search the Bible for a verse that is the opposite of your addiction. A whole selection of verses is provided in appendix 1. Use the specific scripture you chose to bind the strong man every time he tempts you. Write this verse on an index card and memorize it.

Luke 11:22 states the strong man was stripped of his weapons and his belongings were carried off. Matthew 12:29 asserts when Satan was bound his demons could be cast out. After you tie up the strong man with the Word of God—ignore him. He will try to hobble after you because he doesn't give up easily. If he did, he wouldn't be a strong man. Remember, the next time you are tempted, you're facing a critical moment. When you give him (the spirit of addiction) your attention by drinking, eating sugary foods, worrying—whatever addiction it was—you are, in effect, untying the strong man.

5. Praise God and practice gratitude.

When you praise God and thank him for his blessings, the strong man won't hang around. Don't be satisfied with binding the strong man and walking away—punish him.

Fill your mind, heart, and body with the Spirit of God by putting the right things in your spirit. Listen to praise music; read the Bible and pray; memorize scripture; attend church, Sunday school, or a Bible study. Also, start doing more to help others. Performing acts of service and helping others fills your heart with honorable feelings and humility. Every day, write in your journal about all you can praise God for and thank him.

Beat the strong man by declaring Bible verses out loud. Stomp him into the ground by singing praises to God. The devil can't stand to be around someone who worships the Lord.

Become God's warrior by using his mighty unseen weapons. Paul advises, "It is true that I am an ordinary, weak human being, but I don't use human plans and methods to win my battles. I use God's mighty weapons, not those made by men, to knock down the devil's strongholds" (2 Corinthians 10:3–4 TLB). Get ready to knock out and tie up the strong man of addiction in your life. You are God's mighty conqueror!

APPENDIX 9: CURB THE SWEET TOOTH

When the craving for sugar arises, I eat one of these nutritious snacks:

- Slice a green apple, which is low in sugar, and add almond or cashew butter to each slice. It tastes sweet; conversely, the almond butter is high in protein. Both the apple and nut butter provide fiber and fill me up.
- Melt 70-percent dark chocolate in a pan on the stove and add different types of nuts until well coated with the chocolate. Place mounds of nut clusters on wax paper. After an hour they harden. Keep in an airtight container on the counter or refrigerator for a week. Nuts contain fiber and are filling.
- Sparingly eat one date along with seven pecan halves. Dates are high in natural sugar, so you only need a smidgen to attain the sweetness. Don't eat too many dates, which are high in sugar, but instead fill up on the pecans, which are high in protein.
- I grow fruit trees in my yard, so from June through December I pick fresh blueberries, apples, grapes, pears, and

oriental persimmons. I eat one serving of fruit each day either for breakfast or as an afternoon snack.

- Curb sweet cravings by adding a teaspoon of raw, unfiltered, unpasteurized apple cider vinegar in a cup of water with a couple of drops of stevia.

APPENDIX 10: FOOD ADDICTION BATTLE STRATEGIES

1. Record pertinent information listed in appendix 3 in your journal.
2. Find a specific Bible verse to oppose your food issue and write it on an index card. Keep it with you until you memorize it. Speak the verse out loud every time you feel the urge to eat unhealthy foods.
3. Ask a friend to be your accountability and prayer partner.
4. Join a Christian weight loss program or an online food addiction program.
5. Determine food triggers and eliminate them.
6. Implement the Five Steps to Binding the Strong Man Plan:
7. Name the thing controlling you—your food addiction, anxiety, eating disorder, depression, etc.—whatever it may be, and declare (out loud) Jesus Christ is your Lord in its place!
8. Submit yourself completely to God.
9. Bind the strong man (evil spirit of addiction) with the name of Jesus.
10. Use the Word of God to bind the strong man.
11. Punish the strong man by praising God.

Do you have an accountability/prayer partner, yet? Acquiring a support system is integral to successfully make this lifestyle change. Have you joined a Christian weight loss program or one of the online food addiction programs? A list of these programs is provided in appendix 2. If you need to, reread step 2 about how to create your support system.

When you eat any unhealthy food, be sure to journal afterward—every single time. Figure out what you told yourself that validated why it was okay to eat the item. Then go through the Five Steps to Binding the Strong Man Plan (appendix 8). If you journal and implement this five-step plan every time you binge, you will experience success. Retraining your mind is like disciplining a child; consistency is vital to conformity.

NOTES

Step 1

1. William Davis MD, *Wheat Belly* (New York: Rodale Inc., 2011), 8–9, 48–49.
2. Fiona MacDonald, "Watch: This is How Sugar Affects Your Brain," *Science Alert*, November 3, 2015, https://www.sciencealert.com/watch-this-is-how-sugar-affects-your-brain.
3. Rick Warren, Daniel Amen MD, and Mark Hyman MD, *The Daniel Plan: 40 Days to a Healthier Life* (Grand Rapids: Zondervan, 2013), 106–7.
4. Donna Gates, *The Body Ecology Diet* (New York: Hay House, Inc., 2010), 3.
5. Fran Smith, "The Addicted Brain," *National Geographic*, September 2017, 36–37, 42–43.

Step 2

1. Erin Schumaker, "Surgeon General Vivek Murthy:

Addiction is a Chronic Brain Disease, Not a Moral Failing,"
Huffington Post, November 17, 2016.

2. Deane Alban, "How to Increase Dopamine Naturally," Be
   Brain Fit, Bebrainfit.com/increase-dopamine/.
3. Smith, "Addicted Brain," 36–37, 42–43.
4. Ibid., 36.
5. Ibid., 36–37.
6. "Candida Yeast Infection, Leaky Gut, Irritable Bowel and
   Food Allergies," National Candida Center,
   https://www.nationalcandidacenter.com/Leaky-Gut-and-
   Candida-Yeast-Infection-s/1823.htm.
7. Davis, *Wheat Belly,* 24.
8. Hetty C. van den Broeck, Hein C. de Jong, Elma M. J.
   Salentin, Liesbeth Dekking, Dirk Bosch, Rob J. Hamer,
   Ludovicus J. W. J. Gilissen, Ingrid M. van der Meer, and
   Marinus J. M. Smulders, *"Prescence of celiac disease epitopes in
   modern and old hexaploid wheat varieties: wheat breeding my
   have contributed to increased prevalence of celiac disease,"*
   Theoretical and Applied Genetics 121(8), (November 2010):
   1527–39,
   https://www.ncbi.nlm.nih.gov/pmc/articles/PMC2963738/.
9. Ibid.
10. "Candida Yeast Infection, Leaky Gut, Irritable Bowel and
    Food Allergies."
11. Davis, *Wheat Belly,* 60–63.
12. John Brennan, "What is Roundup Ready Corn," Sciencing,
    April 25, 2017, https://sciencing.com/roundup-ready-corn-
    6762437.html.
13. Rebecca Boyle, "How to Genetically Modify a Seed, Step By
    Step," *Popular Science,* January 24, 2011.
14. Gates, *Body Ecology Diet,* 59–63.
15. Mark Water, *Scripture Memory Made Easy* (Peabody:
    Hendrickson Publishers, 1999), 9–11.
16. Davis, *Wheat Belly,* 8.

Step 3

1. Smith, "Addicted Brain," 37, 43–44.
2. Davis, *Wheat Belly*, 25–26.
3. Smith, "Addicted Brain," 50.
4. Tom McKay, "What Happens to Your Brain on Sugar: Explained by Science," Mic.com, April 21, 2014, https://mic.com/articles/88015/what-happens-to-your-brain-on-sugar-explained-by-science-.rAKas1ERY.
5. John Brennan, "What is Roundup Ready Corn," Sciencing, April 25, 2017, https://sciencing.com/roundup-ready-corn-6762437.html.
6. Alexandra Sifferlin, "Artificial Sweeteners are Linked to Weight Gain—Not Weight Loss," Time, July 17, 2017, http://time.com/4859012/artificial-sweeteners-weight-loss/.
7. Susan Scutti, "Dangerous Effects of Artificial Sweeteners on Your Health," Medical Daily, July 10, 2013, http://www.medicaldaily.com/4-dangerous-effects-artificial-sweeteners-your-health-247543.
8. Stacy Simon, "World Health Organization Says Processed Meat Causes Cancer," *American Cancer Society*, October 26, 2015, https://www.cancer.org/latest-news/world-health-organization-says-processed-meat-causes-cancer.html.
9. Kris Gunnars, "Why is Coconut Oil Good for You? A Healthy Oil for Cooking," *Health Line*, May 26, 2017, https://www.healthline.com/nutrition/why-is-coconut-oil-good-for-you - section4.
10. Jennifer Hartle, Ana Navas-Acien, Robert Lawrence, "The consumption of canned food and beverages and urinary Bishpenol A concentrations in NHANES 2003–2008," *Environmental Research* Volume 150, (October 2016): 375–76, Sciencedirect.com/science/article/pii/S0013935116302407.
11. "U.S. Food and Drug Administration," "Bishpenol A (BPA):

Use in Food Contact Application" (November 2014),
www.fda.gov/newsevents/publichealthfocus/ucm064437.

12. Tom Valentine, "The Proven Dangers of Microwaves,"
Nexus Volume 2, #25 (April-May 1995),
http://www.mercola.com/article/microwave/hazards2.htm.

13. "What's in Your Pantry?" by Tana Amen BSN, RN and Dr.
Daniel Amen, YouTube, https://www.youtube.com/watch?
v=VqoWO0-RSAI.

Step 4

1. Keri Gardner, "How Acids Affect Calcium in the Teeth &
Bones," *LiveStrong*, August 14, 2017.

2. James Colquhoun, "The Truth About Calcium and
Osteoporosis," *Food Matters*, November 24, 2009,
http://www.foodmatters.com/article/the-truth-about-
calcium-and-osteoporosis.

3. Rick Warren, Daniel Amen MD, and Mark Hyman MD, *The
Daniel Plan Cookbook* (Grand Rapids: Zondervan, 2014),
16–17.

4. Brenda Davy, "Clinical Trial Confirms effectiveness of
Simple Appetite Control Method," *American Chemical
Society*, August 23, 2010, http://www.acs.org.

5. Alexa Fleckenstein, MD, "The Top Foods Inflaming Your
Body," *Rodale Wellness*, November 11, 2014.

6. Donna Gates, *Body Ecology Diet*, 3–8.

7. Perlmutter, *Grain Brain*, 224.

Step 5

1. Darren Warburton, Crystal Nicol, and Shannon Bredin,
"Health Benefits of Physical Activity: The Evidence," *Canada
Medical Association Journal* 174, (March 14, 2006): 801–9.

2. Miriam Reiner, Christina Niermann, Darko Jekauc, and
Alexander Woll, "Long-term Health Benefits of Physical

Activity—A Systematic Review of Longitudinal Studies," *BioMed Central Public Health*, September 8, 2013.

3. Smith, "Addicted Brain," 51.

4. "Bible Commentary," Adam Clarke Commentary, https://www.studylight.org/commentaries/acc/matthew-12.html.

5. Larry Lea, *The Weapons of Your Warfare: Equipping Yourself to Defeat the Enemy* (Reading: Cox and Wyman, Ltd. 1990), 126, 182.

Step 7

1. James Allen, *As a Man Thinketh* (Orig. pub. 1903; London: Value Classic Reprints, 2017).

2. Smith, "Addicted Brain," 36–37.

Appendix 4

1. "Kim's Gluten Free, Dairy Free, Whole Grain Bread," Gluten Free Real Food, https://gfrealfood.com/2009/06/10/kims-gluten-free-dairy-free-whole-grain-bread/.

ABOUT THE AUTHOR

Susan U. Neal, RN, MBA, MHS, is an award-winning author, speaker, and certified health and wellness coach whose background in nursing and health services led her to seek new ways to educate and coach people to overcome health challenges. She published *Christian Study Guide for 7 Steps to Get Off Sugar and Carbohydrates* and the *Healthy Living Journal*. Her passion and mission is to improve the health of the body of Christ. To learn more about Susan visit her website at Susan-UNeal.com.

Susan is the creator of Scripture Yoga™ and published *Scripture Yoga*, a #1 Amazon best-selling yoga book, and *Yoga for Beginners*. These products are available on Amazon and ChristianYoga.com.

Susan has been interviewed on the *Bridges Show* on Christian Television Network (CTN), Moody Radio, Blog Talk Radio, and Premier Christian Radio from the UK.

Susan founded Scripture Yoga™, a form of Christian yoga, and enjoys leading classes at her church and fitness club. She is a speaker and enjoys teaching Scripture Yoga™ sessions at women's retreats, Christian conferences, and yoga retreats.

Previously Susan worked as a kidney transplant nurse at Shands Hospital in Gainesville, Florida; assistant administrator at Mayo Clinic Jacksonville; and quality assurance nurse at Blue Cross Blue Shield of Florida. Currently, she owns her own business, Christian Yoga, LLC, and publishes Christian products, along with teaching group fitness classes.

Connect with Susan Online

Susan created the Healthy Living Series blog to provide healthy lifestyle tips and the latest scientific findings regarding foods and health. She also posts her weekly menu and grocery shopping list to help with planning healthy menus. You can subscribe to the blog at SusanUNeal.com/healthy-living-blog.

Please follow Susan on BookBub and get an email when she releases a new book or when her books go on sale at Bookbub.com/authors/susan-u-neal.

You can follow Susan on:
Facebook.com/SusanUllrichNeal
Facebook.com/ScriptureYoga/
Facebook.com/HealthyLivingSeries/
Twitter.com/SusanNealYoga
Youtube.com/c/SusanNealScriptureYoga/
Pinterest.com/SusanUNeal/

Instagram.com/healthylivingseries/
Linkedin.com/in/susannealyoga/

SusanUNeal.com and ChristianYoga.com
SusanNeal@bellsouth.net

OTHER PRODUCTS BY SUSAN NEAL

HEALTHY LIVING SERIES COURSE & BOOKS
7 Steps to Reclaim Your Health and Optimal Weight Online Course

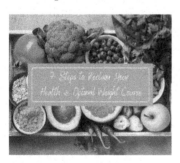

If you need additional support making this lifestyle change, purchase my course, 7 Steps to Reclaim Your Health and Optimal Weight at Susan-UNeal.com/courses/7-steps-to-get-off-sugar-and-carbs-course. In this course I walk you through all the material covered in my Healthy Living Series.

I teach you the root causes of inappropriate eating habits and help you resolve those issues. One solved, taming your appetite is much easier. Learn how to change your eating habits successfully once and for all.

Christian Study Guide for 7 Steps to Get Off Sugar and Carbohydrates

More than half of Americans suffer with a chronic disease and 40 percent are obese. Struggling with health problems is not our true

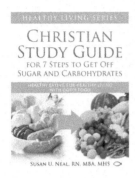

destiny. Jesus promised us a life of abundance. He also told us, "The thief's purpose is to steal, kill, and destroy" (John 10:10 TLB). Shortening our lifespan through our unhealthy food patterns is the enemy's perfect scheme.

Many of the health problems we suffer are connected to eating habits. Change your life by changing the types of food you eat. Learn which foods are beneficial and which foods make you sick. Don't struggle on your own to make necessary lifestyle changes. Learn how to mobilize God's power. Through the Holy Spirit, you become strong and able to accomplish what you cannot achieve by your own efforts. When you apply God's wisdom, along with accurate knowledge about today's food, you will improve your health and weight and defeat the enemy.

This study guide provides a group experience to help implement the plans in *7 Steps to Get Off Sugar and Carbohydrates*. Accountability and encouragement improve your chance for success as you learn to become a healthy steward of the resources you've been given. You only have one body, and you want it to carry you through this life gracefully. Reclaim the abundant life God wants you to live. Take this journey to recover your health and achieve all the blessings the Lord has in store for you. You can purchase this book on Amazon or Susan-UNeal.com/books.

Healthy Living Journal

Have you tried to decrease your weight and improve your health without success? Or maybe you lost weight but gained it back. Don't allow frustration to take over. This journal will help you make and maintain healthy lifestyle changes.

During the next six weeks, commit to spend a few minutes daily recording your eating choices and how your body responds. With time you will see how different foods affect you physically and

HEALTHY LIVING SERIES

HEALTHY LIVING
JOURNAL

TRACK YOUR HEALTHY EATING AND LIVING HABITS
FOR IMPROVED HEALTH AND WELL-BEING

SUSAN U. NEAL, RN, MBA, MHS

emotionally. As you record and reflect in this journal, you will begin to solve your personal health puzzle.

As you discover each new puzzle piece, you will learn how to make your body feel good again. Each day you'll record water and food intake, exercise, energy level, and corresponding moods. Through journaling you will discover more about yourself and any negative eating patterns, draw closer to God, and experience better health.

Jesus wants you to live life in all its fullness, not in a worn-out, sick body. So let's determine the root causes and solutions for your ill health or excessive weight so you can experience a more abundant life as you:

• feel and look better
• increase your energy
• sharpen your clarity of mind
• harness God's strength to make changes
• identify and eliminate unhealthy behaviors
• lose weight naturally without fad diets, prepared meals, or supplements

Reclaim the abundant life Jesus wants you to experience. Your body will thank you. You can purchase this book on Amazon or Susan-UNeal.com/books.

Healthy Living Series: 3 Books in 1

Determine the root causes and solutions for your ill health or excessive weight so you can experience a more abundant life and feel good again.

Healthy Living Series: 3 Books in 1 contains the following three books:

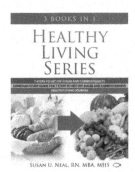

7 Steps to Get Off Sugar and Carbohydrates provides a day-by-day plan to wean your body off these addictive products and regain your health. The changes in your eating habits will start your lifestyle journey to the abundant life Jesus wants you to experience, not a life filled with disease and poor health.

Christian Study Guide for 7 Steps to Get Off Sugar and Carbohydrates provides a group experience to help implement the plans in *7 Steps to Get Off Sugar and Carbohydrates*. Accountability and encouragement improve your chance for success as you learn to become a healthy steward of the resources you've been given.

Healthy Living Journal will help you make and maintain healthy lifestyle changes. Have you tried to decrease your weight and improve your health without success? Don't allow frustration to take over. During the next six weeks, commit to spend a few minutes daily recording your eating choices and how your body responds to solve your personal health puzzle.

Take this journey to recover your health and achieve all the blessings the Lord has in store for you.

Solving the Gluten Puzzle

Are you experiencing symptoms that you or your doctor don't understand? Ruling out a gluten-related diagnosis may move you one step closer to wellness. Discovering whether you have celiac disease, gluten sensitivity, wheat sensitivity, or a wheat allergy is like piecing together a puzzle. Random pieces don't make sense and won't until the whole picture fits together. *Solving the Gluten Puzzle* explains the symptoms, diagnostic tests, and treatment for these ailments.

Nearly 10 percent of the population is affected by one of four gluten-related disorders, which can cause more than two hundred symptoms, most of which are not digestive. These disorders can strike at any age. Unfortunately, a single diagnostic test to determine gluten sensitivity does not exist. Consequently, up to 80 percent of individuals go undiagnosed. Determine whether you suffer from one of these conditions and how to cure your symptoms by embracing a gluten-free lifestyle.

HOW TO PREVENT, IMPROVE, AND REVERSE ALZHEIMER'S AND DEMENTIA

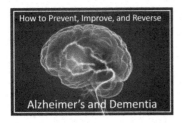

This pamphlet provides twenty-four interventions you can do to prevent, improve, or even reverse Alzheimer's and dementia. To order this pamphlet go to SusanUNeal.com/ALZ.

YOGA BOOKS

Scripture Yoga

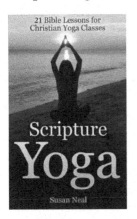

Scripture Yoga assists yoga students in creating a Christian atmosphere for their classes. Choose from twenty-one lessons, each a mini–Bible study that will deepen the participants' walk with God.

Each lesson contains a scriptural theme designed to facilitate meditation on God's Word. The Scripture verses are arranged progressively to facilitate an understanding of each Bible study topic.

The Bible lessons will enhance the spiritual depth of your yoga class and make it appropriate and desirable for Christians.

Check your poses with photographs of over sixty yoga postures taken on the sugar-white sands of the Emerald Coast of Florida. A detailed description of each pose is provided with full-page photographs so postures are easily seen and replicated. You can purchase this book on ChristianYoga.com.

Yoga for Beginners

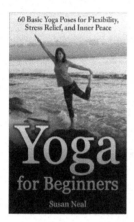

Yoga for Beginners eases you into the inner peace you long for at an easy, step-by-step beginner's pace. Through Susan's gentle encouragement, you will learn how to improve your flexibility and relieve stress. A broad range of yoga poses provides many options for the beginner- to intermediate-level student.

In *Yoga for Beginners* you get it more than basic yoga postures. You will begin to breathe a new sense of well-being when you follow Susan's life-changing eating practices. Learn not only what to eat but also why. This book includes:

- Sixty basic yoga poses with full-page photographs and detailed explanations
- Three different routines to give variety
- Warm-up stretches
- Injury prevention and posture modification suggestions
- How to ease pain and anxiety
- Essential components of yoga such as breathing and stretching
- Meditation techniques to reduce stress
- Low-glycemic diet guidelines to obtain optimal weight
- Causes of sugar cravings and solutions for controlling them

To purchase *Yoga for Beginners* go to ChristianYoga.com.

CHRISTIAN YOGA CARD DECKS

Scripture Yoga Card Decks include a yoga pose on one side and a theme-based Bible verse on the other. The decks assist Christian yoga instructors and students in creating a Christian atmosphere for their classes through meditating on the Word of God. You can order the card decks at ChristianYoga.com.

The Fruit of the Spirit Deck

This lesson, "The Fruit of the Spirit," describes each of the fruits of the spirit including love, joy, peace, patience, kindness, goodness, gentleness, faithfulness, and self-control. It is a mini Bible study that will deepen the participant's walk with God.

The Scripture verses are arranged progressively to facilitate a complete understanding of the Bible study topic. The Bible lesson will enhance the spiritual depth of your yoga class, and make it appropriate and desirable for Christian participants.

How to Receive God's Peace Deck

This lesson, "How to Receive God's Peace," walks the participant through the steps needed to cast fear and anxiety on God and receive his peace. It is a peace the world cannot give. This mini Bible study will deepen the participant's walk with God.

SCRIPTURE YOGA DVDS

What The Bible Says about Prayer Scripture Yoga DVD

In this session, we explore different aspects of prayer. We look at the "when, where, and how" of prayer illustrated through Bible verses and stories. For example, when Jesus prayed:

"Before daybreak the next morning, Jesus got up and went out to an isolated place to pray" (Mark 1:35). A friend once told me all you need is faith, and your prayers will be answered. So I prayed and prayed that my daughter's asthma would be healed. When healing did not occur, I began to investigate God's Word specifically about prayer. I learned that faith is only one component of prayer, but there are many others. In this DVD, I share with you many facets of prayer. Prayer is more powerful than we can imagine. This DVD will help your prayer life. To purchase go to ChristianYoga.com.

God's Mighty Angels Christian Yoga DVD

Enter the realm of God's mighty angels and find out how they intercede in our lives. Angels are God's messengers and he sends them to protect you wherever you go (Psalm 91:11). Over twenty verses about angels are recited during the class. This is a gentle yoga class that includes 25 minutes of stretching and 55 minutes of yoga postures for an 80-minute class. To purchase God's Mighty Angels DVD go to ChristianYoga.com.

Regulating Tobacco

5/8

REGULATING TOBACCO

Edited by
Robert L. Rabin &
Stephen D. Sugarman

OXFORD
UNIVERSITY PRESS

2001

OXFORD
UNIVERSITY PRESS

Oxford   New York
Athens   Auckland   Bangkok   Bogotá   Buenos Aires   Cape Town
Chennai   Dar es Salaam   Delhi   Florence   Hong Kong   Istanbul   Karachi
Kolkata   Kuala Lumpur   Madrid   Melbourne   Mexico City   Mumbai   Nairobi
Paris   São Paulo   Shanghai   Singapore   Taipei   Tokyo   Toronto   Warsaw

and associated companies in
Berlin   Ibadan

Copyright © 2001 by Oxford University Press

Published by Oxford University Press, Inc.
198 Madison Avenue, New York, New York 10016

Library of Congress Cataloging-in-Publication Data
Regulating tobacco / edited by Robert L. Rabin and Stephen D. Sugarman.
     p.   cm.
Includes bibliographical references and index.
ISBN 0-19-513907-0; ISBN 0-19-514756-1 (pbk.)
1. Tobacco industry—Government policy—United States.   2. Cigarette industry—
Government policy—United States.   3. Tobacco habit—Health aspects—United States.
4. Tobacco habit—Prevention—Government policy—United States.   5. Cigarette smoke—
Health aspects—United States.   6. Advertising—Cigarettes—Government policy—
United States.   7. Youth—Tobacco use—Prevention—Government policy—United States.
8. Medical policy—United States.   9. Tobacco industry—Law and legislation—
United States.   10. Smoking—Law and legislation—United States.   I. Rabin,
Robert L.   II. Sugarman, Stephen D.
HD9136 .R43 2001
362.29'66'0973—dc21   00-053734

9 8 7 6 5 4 3 2

Printed in the United States of America
on acid-free paper

Acknowledgments

We would like to express our appreciation to the Robert Wood Johnson Foundation for funding the research and writing of this book. The contributors to this volume also received valuable research assistance from Kirstin Ault, Jennifer Jackson, Nushin Kormi, Carla Levy, Shelley Mack, and Nina Rabin.

Stanford California   R. L. R.
Berkeley, California   S. D. S.
March 2001

Contents

About the Contributors

Robert L. Rabin is A. Calder Mackay Professor of Law, Stanford University

Stephen D. Sugarman is Agnes Roddy Robb Professor of Law, University of California, Berkeley

Frank J. Chaloupka is Professor of Economics, University of Illinois at Chicago, and Research Associate, National Bureau of Economic Research; Melanie Wakefield is Visiting Research Scientist, Health Research and Policy Centers, University of Illinois at Chicago; Christina Czart is a Ph.D. Candidate, Department of Economics, University of Illinois at Chicago

Peter D. Jacobson is Associate Professor, University of Michigan School of Public Health; Lisa M. Zapawa is Research Associate, University of Michigan School of Public Health

Robert A. Kagan is Professor of Political Science and Law, University of California, Berkeley; William P. Nelson is a Ph.D. Candidate, Jurisprudence and Social Policy Program, University of California, Berkeley

Nancy A. Rigotti, M.D., is Associate Professor of Medicine, Harvard Medical School, Director, Tobacco Research & Treatment Center, Massachusetts General Hospital

John Slade, M.D., is Professor at the University of Medicine and Dentistry of New Jersey, School of Public Health, Program in Addictions

Kenneth E. Warner is Richard D. Remington Collegiate Professor of Public Health and Director, University of Michigan Tobacco Research Network, Dept. of Health Management and Policy, School of Public Health, University of Michigan

Regulating Tobacco

1

Perspectives on Policy: Introduction

Robert L. Rabin & Stephen D. Sugarman

Tobacco policy has assumed center stage in recent years. A product responsible for more than 400,000 premature deaths annually in the United States alone clearly raises a serious public health concern. Yet in our society there is a strong presumption that freedom of choice to engage in risky activities ought to be protected from paternalistic regulation (at least so long as the activities result in no harm to others). As a consequence, it does not follow inexorably that public health concerns require governmental action. Perhaps the clearest evidence in support of this proposition is the lack of any discernible current support for an absolute prohibition on the sale and consumption of tobacco products. Correspondingly, until very recently, the tobacco industry relied, with unbroken success, on this same personal responsibility theme in the judicial forum as the foundation of its defense to smokers' compensation lawsuits.

Nevertheless, over the course of almost four decades, since the surgeon general's famous 1964 report on smoking, a consensus has arisen that governmental intervention to control tobacco use is not only legitimate but essential. Indeed, the tobacco industry itself, in the face of unassailable evidence and public indignation, no longer contests the need to curtail youth access and ensure adult awareness of the dangers of smoking. But there has been and remains intense controversy over precisely what tobacco control policy should include.

There is, after all, a broad continuum of potential tobacco control strategies that lie between prohibition as a proactive extreme at one end and health risk warnings as a minimalist measure at the other. This book is aimed at assessing the strategies that have been adopted and exploring the question of what more or different might be done. After a cross-cutting chapter surveying the political culture of tobacco regulation (chapter 2 by Robert Kagan and William Nelson), the remaining chapters are organized around specific tobacco control strategies: tobacco product taxation, marketing constraints, tobacco harm reduction (including smoking cessation), checks on youth access, tobacco litigation, curbs on secondhand smoke, and global regulation through the World Health Organization's (WHO) proposed tobacco control treaty.

This wide array of strategies tracks the real world of tobacco control advocacy in which action has proceeded simultaneously on a number of fronts. Of course, if a national consensus existed that tobacco use imposes intolerable social costs, a *package* of regulatory initiatives might not necessarily be called for—perhaps prohibition alone might then be the preferred approach. But our national experience with the failure of alcohol prohibition in the early twentieth century, as well as the normative commitment to freedom of choice mentioned previously, has counseled against branding tobacco use as an illegal activity.

To explain the multiple-strategy approach, one must examine more closely the dimensions of the public health problem posed by tobacco. Most fundamentally, tobacco control policy is targeted at a number of distinct populations—in particular, youths who may take up smoking, youth and adult smokers who might quit smoking (or avoid relapse), and nonsmokers who are exposed to environmental tobacco smoke. Disregarding some form of taxation that would be tantamount to prohibition, no single policy speaks directly to all of these objectives. Moreover, each of the strategies has fallen short of what might be accomplished on its own terms in an ideal world.

Consider, initially, what could be regarded as the least intrusive regulatory strategy (most consonant, that is, with respect for individual autonomy): providing information about the dangers of smoking. This approach might include, for example, required warnings on tobacco product packaging and advertising that conveys risk information, as well as mandatory education in elementary and secondary schools about tobacco's dangers. It would rely on the idea that most people will simply choose not to smoke (or they will quit if they are current smokers) once society assures that they are well informed of the risks. In fact, information-based government interventions (including the issuance of the surgeon general's initial and subsequent reports) have effectively brought home the risks of tobacco to much of the public and have contributed to the sharp reduction in tobacco use over the past forty years. But this approach has just as clearly now reached the point of diminishing returns—barring some breakthrough in making teenagers much more time-sensitive to risk.

As a consequence, tobacco control advocates have promoted more proactive forms of addressing the consumer demand side of the tobacco equation. A notable example has been tobacco tax policy, which is addressed in chapter 3 by Frank Chaloupka, Melanie Wakefield, and Christina Czart. Higher tobacco taxes seek to change smoking behavior through a price effect, on the assumption that increased taxes will be passed on to smokers through an increased cost of tobacco products. Higher prices simultaneously seek to discourage some people (especially teens) from taking up smoking, to encourage some to make good on their promise to themselves to quit, to deter recent quitters from relapse, and to persuade continuing smokers to smoke less. This policy approach assumes a certain existing demand for cigarettes and postulates that, as with most products, increasing the price will push at least some individuals to quit—and hence will result in a reduced level of consumption for society as a whole.

But many will not respond to price increases in the desired ways. They might just pay more to smoke and have less money left for other things; or they might switch to cheaper brands of cigarettes; or they might smoke fewer cigarettes but in more dangerous ways (like smoking more carefully down to the end or inhaling each puff more deeply). Hence, even though substantially increasing the cigarette tax is highly regarded as a tobacco control policy in many quarters, any politically acceptable tobacco excise tax will still leave more people smoking than most public health leaders find desirable.

Moreover, critics of the strategy also point to what they see as its increasingly regressive character; as smoking has come to be disproportionately a lower-income activity in our society, poorer people who continue to smoke would actually bear the heaviest burden of a tax increase. Also, the greater weight one attaches to the power of addiction, the stronger the equitable argument that tobacco taxation is a form of punishment for those who simply cannot quit. And finally, in pragmatic terms, there is the concern that both increased smuggling, and the organized crime activities that often accompany a significant level of black market activity, would result from single-minded (and successful) reliance on the tax increase strategy. It comes as no surprise, then, that tobacco control advocates seek to combine higher taxes with other policies.

While tobacco tax strategy starts with existing demand for smoking, tobacco advertising controls, by contrast, seek to change people's "taste" for smoking. This policy approach, addressed in chapter 4 by John Slade, tries to alter people's demand curves and thereby reduce consumption, quite apart from any increase in price. The underlying objective here—to make people simply less interested in smoking—rests on a model positing that demand for tobacco products is shaped (at least in part) by the persuasive powers of advertising. In a sense, then, advertising bans (or limitations) can be regarded as "disinformation" initiatives—efforts to filter out the imagery that makes smoking appear to be a pleasurable (and implicitly benign) activity. The opposite side of the strategic coin, counteradvertising, relies on both counter-imagery and hard facts about health risks to similarly address the "taste" for smoking. It is an informational strategy and more. In tandem, restrictions on advertising and reliance on counteradvertising aspire to the same outcomes. If they are successfully employed, some people will be less interested in smoking in the first place, fewer will relapse after quitting, and others will find it less attractive to continue smoking. This approach rests generally on the belief that self-image plays an important role in smoking behavior, and more precisely on the notion that if people think of themselves as "uncool" rather than "cool" for smoking, then smoking will lose its appeal.

At best, this strategy, too, only goes so far. For one thing, many smokers are motivated by reasons other than advertising—among others, the behavior of friends and family. And those influences will outweigh even a dramatically altered promotional scene. In addition, the tobacco industry has been re-markably inventive in devising new promotional techniques, usually staying a step or two ahead of each round of marketing controls. Besides, as with tobacco tax policy, there is also a down side to pushing tobacco advertising policies too far. On one hand, excessive controls on the marketing efforts of tobacco companies can run afoul of the protections guaranteed to "commercial speech" by the First Amendment of the Constitution. On the other, excessively propagandistic antismoking ads (even if effective) can begin to look like an unseemly activity of government.

To the extent that strongly addicted smokers are largely impervious to higher taxes (they just stoically bear the higher costs) and unfazed by anti-smoking ads, still other techniques exist for reducing demand. The main tobacco control strategy for these smokers is to try to help them overcome their addiction by providing financial support for smoking cessation and other programs, a topic addressed in chapter 5 by Kenneth Warner. Tradi-tionally, the outlook of tobacco control advocates has mimicked that of the mainstream approach taken by illegal-drug control strategists—"just say no." In short, the goal has been to get people to abstain completely. To be sure, the techniques for achieving that goal have been different. Confiscation and criminalization (i.e., prohibition), the hallmarks of U.S. drug policy, have not, as noted already, been the favored tools of tobacco control. Instead, tobacco control has sought to promote cessation through other means, in-cluding public support for "step" programs, regular admonitions by physi-cians, and nicotine replacement therapy (e.g., gum and the patch).

Recently, some have argued that "harm reduction" (the European ap-proach to illegal drugs) is an appropriate outlook on smoking too, at least so long as the policies adopted yield more good (getting people to smoke less) than harm (having people smoke some, who would otherwise have quit or never started). Harm reduction proponents urge that public health attention should also be given to smokers for whom cessation seems beyond reach, at least for the present. The use of alternative devices for the delivery of nicotine (like the patch or gum or newly developing quasi-cigarettes), combined with substantially reduced smoking, serves as an example of how harm reduction might be achieved. Of course, not all strongly addicted smokers will be responsive to these techniques of quitting (or smoking less), as years of experience with alcohol and drugs has shown. Still, there is reason to think that a positive public health payoff can be achieved from sensible public investment in subsidizing cessation and other harm reduction approaches.

In contrast to the demand-side strategies discussed to this point, the seemingly intractable problem of combating youth smoking has been addressed on the supply side as well, principally through outright bans on the sale of tobacco products to minors, as well as bans on cigarette vending machines (or restricting their location to "adult only" premises). This policy approach is addressed in chapter 6 by Nancy Rigotti. The simple idea is that the harder cigarettes are for children to obtain, the fewer of them will smoke. This aspiration rests, in turn, on the premise that if public policy can prevent people from smoking when they are children, it will have a strong lifelong impact—for studies now show that a very high proportion of adult smokers began as children.

Of course, not all minors currently obtain their cigarettes from retailers, and more would resort to "secondary markets" if regular commercial sales to minors were much more effectively policed than they are today (e.g., obtaining cigarettes from friends, older siblings, parents, high school playground sellers, and the like). Besides, a truly effective "forbidden fruit" policy would probably make some rebellious teens even more interested in smoking than they are today. Still, inconvenience can make something of a difference with youths, who are also affected when school "smoking lounges" are closed and when smoking is no longer permitted at the commercial "hang-outs" where teens gather after school and in the evenings. That supply-curtailing strategies aimed at children will surely not be completely effective simply reinforces the basic observation throughout this discussion: tobacco control advocates have not wanted to put all of their eggs in a single policy basket.

But as mentioned at the outset, it is not just the limited efficacy of any single strategy that has led to a multi-initiative approach. Rather, it is the essential circumstance that the problem itself can be viewed from a number of perspectives. Thus, youth-access proscriptions, for example, view the tobacco control problem from the vantage point of protecting vulnerable minors, whereas informational strategies, by contrast, focus on assuring fully informed consumers.

Although policies aimed at controlling tobacco marketing and promoting smoking cessation are somewhat based on notions of the "smoker as victim," this perspective is central to the widely publicized litigation strategy, which is addressed in chapter 7 by Robert Rabin. This is clearly the case for tobacco-related lawsuits seeking financial compensation that have been brought both by individual smokers and by groups of smokers in class actions. Yet litigation against the tobacco industry has, in fact, proceeded on a number of additional fronts. These other cases include third-party reimbursement efforts brought by payors of smokers' medical costs and nonsmokers' suits for exposure-related harm from tobacco use. Like tort litigation generally, the full range of these lawsuits is aimed at both compensating victims of harm and, at the same time, deterring harmful conduct by assigning the costs to the source. Indeed, the recent litigation has had special bite on the cost-assignment side through the threat of massive punitive damage awards. But the litigation strategy, too, has in practice fallen short of its full potential—until now, at least. The tobacco industry has demonstrated great ingenuity in contesting compensation claims, and the long-term deterrent impact of litigation remains clouded in uncertainty.

Regulatory initiatives aimed at protecting nonsmokers from tobacco-related harm, just alluded to in the litigation setting, have been most fully realized in the continuing proliferation of restrictions on smoking in the workplace and public places of recreation and commerce. These restrictions, addressed in chapter 8 by Peter Jacobson and Lisa Zapawa, are grounded in a long-recognized foundation for regulatory action: capturing the "externalities"—costs imposed on third parties—generated by production processes that would, in the absence of such regulation, exceed optimum levels of activity.

In the case of tobacco, antismoking advocates have noted an additionally promising dimension to the strategy: that "zoning out" workplace tobacco use, by creating substantial obstacles to smoking whenever and wherever the smoker might please, has in itself the benefit of reducing smoking prevalence—by helping some smokers who want to stop accomplish this objective and by making smoking sufficiently inconvenient as to cause others to quit. This impact, however, is quite unlikely to yield a sufficiently reduced level of tobacco consumption to make tobacco control advocates want to rely upon clean indoor air policies alone. Moreover, critics of sweeping clean indoor air laws, who favor relying on the market to determine which indoor areas are smoke free and which are not, increasingly claim that this policy initiative is, at base, driven by improper paternalistic motives rather than from a concern with third-party victims. Feeling themselves perhaps vulnerable on just such charges, clean indoor air advocates tend to respond that, in fact, their "real" goal is only to protect involuntary passive smokers. In that posture, surely clean indoor air laws can be but part of an overall tobacco control package.

Smoking is a public health problem not only in America but around the world. Indeed, smoking rates are much higher in many other nations, and it is projected that thirty years from now more than two-thirds of the worldwide death toll from tobacco products will occur in what today are developing nations. In response to the global tobacco epidemic, the WHO has been charged with the responsibility of drafting and assisting in the adoption of an international tobacco control treaty. Discussed in chapter 9 by Stephen Sugarman, the planned "framework convention on tobacco control" has been set on a path for eventual adoption in 2003. Although it is now too early to know precisely what provisions might be contained in a successful "convention" and accompanying binding "protocols," it seems clear that those behind the WHO effort have several objectives in mind. First, they want an agreed upon set of tobacco policy provisions that all nations signing the treaty would impose in their own countries. Second, they want several cross-border problems tackled through multinational cooperation—such as smuggling and the leakage of advertising campaigns (via television, magazines, the Internet, and so on). Third, they want cooperative information exchanges, training sessions, mutual reporting arrangements, and the like that will both allow nations to learn from each other and facilitate the build-up of a sophisticated tobacco control infrastructure in countries that currently have limited expertise. Fourth, they want a united world public health community to link arms in opposition to an international tobacco industry whose economic power is increasingly concentrated in a few giant multinational corporations.

Although the WHO framework convention strategy is aimed at improved public health in developing nations, it could have some impact in the United States—even if the United States refuses to adopt the treaty, a not unlikely result given America's reluctance to sign many other global treaties. If nothing else, a package of agreed upon international tobacco control provisions might strengthen the hands of domestic advocates in their political and regulatory efforts to ratchet up tobacco control in the United States.

In the end, just as the proposed WHO treaty envisions a multifaceted approach to tobacco control, so too within any nation the resort to a multiplicity of initiatives is a recognition of the complex set of values and norms that tobacco control calls into play. As we have seen, if pushed too hard, advertising controls and clean indoor air laws trigger objections from a paternalism perspective. Tobacco litigation claims engender opposition based on norms of personal responsibility. Youth access restrictions must cope with lukewarm enthusiasm for robust enforcement activity. Informational strategies raise doubts about marginal efficacy. And the list goes on. The prospects for getting the mix right turn on at least two important considerations: first, taking careful account of what has worked until now and what is likely to work in the future, and second, appreciating how far the public is prepared to accept measures that move away from the norm of autonomy and along the continuum toward paternalism and prohibition.

As Kagan and Nelson conclude in the next chapter of this volume, the American public may now have roughly attained the mix of tobacco controls it wants—albeit the fit is not perfect. The implication of this analysis is that if tobacco control advocates are to achieve substantially greater legal regulation in the future, they will probably first have to win over public opinion. We would hope that the ideas and analyses offered in the following chapters will contribute to the ongoing process of shaping that policy debate.

2

The Politics of Tobacco Regulation in the United States

Robert A. Kagan & William P. Nelson

During the 1940s and 1950s, cigarette smoking rivaled baseball as America's national pastime. On motion picture screens, cigarettes were depicted as wholly desirable, smoked by the glamorous and sophisticated, by gritty GIs winning World War II, and tilting up at a jaunty angle from President Franklin Roosevelt's profile. In 1965, 52% of American adult men were cigarette smokers. Now, however, cigarettes are widely castigated as the nation's number one public health problem. Cigarette manufacturers have been besieged by multimillion and even multibillion dollar lawsuits; their shares trade at a record low price-earnings ratio (Norris 2000). In many cities, office workers who want a cigarette break are forced to huddle outside the building's doorway. In 1995, only 25% of American adults were smokers, and in many social circles, smoking is regarded as pathological.

This remarkable transformation is far from complete. Millions of Americans have not quit smoking, hundreds of thousands continue to die from lung cancer and other diseases each year, and teenagers still join the army of the addicted in disturbingly large numbers. Nevertheless, it seems clear that tobacco, once unchallenged, is now on the defensive, and few would bet that in 25 years the proportion of Americans who smoke cigarettes as we know them will be as high as it is today.

If we ask what accounts for this change, the most obvious answer would be the diffusion of scientifically based knowledge about tobacco's carcinogenic properties, a process that began in the 1950s and has since accelerated. Yet the diffusion of scientific findings tells us only part of the story. Thanks to global communications systems, knowledge about tobacco's hazards is widely disseminated. But the response, both by governments and by popular cultures, has not been uniform. Just as contemporary Europeans seem to worry far more about genetically engineered vegetables and hormone-fed beef than Americans, perceptions of the depth and urgency of the smoking problem vary across cultures. National governments have differed in disseminating information about tobacco and in their efforts to discourage smoking. Japanese governments (which have been quite active in regulating certain forms of environmental pollution) have done relatively little to discourage smoking (Levin 1997). Many Western European countries have increased taxes on cigarettes to discourage smoking far more aggressively than has the United States and they have imposed greater restrictions on cigarette advertising, but they have been less aggressive in banning smoking from workplaces and restaurants. And only in the United States has litigation against tobacco companies become a prominent (and sometimes dominant) aspect of national tobacco control efforts.

This chapter explores why American tobacco control efforts have taken such a distinctive course and how the resulting control measures relate to public opinion and to democratic politics. Through the lens of standard accounts of the American political process, we first look at the diverse and shifting array of actors, institutions, and forums that have shaped American tobacco policy across the last four decades. We then suggest, referring to opinion poll data, that this fragmented, freewheeling process has produced a mix of policies that Americans basically want. Hence, those who claim that U.S. policies are too modest because of the power of the tobacco industry and those who claim U.S. policies are too restrictive because of enterprising politicians acting in cahoots with paternalistic antismoking elites may both be wrong.

1. Tobacco Control and Democratic Politics

If tobacco control policies in the United States are distinctive, one might hypothesize that is because the American public—as compared to the French, the Canadians or the Swedes—more strongly endorses the idea of powerful anti-tobacco-company lawsuits and far-reaching protections for nonsmokers' rights to clean air, but prefers relatively modest measures aimed at smokers themselves, such as use-discouraging cigarette taxes, restrictions on advertising, and subsidized cessation programs. That hypothesis, of course, presumes that public policy is directly responsive to public opinion. Most American political scientists, however, question that presumption. They view policy making in American government through the lens of interest group politics. In contrast to parliamentary systems, political authority in the

United States is highly fragmented, both structurally and within the loosely coupled American political parties, which makes it easier for organized interest groups to play a prominent role. In this political structure it is especially difficult for hopeful reformers to assemble legislative majorities to enact potentially popular new policies into law and easier for opponents to find a veto point at which to block the enactment of policies they oppose.

From the standpoint of such interest group–conflict models of policy change, the obstacles to effective governmental tobacco control policies in the United States would seem to be close to insuperable. The tobacco industry is large, extremely profitable, and politically well organized. It can and does contribute lavishly to the political campaigns of individual legislators and parties. The tobacco growing industry exercises considerable political influence in some states. Tobacco company advertising has been an important source of income for magazines, newspapers, and advertising agencies, and tobacco firms have sought additional political allies through generous funding of sporting events, the arts, civil rights organizations, and charities. The tobacco companies can afford the best lobbyists and lawyers to defend their interests, full time, in legislatures and in the courts. Behind them are millions of smokers who, as voters, might be expected to oppose higher cigarette taxes and restrictions on smoking. Although millions of Americans do not smoke, and many of them may prefer tougher controls on smoking, it is notoriously difficult to mobilize highly diffuse populations into an effective political voice (Olson 1965).

Interest-group models are not the only analytic approach to American politics, however. The United States also has a lively tradition of what political scientist James Q. Wilson (1980) has called "entrepreneurial politics," in which politically ambitious or morally committed leaders employ modern techniques of mass communication to propose measures in "the public interest," reframing the way in which social problems are perceived and talked about. In modern times, policy entrepreneurs often emerge from or are closely supported by "epistemic communities"—"networks of professionals with recognized expertise and competence," who share normative commitments as well as a scientific epistemology (Haas 1992). The environmental movement, with its array of advocacy groups and its ties to committed members of the environmental science community, provides one prominent example (Elliott et al. 1985; Farber 1992). The antitobacco movement provides another. Most prominent among the antitobacco advocates in the United States, as in other countries, have been members of what might be called the public health establishment—public health researchers and governmental public health officials. In the United States, prominent antitobacco activists[1] have emerged from time to time in the U.S. Surgeon General's Office, the Department of Health and Human Services, the Food and Drug Administration, and in state and municipal departments of health, as well as at university medical schools and schools of public health. Other antismoking activists have been associated with private, nonprofit public health organizations, such as the American Cancer Society and the American Lung Association, as well as with specialized antitobacco lobbying organizations and local nonsmokers' rights organizations. In addition, some elected politicians have found crusading against smoking morally compelling or politically advantageous. Together, the antitobacco "policy entrepreneurs" have come to be the functional equivalent of a traditional industry-based interest group, except that they are more decentralized and motivated more by idealism than economic self-interest.

Finally, the unusual openness and malleability of the American legal system has opened the door to yet another mode of entrepreneurial action. Thus, the United States is distinctive in that antitobacco leadership has been displayed by *lawyers*, some motivated by idealism, some by the prospect of large contingency fees, who have filed individual tort claims or financially threatening class action suits against tobacco companies.

Against the financial resources of the tobacco companies, this complex of public and private policy entrepreneurs has attempted to deploy the power of ideas, disseminating information about health risks and about tobacco industry conduct, thereby seeking to redefine the social acceptability of smoking and tobacco marketing and to mobilize political support for legal restrictions on both. The tobacco industry responded in kind, trying to influence public opinion by downplaying the hazards of smoking, by emphasizing traditions of individual liberty, and by drawing on populist traditions of antipathy to taxation. Each side has sought to obtain favorable coverage in the mass media and to reframe the public discourse in ways that support its policy preferences.

In many ways, the public health–oriented reformers and lawyers have been remarkably successful, bringing about three broad transformations in public understanding of the nature of the cigarette problem—first as a product harmful to smokers, then as one harmful to nonsmokers as well, and finally as a problem of corporate malfeasance and fraud too. One sign of their success has been the decline in the social popularity of smoking. This decline has had political consequences too, increasing the ratio of nonsmoking to smoking voters; the latter now constitute a political as well as a social minority and are subjected to excise taxes that benefit the public at large.

Nevertheless, to many members of the public health community, progress in tobacco control has been limited by the wealth and political clout of the tobacco industry. As noted earlier, compared to some other economically advanced democracies, American taxes on cigarettes are lower, and its cigarette-package warnings and advertising restrictions are milder. American governments do relatively little to subsidize smoking cessation programs. The United States, generally quick to regulate product safety, does not regulate the content of cigarettes or nicotine levels. Millions of Americans still smoke and millions become addicted every year. The reason for these failures, in this perspective, is that the tobacco industry repeatedly has used massive campaign contributions,[2] together with platoons of high-powered lobbyists and lawyers and public relations firms, to block or dilute potentially popular tobacco control efforts.

From the standpoint of the tobacco industry, in contrast, it is the social and political elites in the antitobacco movement who have warped or defied public opinion. In this perspective, moral entrepreneurs in the "public health community" have pursued their own paternalistic agenda, often in forums that are insulated from public opinion, such as courts and government agencies. Hence, state attorneys general have sought use-discouraging cigarette price increases and funds for antismoking campaigns not through cigarette tax increases enacted by elected legislatures but through coercive "bet your company" litigation, which tobacco companies cannot risk taking to trial in the unpredictable American court system. The most extreme version of this theory is that public health activists have manipulated public attitudes by exaggerating the intensity of the risks posed by "secondhand smoke" and even by smoking (Levy and Marimont 1998),[3] by mounting antismoking ad campaigns that demonize tobacco company executives, and by neglecting the adverse impact of higher cigarette taxes on smokers, who are disproportionately working class or poor.

Yet neither the tobacco industry nor the antitobacco movement, the succeeding sections of this chapter indicate, has molded public opinion entirely to its worldview, and neither has bent legislation entirely to its will. In some policy spheres and arenas, tobacco interests have dominated, in others they have not, and in still others neither side has achieved its goals. This mixed record suggests that there may be limits to how far American public opinion can be molded by either side in the tobacco wars. Many of the distinctive features of American tobacco policy not only appear to be roughly in line with American public opinion, as discussed in section 3, but also in tune with enduring characteristics of American political culture. The American public, in short, may be getting the mix of tobacco control policies that appeals to the majority of citizens.

2. Many Policies, Many Forums

In the United States, the political struggle over tobacco control has not produced total victory for either side partly because it is fought on so many different institutional fronts and around many types of policies. From the start, governmental action to discourage smoking has been sharply constrained by the long-standing ubiquity of tobacco products and the large number of smokers. With the aborted effort to prohibit alcoholic beverages stored in the nation's memory and the ineffective prohibition of narcotic drugs currently filling the nation's prisons, few public health officials or political leaders have argued that cigarettes should be banned. Even today, the vast majority of Americans, when polled, assert that the decision whether or not to smoke cigarettes should be a matter of individual choice (Saad 1998). With across-the-board prohibition politically off the table, antitobacco activists—some favoring one strategy, some another—have sought to enact a wide range of tobacco control policies designed to reduce the prevalence and harms of smoking. These include (1) the promotion of fully informed individual choice (health warnings on cigarette packs and ads); (2) "paternalistic" policies—paternalistic in the sense that they go beyond simply informing smokers of the risks—such as banning sales of cigarettes to minors, increasing cigarette prices via high taxes, restricting advertising and free giveaways by tobacco companies; (3) nonsmokers' rights policies designed to limit exposure to unwanted second-hand smoke, such as bans on smoking in restaurants, offices, stores, and other public places; and (4) redistributive and punitive policies, such as lawsuits that seek to make tobacco companies pay compensatory and punitive damages to those harmed by smoking.

Tobacco control activists also have sought to capitalize on the structural fragmentation of power in the American constitutional system—and the tobacco industry has responded in kind. A brief and necessarily truncated review of governmental tobacco control actions in recent decades, summarized in table 2.1, shows how the policy ball has bounced from one governmental unit to another, including federal regulatory agencies, Congress, state legislatures, city councils, state attorney generals' offices, and both state and federal courts. With this array of authorities to turn to, both control advocates and the tobacco industry often have managed to balance a defeat in one political forum by seeking allies in another. If one city council declines to regulate smoking, tobacco control advocates can search for another willing to enact strict controls, while tobacco industry lobbyists seek out state legislators willing to pass weak smokers' rights laws that preempt local ordinances. If a state legislature declines to enact higher cigarette taxes to discourage smoking, antitobacco activists may be able to achieve the same goal through a ballot initiative, or a state court jury might be willing to impose huge money damages on cigarette manufacturers, stimulating a price increase equivalent to a substantial tax hike.

Table 2.1. Major Tobacco Control Actions by Date and Political Forum

Year	Federal politics	State and local politics	Litigation	Current smoking prevalence
1964	First surgeon general's report.			.53
1965	Cigarette Labeling and Advertising Act (warnings on cigarette packs).			
1967			FCC's Fairness Doctrine applied to cigarette ads.	
1969	Public Health Cigarette Smoking Act bans all cigarette ads on radio and TV, preempts state and local regulation.			.49
1972	Warning label required on cigarette advertisements.			.46
1975		Minnesota enacts first Indoor Clean Air Act.		.43
1983			*Cipollone* suit filed.	
1984	Comprehensive Smoking Education Act requires rotating warning labels.			.36
1980–89		Local restrictions on public smoking surge.		
1985–present		33 states pass "smokers' rights" nondiscrimination legislation.		
1986	Surgeon general's report on secondhand smoke.			
1988		California passes Proposition 99, raising cigarette taxes by $.25.		
1989	Smoking on domestic airline flights banned.			

(*continued*)

Table 2.1. (*continued*)

Year	Federal politics	State and local politics	Litigation	Current smoking preva-lence
1992	"Synar Amendment" ties state ADAMHA block grants to compliance with minimum restrictions on youth cigarette access.	Massachusetts voters approve 25 cent increase in cigarette tax; Arkansas, Nebraska, and Montana reject 25 cent increases.		.28
1993	EPA report designates ETS a Class A carcinogen; proposes regulation of indoor air quality.			
1994	Industry executives deny cigarettes are addictive at Waxman hearings.	Arizona and Michigan voters approve $.40 and $.50 tax increases; Colorado rejects $.50 increase.	'Castano' private class action suits filed. Tobacco industry sues to overturn EPA second-hand smoke ruling. Mississippi AG files suit to recover Medicaid costs.	.25
1995	FDA proposes jurisdiction over marketing of cigarettes and announces regulations aimed at restricting youth access.		46 of 50 states file similar suits.	.24
1996			Tobacco industry challenges FDA jurisdiction; Castano litigation de-certified.	
1997			First proposed settlement of AG suits announced.	
1998	Congress amends but fails to legislate "national settlement" of state AG suits.	California voters narrowly approve $.50 increase in cigarette tax. California becomes first state in nation to ban smoking in bars.	"National Settlement" collapses after Congress fails to approve. U.S. Court of Appeals rejects proposed FDA jurisdiction. 46 of 50 states announce settlement with industry.	

Table 2.1. (*continued*)

Year	Federal politics	State and local politics	Litigation	Current smoking prevalence
2000			U.S. Supreme Court rejects proposed FDA jurisdiction; U.S. Department of Justice initiates lawsuit against industry; several large jury verdicts returned against tobacco industry in Florida and California.	

Such forum-to-forum reversals of fortune began with the first federal antitobacco efforts, beginning in the 1960s. The landmark political event of that decade was the 1964 publication of the U.S. surgeon general's first Report on Smoking and Health, which can be viewed as a product of cooperation among policy entrepreneurs in the private and governmental public health establishment. The report's conclusion that smoking was causally related to lung cancer triggered dramatic press coverage (Kluger 1997, 260) and prompted the Federal Trade Commission (FTC) to draft a regulation requiring strong warning labels (which included the word "cancer") on all cigarette packs and advertising. But the proposed FTC rule also stimulated the political mobilization of the tobacco industry (Kluger 1997, 273–91), which successfully sought support in Congress. The 1965 Cigarette Labeling and Advertising Act displaced the proposed FTC label and required a much weaker warning—"Caution: Cigarette smoking may be hazardous to your health"—on cigarette packages only (Jacobson, Wasserman, and Anderson 1997, 80). Moreover, the act preempted states and federal agencies from imposing sterner warning requirements.

Antismoking activists were quick to open another front in the effort to inform the public about smoking's hazards, again turning to regulatory agencies—and also to the courts. In 1967, John F. Banzhaf successfully petitioned the Federal Communications Commission to compel broadcasters who aired cigarette commercials to provide free time to anticigarette forces for counteradvertisements. Some 1,300 antismoking messages were broadcast by the three major networks through 1968; according to a Gallup poll in that year,

71% of respondents believed that smoking causes cancer (Kluger 1997, 325), and American cigarette smoking rates showed a sharp decline. But tobacco companies again persuaded Congress to dampen a regulatory initiative. In 1969, the federal Public Health Cigarette Smoking Act banned all television and radio ads for cigarette products (ending the free countercommercials) and prohibited state governments from imposing their own advertising and promotion restrictions. It would be 15 years before Congress enacted any further legislation regulating tobacco products (Kluger 1997, 370). The most significant federal actions in the 1970s explicitly exempted tobacco products from otherwise sweeping legislation, including the 1970 Controlled Substances Act, the 1972 Consumer Products Safety Act, and the 1976 Toxic substances Act (Kluger 1997, 375). Indeed, this pattern, in which antitobacco activists achieved more influence in regulatory and public health agencies and in courts, while the tobacco industry has countered them in Congress—a body both more directly responsive to the electorate and more responsive to sources of campaign funds—persisted through the 1990s.

Partly because the tobacco industry's political influence seemed to be dominant on Capitol Hill, antismoking activists began to move the struggle against tobacco to the arena of state government, emphasizing a new policy direction, the protection of individual rights. Drawing on the success of the environmental movement, activists labeled cigarettes a source of indoor air pollution. Minnesota passed the first comprehensive state Indoor Clean Air Act in 1975, which required separation of smokers and nonsmokers in public areas. By the end of the 1970s, some 28 states had enacted some form of restriction on public smoking. But many of these laws also reflected the influence of the tobacco industry, which quickly organized to lobby state legislatures, often managing to win limits on the breadth and enforcement provisions of the state statutes, as well as provisions preempting more stringent regulation by city and county governments (Jacobson et al. 1997, 84). And beginning in the 1970s the tobacco industry pushed state legislatures in at least 30 states to enact "smokers' rights" provisions, which prohibit employment and other discrimination against smokers.

Nonetheless, American smoking rates continued to decline. Whereas nearly half of the adult population smoked in 1970, only 40% did at the decade's end, and smoking desistance was quite pronounced among elites: professional people, sports and television stars, and the well-educated (Zimring 1993). In the 1980s, the public health community kept up the pressure, producing articles in medical journals on the adverse impact of "environmental tobacco smoke" (ETS) on nonsmokers and then, in 1986, another important U.S. surgeon general's report, identifying ETS as a causal agent for lung cancer. The 1986 surgeon general's report provided ammunition for an increasingly active, decentralized network of local grass-roots activist organizations, known then as GASPs (Groups Against Smoking Pollution), which pressed *local* governments for ordinances establishing "nonsmokers' rights." In this campaign, the GASPS simultaneously tapped the American political tradition of individual rights and circumvented the tobacco's industry's financial influence on federal and state legislators, who are hungrier for campaign funds, by and large, than city council members. At the outset of the 1980s, fewer than 100 communities restricted smoking in public places; at its end, more than 500 cities, representing more than half of the nation's midsized or larger cities and 70% of the national population, had enacted antismoking ordinances that segregate or prohibit public smoking across a wide variety of locales[4] (Rigotti and Pashos 1991).

A crucial part of this political story was the relative silence of smokers. Tobacco companies sought to organize them into an effective smokers' rights lobby, analogous to the National Rifle Association (NRA), but met with little success. For the most part, local ordinances restricting smoking evoked a surprisingly high level of voluntary compliance, indicating the spread of norms that branded smoking as socially undesirable (Kagan and Skolnick 1993). The tobacco industry expended a great deal of money on publications that sought to obfuscate the links between smoking and disease, tried to use its leverage as a large advertiser to suppress stories that illustrated those risks, and tried to cultivate a favorable image by contributing generously to civil rights and women's rights organizations, arts organizations, and a program celebrating the Bill of Rights. Nevertheless, by the early 1990s, surveys indicated that over 90% of the electorate believed that smoking tobacco caused lung cancer (Saad 1998) and indeed tended to overestimate the risk (Viscusi 1992).

As the political importance of smokers in the electorate declined, public health advocates also enjoyed some success in the politics of tobacco taxation in state legislatures. From 1980 to 1990, nineteen states raised their excise taxes on cigarettes by more than 100%. In 1988 through 1998, 38 states enacted substantial tax increases—34 through legislative enactments, 4 by means of ballot initiatives (Tobacco Institute 1996, 13). The highest taxing states currently are Alaska and Hawaii at $1.00 per pack, followed by California at $0.87 per pack (up from $0.10 in 1980), Washington at $0.82 per pack (up from $0.16 in 1980), and Michigan at $0.75 (up from $0.11 in 1980). The lowest include the tobacco producing states of Virginia at 2.5 cents per pack, North Carolina at $0.05, and Kentucky at $0.03.

In the 1990s, antitobacco advocates, relying largely on revelations achieved through lawsuits against the tobacco industry, sought to reframe the cigarette problem as a matter of corporate evil. In the *Cipollone* lawsuit, filed in 1983, plaintiffs' lawyers employed the powerful pretrial discovery tools provided by the American civil justice system to dislodge internal tobacco industry documents and then articulated a well-publicized legal narrative focused on the industry's history of lying, distorting, and covering up the truth that cigarettes are addictive and carcinogenic. Although the tobacco industry ultimately won the case, it suffered a serious blow in the battle for public opinion; U.S. District Court Judge H. Lee Sarokin, dismissing the industry's motion for a directed verdict in 1988,[5] wrote that the industry had participated in a conspiracy "vast in its scope, devious in its purpose, and devastating in its results" that had been "organized to refute, undermine, and neutralize information coming from the scientific and medical community and, at the same time, to confuse and mislead the consuming public" (Kluger 1997, 670).

Picking up the deception theme, in April 1994 Congressman Henry Waxman's committee, in the wake of public disclosures indicating that manufacturers had manipulated nicotine levels in cigarettes, subpoenaed the CEOs of seven major tobacco companies and asked each of them, seriatim, whether he believed nicotine is addictive. Congress was not likely to enact legislation regulating nicotine levels, so the question was simply an artfully staged bit of political theater. The tobacco executives' denials, contradicting what "everyone knew" about how difficult it was to stop smoking, became a repeatedly televised dramatization of the idea that the tobacco industry had engaged in an ongoing fraud.

The political effort to reframe tobacco control as a matter of punishing corporate misbehavior reinvigorated litigation against the industry. Private attorneys, a number of whom had accumulated substantial wealth and experience through litigation against asbestos companies,[6] filed a new wave of private class action lawsuits against tobacco companies. They also forged alliances with attorneys general in Mississippi, Florida, and West Virginia, who hired them on a contingency fee basis to file suits on behalf of the states, seeking to recover from the tobacco firms billions of dollars of Medicaid payments for smoking-related diseases. As favorable publicity about the attorneys general suits mounted,[7] the vast majority of states—even those like California, whose Republican attorney general appeared reluctant to sue the industry—felt compelled to initiate suits against the industry (Viscusi 1997). Other organizations and lawyers, too, joined the fray at a frenzied pace (Taylor 1998a), and according to political scientist Lynn Mather (1998, 911),

> By June 1, 1998, there were 807 legal actions pending against the tobacco industry, including the state cases, 55 class action suits, 62 suits brought by union health plans, 613 individual claims, and assorted other suits filed by Blue Cross and Blue Shield, cities, counties, countries, and Indian tribes.

In June 1997, a group of state attorneys general announced a settlement with the industry that called for $368 billion in damages, plus bans on all outdoor advertising and on the sale of cigarettes through vending machines, plus acceptance of FDA authority to regulate the manufacture and sale of tobacco products, including nicotine levels (Bulow and Klemperer 1998; Mollenkamp, Levy, Menn, and Rothfelder 1998). In return for these concessions, the "global settlement" offered the tobacco industry immunity from class action litigation and from punitive damages for its past actions. Moreover, the settlement would have capped the industry's liability for private litigation at $5 billion annually, 80% of which would be paid from increased tax revenues (Bulow and Klemperer 1998). But once Congress began to draft a bill to implement the settlement, antitobacco activists from the public health community (which by and large had maintained a distance from the lawsuits and the settlement negotiations) urged a larger payment, more regulatory restrictions, and fewer protections for the industry (Bloch, Daynard, and Roemer 1998). The Senate Commerce Committee proposed a bill in April 1998 that called for over $500 billion in payments and no prohibition on class action litigation and punitive damages for past conduct (Bulow and Klemperer 1998). At this, the tobacco companies—which had up until then spent millions in lobbying and advertising to generate public support for settlement—announced their opposition to the pending bill and launched an advertising campaign denouncing the planned penalty as an example of greedy and regressive government taxation (Taylor 1998b). The bill died on June 17, 1998. Once again, antitobacco activists, after winning a favorable settlement in a nonlegislative forum—in this instance, the litigation process—had encountered a setback in Congress.

Yet Congress was not the only political forum that mattered. Ultimately, the state attorneys general negotiated a new settlement with the tobacco industry, this time calling for $239 billion in payments, some restrictions on advertising and promotion, but no legal protections for the industry (apart from the dismissal of the state suits). In the late 1990s, as juries were steeped in revelations of industry misconduct, the tobacco companies started losing some private suits, and the uncertain possibility of massive losses sometime in the future continued to depress company stocks (Norris 2000).[8] Moreover, the public health community continued to define the tobacco problem as a matter of the corporate evil. Antitobacco television ads in the late 1990s often featured portrayals of Machiavellian tobacco company executives. Many politicians found it awkward to be publicly associated with the industry in any way. President Bill Clinton and Vice President Al Gore began to use the "bully pulpit" to expound on the smoking problem. In this political context, federal regulatory agencies moved more vigorously against tobacco. In 1992 the EPA designated secondhand smoke a Class A carcinogen, subject to regulation by the Occupational Safety and Health Administration (OSHA)—which thus far had declined to restrict tobacco smoke in the nation's workplaces (and which nonetheless has continued to delay rulemaking). In 1995, the Food and Drug Administration (FDA) proposed rules asserting jurisdiction over the marketing of tobacco products and imposing restrictions designed to further restrict youth access to tobacco.

But it was then the tobacco companies' turn to take to the courts. Within days of President Clinton's approval of the proposed FDA rules, the major manufacturers challenged the FDA's jurisdiction over tobacco products, filing suit in federal court in Greensboro, North Carolina—the heart of American tobacco country. In April 1997, District Court Judge William Osteen upheld the agency's authority to regulate cigarettes under the Food, Drug, and Cosmetic Act, though not its authority to promulgate advertising restrictions. The industry appealed, and in 1998, the U.S. Fourth Circuit Court of Appeals reversed the decision, finding that Congress had not intended to "delegate jurisdiction over tobacco products to the FDA,"[9] a decision affirmed by the Supreme Court in March 2000.[10]

In principle, Congress could have clarified the FDA's regulatory authority at any point in the litigation by enacting a statute explicitly declaring tobacco a drug or otherwise granting the FDA power to regulate it. But public health activists apparently concluded that Congress did not have the political will to do so, particularly after the Republicans acquired a majority in the 1994 elections.[11] Again, it was the tobacco industry's ostensible strength in Congress that left the FDA's regulatory initiatives vulnerable to legal attack in the courts. The Supreme Court's March 2000 opinion stressed the deadly health consequences of tobacco, virtually inviting a congressional response (Clymer 2000). Still, as of April 2001, whereas there is extensive governmental regulation of many other dangerous products in the United States—such as National Highway Safety Administration rules concerning the safe design of motor vehicles, EPA regulation of motor vehicle emissions, and state laws prescribing maximum alcohol content and licensing of sellers of liquor and beer—there are no American regulations concerning nicotine levels or other features of cigarettes and cigars (apart from requirements that the industry disclose tobacco product constituents to the government) nor licensure of vendors.

Yet if federal regulation was stalled at the end of the millennium, the executive branch could try to circumvent Congress by resort to the courts. Denouncing the cigarette industry's "massive fraud," the Department of Justice, prompted by a pledge in President Clinton's State of the Union address, filed a lawsuit against all major tobacco companies in September 1999, seeking damages for governmental expenditures on health care for smokers, a figure placed at $25 billion annually. The cigarette makers derided the suit as a meritless effort to circumvent democratic politics by litigating what could not be legislated and vowed they would never settle. A federal district court in 2000 dismissed several but not all of the DOJ charges.[12] The uncertain legal and political outcome will be left to the future.

3. American Tobacco Control Policy and Public Opinion

This open, fragmented policy process has seen the development of a tobacco control regime in the United States that, as noted earlier, differs from tobacco regulation in other economically advanced countries. Tobacco excise tax rates are lower in the United States than in Canada and most of Western Europe, and cigarette pack warnings and advertising restrictions generally are feebler. American governments do relatively little to subsidize smoking cessation programs. More than elsewhere, however, political discourse in the United States focuses on the rights of nonsmokers to a smoke-free environment, producing stricter restrictions on smoking behavior. Only in the United States has public discourse so strongly framed the tobacco industry as an essentially criminal enterprise and has litigation by private plaintiffs' attorneys and public prosecutors had a major impact on tobacco control.

Does the resulting American policy mix reflect a straightforward "majoritarian democracy" hypothesis—that public policy responds fairly directly to public opinion—or have either tobacco industry or entrepreneurial politicking, using their comparative advantage in different governmental arenas, pushed or pulled American tobacco control policy *substantially* off the course preferred by the electorate? One rough and ready way of addressing that question is to compare U.S. tobacco policies with the relatively limited public opinion poll and some voting data.

Restrictions on Smoking

Viewed in cross-national perspective, American governments are particularly aggressive in protecting nonsmokers from exposure to environmental tobacco smoke. The entrepreneurial politics thesis suggests that American attitudes in this regard have been shaped by tobacco control activists, who sought to reframe the smoking question by emphasizing the risks associated with second-hand smoke. However, even prior to the public health community's focus on ETS exposure, substantial numbers of Americans seemed inclined to support regulatory restrictions on the time, place, and manner of smoking.

About 55% of respondents in 1964 felt that "smoking should be permitted in fewer places than it is now" (U.S. Department of Health 1973). In 1970, 52% of male respondents and 64% of female respondents agreed that it is "annoying to be near a person who is smoking cigarettes." A 1984 Louis Harris and Associates poll found 61% of respondents favoring mandated smoking and nonsmoking areas, compared to 20% in favor of banning all smoking in public places, and 15% in favor of no regulation whatsoever (Louis Harris and Associates 1984).

On the other hand, support for sterner public smoking restrictions appears to have been accelerated by publicity regarding ETS studies, culminating in the 1986 U.S. surgeon general's report. The late 1980s saw a rapid increase in the number of communities enacting nonsmokers' rights laws. In an American Medical Association (AMA) survey in 1987, respondents believed by a margin of nearly 8 to 1 that the "right of nonsmokers to a smoke-free environment" outweighed the "right of smokers to smoke anywhere" (Saad 1998). Only 36% of respondents in a 1989 national survey believed that smokers had a right to smoke "indoors when other people are around" (Document 12, 2024710395/0444). By 1990, polls indicated a widespread nonsmokers' rights norm: 77% of all respondents agreed that smokers should refrain from smoking in the presence of nonsmokers (Gallup Organization 1990). With respect to public preferences for laws restricting smoking in public places, most Americans have consistently supported laws setting up segregated smoking and nonsmoking areas in shared public spaces, with a growing minority favoring complete bans. In a 1990 Gallup survey, more than two-thirds of respondents favored mandating segregated areas for smokers across a wide array of public facilities, including workplaces, restaurants, and hotels. Roughly 25% of respondents favored complete smoking bans in those facilities in 1990, and support for complete bans has continued to grow during the nineties, with 40% of respondents favoring total smoking bans in restaurants in 1999 (Moore 1999).

The decentralized, local character of nonsmokers' rights regulations in the United States also suggests that these laws are roughly consonant with local majority opinion. Some communities and workplaces have enacted restrictions, including total bans on smoking in many settings, that are stricter than the national opinion polls would imply, whereas other communities, where popular opposition presumably has been stronger, have no or weaker restrictions. On the other hand, many state "clean air laws" forbid local ordinances that would impose restrictions tougher than those in the state statute. It seems likely, although not certain, that these preemption laws—which the tobacco industry avidly sought—squelched preferences for tighter restrictions in some cities.[13] Insofar as this is the case, the preemption statutes provide support for the "industry power" theory of tobacco policy.

Taxation

In the United States, public discourse about tobacco in the 1990s often focused on the "youth smoking" issue, stimulated by attacks on R. J. Reynolds's "Joe Camel" advertising campaign, disclosures that tobacco companies had targeted young people, and indications that cigarette use by young people, in contrast to the public at large, had stopped falling and was actually increasing (Johnston 1997). Some other countries have pushed cigarette taxes to high levels in hopes of discouraging young people from taking up smoking (as well as encouraging current smokers to quit). But as indicated by table 2.2, cigarette taxes in the United States, despite the increases of the 1980s, lagged far behind—averaging just 30% of the price of a pack of cigarettes, compared to 65% to 84% in a number of other economically advanced democracies (World Bank 1999). As a result, cigarettes remain far more affordable in the United States, at an average of $1.94 per pack.

Why are American cigarette taxes lower? The "industry power" explanation would emphasize the potency of the tobacco industry in both state and federal legislatures, or the industry's ability to influence public opinion. Another possible explanation, however, would emphasize the broader political culture of the United States, where payroll taxes, gasoline taxes, and sales taxes are far lower than in most economically advanced democracies, and where in recent decades politicians have been reluctant to propose any kinds of tax increases. In addition, the regressive[14] character of high cigarette taxes has led organized labor to oppose higher excise taxes and may have reduced the enthusiasm of liberal Democrats, who otherwise favor paternalistic public health measures.

Recent ballot initiatives in which the public votes directly on cigarette tax increases suggest that the electorate is closely divided on the question of higher special taxes on smokers. In 1992, Massachusetts voters approved a 25 cent tax increase (to 51 cents) by a 54% majority, but Arkansas and Ne-

Table 2.2. Cigarette Taxes in Selected Countries

High income countries	Price per pack (U.S.$)	Tax as % of price
Australia	4.85	65
Belgium	3.32	75
Denmark	5.21	84
Finland	4.49	73
Italy	2.19	73
United Kingdom	4.16	78
United States	1.94	30

World Bank 1999

braska voters rejected similar 25 cent increases, and Montana voters defeated a 25 cent increase that earmarked funds for antitobacco education. In 1994 Arizona voters approved a 40 cent cigarette excise tax increase (to 58 cents) by a slim 51%, while a proposed 50 cent increase in Colorado (to 70 cents) went down to decisive defeat by 61%–38%, and in Michigan, a 50 cent tax increase to 75 cents per pack passed comfortably. In 1996 Oregon voters approved a 30 cent tax increase by a 55% to 45% margin. In 1998, a California ballot initiative increasing cigarette taxes by 50 cents per pack passed by a narrow majority of 50.4%.

Polling data indicate that public perceptions of how tax revenues will be used significantly affect support for cigarette excise tax increases. Surveys of Oregon voters before and after the election showed that support for tobacco tax increases dropped from 65% to 20% when respondents were asked whether they would support a tax that channeled proceeds directly into the general fund, rather than being earmarked for antismoking programs (Bjornson et al. 1997). Voter ambivalence about California's 1998 50 cents-a-pack ballot initiative appears to have centered on the apparent disjunction between smoking behavior and early childhood education, the beneficiary of the tax. Among those who opposed the Oregon tax increase, nearly half (47%) reported their primary reason for doing so was that "tobacco users should not be forced to pay a disproportionate share of health costs [of the poor]" (Bjornson et al. 1987) So in addition to the general American antitax sentiment, there may be a substantial concern about the fairness of taxing smokers for public programs that benefit others.

This theme, of course, is the centerpiece of the tobacco industry's campaigns to defeat excise tax ballot initiatives. In each election from California's 1998 Proposition 99 onward, the tobacco industry outspent proponents of the initiatives by at least a factor of 5 to 1. Industry-sponsored radio, television, and newspaper advertisements portrayed the initiatives as regressive taxes that unfairly singled out smokers and questioned the ability of state legislatures to appropriately administer the revenues. Similarly, when the tobacco companies pulled out of the proposed 1997 global settlement, they attacked the pending federal legislation on grounds that it would impose a large tax on the American people and bloat government coffers, and at least some Republican members of Congress used that argument to explain their opposition to the bill.

Nevertheless, it is impossible to know whether, in the absence of high spending by the tobacco industry, states would have been more willing to increase taxes to Western European or Canadian levels, for it is not clear that tobacco money has been a decisive factor. After all, notwithstanding its expenditures, the industry has lost about as many tax initiatives as it has defeated. And insofar as the tobacco industry simply makes appeals to the public based on arguments that enjoy broad support in other contexts, it is difficult to argue that the democratic political process has been seriously distorted in this policy area. Even though nonsmokers constitute the majority of the electorate, and the tobacco industry is far from popular, the rejection of tax initiatives in some states and the divided vote in others suggest that these kinds of taxes do not enjoy universal popularity and that America's comparatively low taxes on cigarettes roughly represent public preferences.

From this perspective, the state attorneys general suits and the ongoing private class action litigation, if they result in significant cigarette price increases, will have driven the effective tax on cigarettes higher than the taxes that have emerged from democratic legislative and initiative processes—which appears to support the claims of the "entrepreneurial politics" thesis.

Litigation

The nonsmoking majority has benefited from the litigation against the tobacco companies insofar as it yields large payments to state treasuries—partly because the payments have been used, by and large, for general government services rather than only to attack the smoking problem. The public has benefited from litigation, too, insofar as it has produced policies that enjoy broad popular support, such as restrictions on tobacco advertising. Yet the ongoing litigation against the tobacco industry, while not actively opposed, does not enjoy unambiguous public support. The available survey data suggest that while they hold the tobacco industry in low regard, most Americans continue to blame smokers themselves for tobacco-related illnesses—and by extension, for the public burdens they impose. In 1987, prior to the most extensive revelations of tobacco industry misconduct, a survey by Louis Harris and associates, sponsored by the tobacco industry, showed that some 75% of respondents thought that smokers should bear the burden of the risks they take, and two-thirds of respondents felt that warning labels on tobacco products excused the industry from liability. Similarly, national polls by the Gallup Organization showed that in 1989, only 16% of respondents thought the tobacco industry should be held legally responsible for smoking-related diseases incurred by smokers, while 79% felt they should not. In the 1990s, as antitobacco activists achieved widespread publicity about the tobacco companies' denials and deceptions, the number of respondents in the Gallup polls who believe the industry is to blame nearly doubled, to 30%. The percentage of respondents who believed the presence of warning labels on cigarette packs excuses the industry from liability declined to 52% in 1997 from 66% in 1991 (Moore 1997). Nonetheless, a 1998 NBC/Wall Street Journal poll found that 16% of respondents blamed the industry and 72% held smokers responsible (Saad 1998).[15]

Moreover, the state attorneys general litigation and huge settlements did not seem to stimulate enthusiastic public support. About a third of respondents to a 1997 Gallup poll had no opinion on the proposed national tobacco settlement (Newport 1997), and 78% of respondents indicated the success or failure of the bill would have no effect on their voting in the next congressional election (Saad 1998), thus suggesting that entrepreneurial action by plaintiff's lawyers have pushed these "redistributive," litigation-based tobacco policies somewhat off the course endorsed by public opinion. Reaction to the U.S. Department of Justice's suit against the industry to recover federal health costs for smoking-related illnesses was mixed as well, with 51% of respondents favoring the government's position and 41% the tobacco industry's (Moore 1999).

Federal Regulation of Tobacco Products

As we have described, federal regulatory agencies have by and large been only weakly involved in American tobacco control policy. The "industry power" thesis would suggest that this is due primarily to the influence of the tobacco industry and its congressional allies in diverting and frustrating attempts to gain jurisdiction over cigarette products. However, whereas the available opinion evidence is limited, it is not clear that the public will has been frustrated in this instance. During the 1990s, as FDA Commissioner David Kessler tried to place cigarettes under FDA jurisdiction, the public at large seemed unenthusiastic or divided about that prospect. According to a 1996 Gallup poll, only 38% of the public supported classification of tobacco as a drug under the FDA's purview, while 57% preferred the status quo (Saad 1998).[16] Hence, it is difficult to view the congressional failure to grant the FDA clear jurisdiction over tobacco products throughout the 1990s either as flouting public opinion or as caving in to the tobacco industry. On the other hand, public opinion on this issue does not appear to be immovable. In spring 2000, a series of highly publicized jury verdicts and a Hollywood motion picture focused public attention once again on the tobacco industry's efforts to suppress information and mislead the public, and the U.S. Supreme Court, even while striking down FDA regulatory authority over tobacco products, forcefully invited Congress to respond. Presidential candidates Albert Gore and George W. Bush both were pushed to take a public stand, and both advocated some form of regulation (Gore much more strongly). Amid all this publicity, an April 2000 poll indicated that 77% of Democratic voters and 70% of Republicans wanted Congress to empower the FDA to regulate tobacco. In the face of this shift in public opinion, which might be attributed to the efforts of antitobacco activists of various kinds, the merits of the "industry power thesis" will be revealed by whether Congress nevertheless fails to act—or enacts legislation that grants the FDA some regulatory authority but also provides the tobacco industry significant statutory protections against the FDA.

Youth Access Restrictions

In contrast to excise taxation, the American public has expressed strong support for other kinds of restrictions aimed at reducing or preventing teen smoking. More than 87% of respondents in a 1997 survey favored stronger enforcement of the existing laws prohibiting the sale of tobacco to minors, and 74% of respondents in a 1995 survey indicated they would support measures requiring the tobacco industry to spend millions of dollars in antismoking initiatives aimed at youths (Saad 1998). From this perspective, although some cities have restricted the placement of cigarette vending machines and conducted some crackdowns on merchants who fail to demand identification from youthful cigarette customers, it is interesting that neither state legislatures nor most local legislatures have matched the public's apparent sense of urgency about restricting sales to youths. In fact, the single largest factor behind increased state and local regulatory activity aimed at youths' access to tobacco has been the Synar amendment, a *federal* law that stemmed from entrepreneurial politics by public health activists requiring states to implement youth access restrictions and monitor compliance. The mixed record of local governmental *enforcement* of restrictions on sales, therefore, may suggest a reading of public opinion that is more complicated than the rough gauge reflected in opinion poll questions. Perhaps most communities would prefer scarce law enforcement resources to be devoted to fighting street crime than to policing and punishing small merchants who are less than vigilant in demanding proof of age from younger customers.

Advertising and Promotion Restrictions

Unlike the United States, at least 27 countries, including France, Canada, and New Zealand, have enacted total bans on cigarette advertising. Roughly the same number of countries completely ban tobacco industry sponsorship of sporting and cultural events. Most European Union (EU) member states are expected to follow, as they phase in an EU directive mandating a total ban on almost all forms of tobacco advertising and promotion. Thus, despite the state attorneys general settlement, which calls for elimination of outdoor advertising, and limits event sponsorship to one cultural or sporting event per year, the United States lags behind many economically advanced democracies in this policy area. Cigarette ads still appear in newspapers, magazines, and on the Internet, as well as in places where cigarettes are sold.

Public support in the United States for severe restrictions on cigarette advertising and promotion has increased substantially throughout the 1990s. A number of big city governments—including New York City, Chicago, and St. Louis—banned outdoor cigarette advertising, and 60% of respondents to a national Gallup poll in 1997 supported a total ban on all cigarette advertising, up from less than half in 1994 (Siegel and Wertheimer 1998). California surveys show a rise in support for a total ban in that state from 55% in 1990 to 65% in 1996. Based on these data, the restrictions on advertising and sponsorship agreed to in settlement of the state attorneys general lawsuits appear consistent with popular preferences. Why, then, hasn't Congress enacted such bans or encouraged state legislatures to do so? Judicial precedents establishing Constitutional protections for commercial freedom of speech (in nontobacco cases) have been one major obstacle. Moreover, public support for advertising restrictions may be more superficial than deep, viewing advertising restrictions and other "inform and educate measures" as largely irrelevant to smoking behavior in adults and minors alike (Saad 1998). In a 1997 national Gallup poll, 85% of respondents thought that sterner warnings on cigarette packs would not substantially reduce teen smoking, and nearly 75% thought they would not encourage current adult smokers to quit (Moore 1997). So although tobacco industry political clout may have played some role in blunting a preferred policy option of the public health community, it is not clear that it has frustrated a strong public mandate to eliminate tobacco advertising and promotion.

Conclusion

On balance, contemporary U.S. tobacco policy seems to reflect American public opinion much more than it does the preference set of either the tobacco industry, public health activists, or antitobacco lawyers. That does not mean that the conflicting efforts of antitobacco policy entrepreneurs and the tobacco industry have been unimportant in influencing public policy, or that their activities had no effect on public opinion. By aggressively publicizing research concerning smoking's deadly consequences, public health activists energized a diverse array of antitobacco advocacy groups and transformed the public acceptability of cigarette smoking. By using the tools of pretrial discovery, plaintiffs' lawyers and state attorneys general helped transform the public dialogue about tobacco companies. By appealing to values of free choice and personal responsibility, the tobacco industry has been largely able to deflect potentially devastating lawsuits and perhaps helped dampen public support for higher taxes. Tobacco industry money undoubtedly has influenced many a politician's vote.

But neither the tobacco companies nor the antitobacco policy entrepreneurs have dominated public opinion formation or have achieved all the legislation they sought. For example, when Congress took up the "global settlement" arising from the massive state attorneys general lawsuits in 1998, public health activists prevented the tobacco companies from obtaining their primary objective—statutorily granted immunity from future class action lawsuits and punitive damages. But the public health activists were unable to obtain *their* primary objective—a much larger tax and advertising restriction package. As we stated earlier, in some policy spheres and arenas, tobacco interests have dominated, in others they have not, and in still others neither side has achieved its goals.

The rough correspondence between U.S. tobacco policy and public opinion suggests that neither the industry power nor the entrepreneurial politics theories can satisfactorily explain the distinctive features of American tobacco policy—far-reaching protections for nonsmokers' rights to clean air and powerful antitobacco lawsuits, but relatively modest "paternalistic" measures (use-discouraging cigarette taxes, restrictions on advertising, subsidization of cessation programs). Rather, those distinctive features reflect enduring characteristics of American political culture. If American cigarette taxes are lower than those in most economically advanced democracies, that is in keeping with a political culture that generally has been unenthusiastic about high excise taxes for gas, alcohol, and other consumption goods. The marked potency of restrictions on where smokers can light up in the United States reflects a strain in American political culture that values individual rights to legal protection from neighbors who project noxious substances into one's property or personal space. Spotty enforcement of restrictions on cigarette sales to minors also seems in keeping with American individualism, which might be reluctant to punish hard-working small retailers for failing to police their customers. It should not be surprising that a polity that is ambivalent about welfare state measures has not invested heavily in subsidizing universally accessible smoking cessation programs. The distinctive role of litigation in shaping American tobacco controls reflects a legal tradition and populist culture that is unique, in comparative terms, in fostering novel tort claims and fearsome class actions in order to sanction corporate malfeasance or harm-causing products.

The unique role of litigation in the United States, however, has produced outcomes that arguably conflict with or frustrate public sentiment. Courts are somewhat "undemocratic" institutions, in which judges are not supposed to bend to the public will. The antitobacco litigation by private litigants and state actors alike has been based on asserted norms that do *not* seem to be in accord with American public opinion: as one might expect from the traditions of American individualism, a majority of Americans reject the notion that the tobacco companies, rather than smokers, are primarily responsible for smokers' tobacco-related diseases—even though good plaintiffs' lawyers can sometimes persuade a particular jury to decide otherwise. The ongoing settlements of litigation will likely raise prices on cigarettes, de facto or de jure, despite the fact that American public opinion has been ambivalent about use-discouraging tax hikes and American legislatures have been reluctant in recent years to enact them. If one has a majoritarian or legislature-centered view of democracy, therefore, the American antitobacco litigation and its consequences could be viewed as undemocratic—a kind of public policy forged by an unrepresentative cohort of lawyers employing the coercive techniques of class action litigation in an erratic and unpredictable court system.

On the other hand, American democracy has long been characterized as pluralistic rather than majoritarian. By fragmenting political authority, both the U.S. and state constitutions intentionally seek to dampen automatic governmental reaction to the public opinion of the moment. Instead, those constitutions foster policy making in multiple, overlapping governmental units, including the courts, each with some capacity to override the others' choices. American political structures also are designed to be open to interest group pressures, whether by tobacco lobbyists, entrepreneurial trial lawyers, or idealistic public health advocates. From the standpoint of pluralistic democracy, the formation of concentrated interests that pursue their goals across a variety of political fora, including the courts, is to be expected. On this view, as long as the tobacco industry (or a highly aroused public backlash) cannot persuade state or federal legislatures to close off the litigation threat by legislation, then the pursuit of policy objectives—including punitive and redistributive measures—through litigation does not fail the test of democratic legitimacy. Although the tobacco litigation system can justly be criticized as legally unpredictable and erratic, and some claims and settlements can be criticized on policy grounds, the litigation has been democratic in the sense that it has further decentralized tobacco control efforts in the United States, bringing new information, policy entrepreneurs, and ideas into the arena.

Finally, even if the litigation against tobacco companies does not coincide with today's majority sentiment, public opinion is notoriously unstable on many issues. If the next 5 years bring more jury verdicts and postverdict news reports that emphasize tobacco company malfeasance, opinion poll majorities may begin to endorse the view that tobacco companies, not smokers, should be held responsible and might also come to endorse higher taxes or new legislative and regulatory restrictions on tobacco products. Hence, as in the past few decades, the crucial struggle between the tobacco industry and public health advocates will continue to revolve around diverse efforts by both camps to reshape public opinion. In the year 2000, for example, tobacco companies publicly proclaimed that they have changed and ran television ads about their efforts to discourage youths' access to cigarettes. Antismoking activists, drawing on funds from tobacco industry settlements, promoted counterads and sought new ways of stigmatizing the tobacco industry, such as urging pension funds to announce "divestment" of their holdings in tobacco company stocks.

Yet American public opinion seems to be remarkably stable on one fundamental point—the right of adults to choose to smoke if they wish. There is no sign that most Americans wish to prohibit the manufacture and sale of tobacco products, except for sales to juveniles, and no sign that politicians, courts, or regulatory officials seek prohibition either. Thus, even if smoking rates continue to decline, in the foreseeable future cigarettes will be a legal product and their hazards will still be with us. Tobacco control policy will continue to be mired in political controversy, influenced by the struggle between the individualistic and the moralistic strains in American political culture. The debate will continue to be about the appropriate balance between freedom and paternalistic control, how high cigarette taxes should be, the extent of tobacco company responsibility for citizens' (and teenagers') risky choices, and the extent to which governments should seek to mold smokers' behavior.

NOTES

1. The word "activist" may connote to some readers an "unscientific" approach to tobacco regulation, rather than one rooted in the evidence of smoking's harms. By "activist" in this chapter, we intend no such connotation but mean only taking a proactive or leadership role in publicizing tobacco's hazards or in formulating and proposing restrictions on tobacco.

2. In one 2-year election cycle, January 1995 to December 1996, tobacco companies donated over $6 million to political parties and candidates, most of it to Republicans, making it perhaps the single most important contributor to that party; by comparison, the Association of American Trial Lawyers, one of the single largest contributors to the Democratic Party, donated $800, 000 in the same period (Ingersoll and Stout 1997).

3. Levy and Marimont's empirical analysis, it should be noted, has been contested by a number of public health analysts. See Lucachko & Whelan 2000.

4. By 1997, according to the Americans for Nonsmokers' Rights database of smoking restrictions, at least 782 communities had put in place such restrictions.

5. *Cipollone v. Liggett*, 683 F. Supp. 1487 (1988).

6. The lawyers in the Castano group pledged $100,000 each to raise a litigation fund of $6 million (Mather 1998).

7. The industry's defense in the attorneys general suits was that since state governments and almost all smokers had repeatedly been informed that smoking could

cause cancer, few smokers, if any, had been misled, and hence damaged, by the tobacco companies' alleged deception. In addition, the tobacco companies could point to other research indicating that because sick smokers died young, they cost the state *less* in total Medicaid costs than nonsmokers, and that smokers, by paying high excise taxes, had "paid their own share" of tobacco-related health costs (Viscusi 1997, 27–32). Nevertheless, news accounts tended to ignore these issues. Lynn Mather (1998, 917–923) found that in a sample of news articles on antitobacco lawsuits from 1993 to 1996, 79% were primarily unfavorable toward the tobacco industry, 2.6% were favorable, and 18.4% were neutral or uncodable.

8. The possibility that private class action judgments entailing punitive damages could drive large tobacco companies into bankruptcy also triggered a split in the antitobacco legal community. In 2000, some attorneys general who had won huge settlements in 1999, to be paid out of company earnings over many years, became concerned that the private lawsuit-to-bankruptcy scenario would halt the flow of funds. They joined with tobacco companies to lobby state legislatures for laws that would provide some liability and procedural protections for the companies (Jenkins 2000).

9. *Brown & Williamson v. FDA*, 153 F. 3d 155 (1998).

10. *FDA v. Brown & Williamson*, 529 U.S. 120 (2000).

11. In the 1990s, the tobacco industry, which had previously donated generously to politicians of both parties, began to favor Republicans, particularly after that party achieved a congressional majority.

12. *U.S. v. Philip Morris, Inc.* 116 F. Supp. 2d 131 (2000).

13. It is also conceivable that the state laws that preempt local regulatory action, however mild, may have established nonsmoker protections that were sterner than at least some cities would have imposed.

14. Excise taxes on tobacco products may not be "classically" regressive as economists define it, given the apparent greater responsiveness to changes in price by the poor (Townsend 1989). Because the less well off will decrease their consumption by more than the better off for a given marginal price increase, they in this sense do not bear a greater load of the tax. However, this fails to capture lay concerns over unfair tax burdens: to suggest that a tax on meat or other staples is not "regressive" because the poor will simply consume less of them hardly constitutes an adequate dismissal of the concern.

15. Recent jury verdicts imposing liability on the tobacco companies suggest that members of the public, when exposed to seriously sick smokers, days of testimony about tobacco industry deceptions, and intense advocacy (albeit by both sides), can shift their positions on this issue, or the verdicts may suggest that general "antiliability" attitudes are not deeply held.

16. The California CTS survey in 1996, however, found 60% of Californians polled supported FDA regulation.

REFERENCES

Bjornson, W., R. C. Sahr, et al. 1997. Tobacco tax initiative—Oregon, 1996. *Morbidity and Mortality Weekly Report* 46 (12):246–46.

Bloch, M., R. Daynard, and R. Roemer. 1998. A year of living dangerously: The tobacco control community meets the global settlement. *Public Health Reports* 13: 488–97.

Bulow, J., and P. Klemperer. 1998. The Tobacco Deal. Economics Working Paper Archive at Washington University, St. Louis. http://ideas.uqam.ca/ideas/data/Papers/wpawuwphe9904002.html

Clymer, A. 2000. Legislators planning response to justices' ruling. *New York Times,* 24 March, A19.

Document ID 2024710395/0444. Date unknown. Attitudes regarding restrictions upon smoking/smokers. Philip Morris Tobacco Documents Archive. http://www.pmdocs.com/PDF/20204710395_0444.PDF

Elliott, E. D., B. Ackerman, and J. Millian. 1985. Toward a theory of statutory evolution: The federalization of environmental law. *Journal of Law, Economics & Organization* 1:313–40.

Farber, D. 1992. Politics and procedure in environmental law. *Journal of Law, Economics & Organization* 8:59–81.

Gallup Organization. 1990. 18 July Gallup Poll.

Haas, P. 1992. Introduction: Epistemic communities and international policy coordination. *International Organization* 46:1–35.

Ingersoll, B., and H. Stout. 1997. The politics of tobacco: Capitol Hill approval may be clouded by big campaign contributors. *Wall Street Journal*, 22 April, A24.

Jacobson, P. D., J. Wasserman, and J. R. Anderson. 1997. Historical overview of tobacco legislation and regulation. *Journal of Social Issues* 54:75–95.

Jenkins, H. 2000. Look who's falling in love with tort reform. *Wall Street Journal*, 26 April, A27.

Johnston, L. 1997. Monitoring the future. Ann Arbor: University of Michigan.

Kagan, R. A., and J. H. Skolnick. 1993. Banning smoking: Compliance without enforcement. In *Smoking Policy: Law, Politics, Culture.* Edited by R. L. Rabin and S. D. Sugarman. New York: Oxford University Press.

Kluger, R. 1997. *Ashes to Ashes: America's Hundred-Year Cigarette War, the Public Health, and the Unabashed Triumph of William Morris.* New York: Alfred A. Knopf.

Levin, Mark A. 1997. Smoke around the rising sun: An American look at tobacco regulation in Japan. *Stanford Law & Policy Review* 8:99–123.

Levy, R., and R. Marimont. 1998. Lies, damned lies, & 400,000 smoking-related deaths. *Regulation* 21:24–29.

Louis Harris and Associates. 1984. Prevention in America: A Prevention Magazine survey. Prevention, November.

Lukachko, A., and E. Whelan. 2000. A critical assessment. *Regulation* 23:2–11.

Mather, L. 1998. Theorizing about trial courts: Lawyers, policymaking, and tobacco litigation. *Law and Social Inquiry* 23 (4):897–940.

Mollenkamp, C., A. Levy, J. Menn, and J. Rothfeder. 1998. *The People vs. Big Tobacco.* Princeton: Bloomberg Press.

Moore, D. 1997. Most Americans feel tobacco companies not liable for smoking-related deaths. Gallup Organization. 24–26 March Gallup Poll.

———. 1999. Public blames smokers more than tobacco companies for smoking-related health problems. Gallup Organization. 7 October Gallup Poll.

Newport, F. 1997. Tobacco pact generates mixed reactions. Gallup Organization. 28 June Gallup Poll.

Norris, F. 2000. Confused markets: Tobacco stocks crumble, bonds don't. *New York Times*, 18 February, C1.

Olson, Mancur. 1965. *The Logic of Collective Action: Public Goods and the Theory of Groups*. Cambridge, MA: Harvard University Press.

Rigotti, N., and C. L. Pashos. 1991. No-smoking laws in the United States: An analysis of state and city actions to limit smoking in public places and workplaces. *JAMA* 266:3162–67.

Saad, L. 1998. The survey data reviewed; Smoking and American values. *Public Perspective* 9:1.

Siegel, R., and L. Wertheimer. 1998. Tobacco: Public opinion. *All Things Considered*. National Public Radio, 19 June.

Taylor, J. 1998a. Getting aboard: Lawyers, once chary of Big Tobacco, rush to line up plaintiffs. *Wall Street Journal*, 1 April, A1.

———. 1998b. Is tobacco industry playing politics with issue ads? *Wall Street Journal*, 1 September, A20.

Tobacco Institute, 1996. *The Tax Burden on Tobacco*. Washington, D.C. P. 13. Townsend, J. 1987. Cigarette tax, economic welfare, and social class patterns of smoking. *Applied Economics* 19:355–65.

U.S. Department of Health, Education, and Welfare, National Clearinghouse for Smoking and Health. 1973. *Adult use of tobacco: 1970*. Washington, D.C.: U.S. Department of Health, Education, and Welfare.

Viscusi, W. K. 1992. *Smoking: Making the Risky Decision*. Oxford: Oxford University Press.

———. 1997. From cash crop to cash cow: How tobacco profits state governments. *Regulation*, Summer: 27–32.

Wilson, James Q. (1980) *The Politics of Regulation*. New York: Basic Books. World Bank 1999. *Curbing The Epidemic: Governments and the Economics of Tobacco Control*. Washington, D.C. World Bank.

Zimring, F. E. 1993. Comparing cigarette policy and illicit drug and alcohol control. In *Smoking Policy: Law, Politics, and Culture*. Edited by R. L. Rabin and S. D. Sugarman. New York: Oxford University Press.

3

Taxing Tobacco: The Impact of Tobacco Taxes on Cigarette Smoking and Other Tobacco Use

Frank J. Chaloupka, Melanie Wakefield, & Christina Czart

For centuries, governments at all levels have taxed tobacco and tobacco products. Historically, these taxes have been used because of their relatively low administrative costs and their substantial revenue-generating potential. This potential was based, in large part, on the perception that tobacco use was insensitive to price. However, over the past several decades, numerous studies using a wide variety of data and statistical methods have found that tobacco use is no exception to the basic principles of economics. These studies clearly show that increases in the prices of tobacco products, including those that result from increased taxation, lead to significant reductions in cigarette smoking and other tobacco use. With this evidence, more recent increases in tobacco taxes have been motivated, at least in part, by their potential to reduce tobacco use and its health consequences. Critics of these taxes, however, argue that increases in taxes are inappropriate and will have harmful economic effects, including increased smuggling and significant job losses.

This chapter explores the use of tobacco taxes in the United States. The history of federal and state tobacco taxes and the administration of these taxes are briefly reviewed, followed by a discussion of the impact of increases in taxes on the prices of tobacco products, including a discussion of industry responses to higher taxes. We then describe the evidence from the large and growing literature examining the effects of tobacco taxes on cigarette smoking and other tobacco use. Rationales for tobacco taxation and a short discussion of barriers to tobacco taxation follow. Finally, the chapter concludes by highlighting the potential for higher tobacco taxes as part of a comprehensive set of policies and programs aimed at reducing the toll associated with cigarette smoking and other tobacco use.

1. A Brief History of Tobacco Taxation in the United States

Federal Tobacco Taxation

Tobacco taxation in North America began in colonial times when the British government first taxed tobacco products. After the Revolutionary War, the U.S. government imposed its first tobacco tax, in 1794, in part to raise revenues to cover the costs of the war. These taxes periodically rose and fell with revenue needs, often increasing in wartime and falling again in times of peace and prosperity. Since 1864, when employed as one part of a package to finance the Civil War, tobacco taxes of one type or another have been a permanent part of the federal tax system.

These taxes have continued to rise over time, at least in nominal terms. As table 3.1 illustrates, cigarette taxes often rose when a ready source of revenues was needed to finance wars (i.e., the Spanish-American War, World Wars I and II, and the Korean War). The last of these war financing tax hikes occurred during the Korean War when the tax increased from 7 to 8 cents per pack, effective November 1, 1951. After remaining at that level for over 30 years, federal taxes were doubled January 1, 1983, as part of the Tax Equity and Fiscal Responsibility Act of 1982. This increase was originally intended as a temporary measure to help reduce the unprecedented budget deficits of the early 1980s. However, after several extensions, the increase was made permanent in 1986. Another deficit-reducing 8 cent increase in the federal tax, in two 4 cent increments, was contained in the Omnibus Budget Reconciliation Act of 1990. Finally, as a result of the 1998 budget agreement, the federal cigarette tax rose to 34 cents per pack on January 1, 2000, and is scheduled to rise by an additional 5 cents per pack 2 years later.

As with cigarette taxes, federal taxes on other tobacco-related products have been raised infrequently, with recent increases motivated largely by the need for new revenues to reduce federal budget deficits. For example, as part of the Consolidated Omnibus Budget Reconciliation Act of 1985, taxes of 8.0, 24.0, and 45.0 cents per pound were imposed on chewing tobacco, snuff, and pipe tobacco, respectively, the first increases in these taxes since 1965. Current taxes are 12.0, 36.0, and 67.5 cents per pound, as a result of 1991 and 1993 increases resulting from the Omnibus Budget Reconciliation Act of 1990. These taxes amount to approximately 2.7 cents per 1.2 ounce tin of snuff, 2.3 cents per 3 ounce pouch of chewing tobacco, and 6.3 cents per

Table 3.1. Federal Cigarette Excise Taxes, 1864–2002

Effective date	Tax (cents per pack of 20)
June 30, 1864	0.8 (valued at not over $6.00 per 100 packs of 25)
	2.4 (valued at more than $6.00 per 100 packs of 25 each
April 1, 1865	2.4 (valued at not over $5.00 per 100 packs of 25)
	4.0 (valued at more than $5.00 per 100 packs of 25 each)
August 1, 1866	4.0 (valued at not over $8.00 per 1000)
	8.0 (valued at more than $8.00 and not over $12.00 per 1000)
	8.0 + 20% (valued at over $12.00 per 1000)
March 2, 1867	10.0
July 20, 1868	3.0
March 3, 1875	3.5
March 3, 1883	1.0
August 15, 1897	2.0
June 14, 1898	3.0
July 1, 1901	1.08 (valued at not over $2.00 per 1000)
	2.16 (valued at more than $2.00 per 1000)
July 1, 1910	2.5
October 4, 1917	4.1
February 25, 1919	6.0
July 1, 1940	6.5
November 1, 1942	7.0
November 1, 1951	8.0
January 1, 1983	16.0
January 1, 1991	20.0
January 1, 1993	24.0
January 1, 2000	34.0
January 1, 2002 (scheduled)	39.0

Source: Tobacco Institute 1999; Budget Reconciliation Act of 1997.

1.5 ounce container of pipe tobacco. No federal taxes are applied to the loose tobacco used for roll-your-own cigarettes.

In recent years, several large increases in federal cigarette taxes have been proposed. The first was the 75 cent per pack increase contained in the Clinton administration's Health Security Act. Revenues from this tax hike would have been used to partially finance the administration's unsuccessful proposal for health care reform. Similarly unsuccessful were cigarette tax increases of up to $2.00 per pack contained in proposals for national tobacco legislation. These proposed increases failed, at least in part, because of a well-orchestrated campaign by the tobacco industry's characterizing of the tax increases as regressive and likely to lead to substantial smuggling. Most recently, the Clinton administration proposed a 55 cent increase in the federal cigarette tax as part of its fiscal year 2000 budget. However, this proposal failed, given the opposition of congressional Republicans.

State and Local Tobacco Taxation

Iowa, in 1921, adopted the first state cigarette excise tax, followed by Georgia, South Carolina, South Dakota, and Utah in 1923. By 1960, nearly all states and the District of Columbia taxed cigarettes, with North Carolina, in 1969, the last state to do so. At the start of 1999, state cigarette taxes range from a low of 2.5 cents per pack in Virginia to a high of $1.00 per pack in Alaska and Hawaii (see table 3.2). In contrast, states have been slower to tax other tobacco products. In 1964, only 17 states taxed any other tobacco product; as of January 1, 1999, six states and the District of Columbia still do not tax other tobacco products. In some states that do tax other tobacco products, not all products are taxed and the taxes imposed are typically far below the levels needed for equalization with cigarette taxes. Similarly, general sales taxes in most, but not all, states are applied to cigarettes and other tobacco products, with the base for the sales tax inclusive of excise taxes in most states. As of November 1, 1998, sales taxes in these states add an additional 6 to 18 cents per pack to cigarette prices. Finally, during fiscal year 1998, 399 cities and 51 counties in 8 states imposed further cigarette taxes, with 84 of them also taxing other tobacco products. Notable among these local taxes are the 8 cent per pack tax in New York City and the 24 cent tax per pack in Chicago (reflecting both the city and county tax).

In contrast to federal government tobacco taxes used mainly to provide revenues, states have been more active in using tobacco taxation as a means for reducing tobacco use. The first evidence of this appeared in the mid-1950s, following the release of the earliest reports on the health consequences of cigarette smoking. In the early 1950s, fewer than three states per year, on average, increased cigarette taxes; by the late 1950s, this had increased to an average of more than eight states per year. This activity peaked after the release of the landmark 1964 surgeon general's report, with a record 22 states raising cigarette taxes in 1965. Because of these increases, the once negligible differences between cigarette taxes in tobacco-growing and other states have grown significantly. Currently, in the six largest tobacco growing states— North Carolina (5 cents per pack), Kentucky (3), Tennessee (13), South Carolina (7), Virginia (2.5), and Georgia (12)—the average tax per pack is just over 7 cents, whereas the average in the remaining 44 states and Washington, D.C., is nearly 40 cents per pack higher.

States' use of tobacco tax increases as a public health policy tool has become particularly clear over the past decade as several states, beginning with California, have passed relatively large tax increases that have earmarked a portion of the resulting revenues for tobacco control activities. In November 1988, California voters approved Proposition 99, the California Tobacco Tax and Health Promotion Act. The act increased California's cigarette excise tax

Table 3.2. State Cigarette Excise Tax Rates, January 1, 1999

State	Tax	State	Tax
Alabama	16.5	Montana	18
Alaska	100	Nebraska	34
Arizona	58	Nevada	35
Arkansas	31.5	New Hampshire	37
California	87	New Jersey	80
Colorado	20	New Mexico	21
Connecticut	50	New York	56
Delaware	24	North Carolina	5
D.C.	65	North Dakota	44
Florida	33.9	Ohio	24
Georgia	12	Oklahoma	23
Hawaii	1.00	Oregon	68
Idaho	28	Pennsylvania	31
Illinois	58	Rhode Island	71
Indiana	15.5	South Carolina	7
Iowa	36	South Dakota	33
Kansas	24	Tennessee	13
Kentucky	3	Texas	41
Louisiana	20	Utah	51.5
Maine	74	Vermont	44
Maryland	36	Virginia	2.5
Massachusetts	76	Washington	82.5
Michigan	75	West Virginia	17
Minnesota	48	Wisconsin	59
Mississippi	18	Wyoming	12
Missouri	17		

Source: Tobacco Institute 1999.

from 10 cents per pack to 35 cents per pack and earmarked 20% of the new revenues for programs to reduce and prevent tobacco use. These funds are allocated for a number of activities. On average, about 15% of the total is used to coordinate local tobacco control activities and to provide technical assistance. Twelve percent has been used, on average, to fund mass media counteradvertising on television and radio and in outdoor and print media. Another 15% has been used to fund community tobacco-prevention efforts, particularly those targeting ethnic minorities, while 22%, on average, has been allocated to local school districts and county education offices for implementing school-based tobacco prevention, education, and cessation programs. The remainder has been used for a variety of administrative activities, to fund tobacco-related research, and to finance medical care programs. Although significant funding for tobacco control has been provided from the tax, the California legislature has generally not fully implemented the funding mandated by the act. In 1998, voters, by a small margin, passed further tobacco tax increases as part of Proposition 10. Effective January 1, 1999, cigarette taxes were raised by 50 cents per pack, and taxes on other tobacco products were also increased. Funds from this tax increase were earmarked for childhood development programs; in addition, funding for the California Tobacco Control Program created by Proposition 99 was to be maintained.

California's success encouraged tobacco control advocates in Massachusetts to put a similar referendum on the ballot in November 1992. The referendum, known as Question 1, strongly endorsed earmarking part of the funds generated by tax increases for activities aimed at reducing tobacco use and won easy acceptance. Effective January 1, 1993, the Massachusetts cigarette tax increased from 26 to 51 cents per pack, while the state tax on chewing tobacco was raised by 25%. Massachusetts law prohibited the earmarking of the new revenues generated by the tax increases for tobacco control activities. Instead, the funds are put into the Health Protection Fund that supports the Massachusetts Tobacco Control Program. The program supports a mass media counteradvertising campaign, cessation services, community- and school-based education efforts, and more. The success of the program led to an additional 25 cent increase in the state cigarette tax in October 1996, an increase in the smokeless tobacco tax, and the adoption of a new state tax on cigars.

In 1994, voters in both Michigan and Arizona approved significant tax increases. The Michigan initiative, Proposal A, included a 50 cent per pack increase in the state cigarette excise tax, the largest single increase in cigarette taxes in the United States to that point, as well as new taxes on other tobacco products. Although Proposal A focused on changing the financing of Michigan public schools, it included provisions earmarking 6% of the new revenues for health improvement activities, including tobacco-related education and prevention. In November 1994, Arizona voters adopted Proposition 200, increasing the state cigarette tax from 18 to 58 cents per pack, proportionally increasing state taxes on other tobacco products, and earmarking 23% of the new revenues for tobacco education programs.

Oregon voters followed by approving Ballot Measure 44 in November 1996. This measure increased the state cigarette excise tax from 38 to 68 cents per pack and earmarked 10% of the new revenues for tobacco prevention and education efforts. These ongoing efforts include a mass media counteradvertising campaign, the creation of a tobacco quit line, funding for community-based programs, including tribal tobacco and multicultural programs, school-based education and prevention activities, and more.

In 1997, the Maine legislature followed the example of these other states by doubling its cigarette excise tax to 74 cents per pack, effective November 1, 1997. Of the new revenues, $3.5 million helped to create the Partnership for a Tobacco-Free Maine with the state's Department of Health and Human

Services. This program has funded a mass media campaign, school- and community-based efforts, and other activities aimed at reducing tobacco use. Similarly, in 1999, Maryland raised its cigarette tax by 30 cents per pack, with part of the new revenues generated by the tax increase targeted for programs aimed at reducing tobacco use.

In addition, several recent state cigarette and other tobacco tax increases, including those in Alaska, Hawaii, New Hampshire, New Jersey, and Vermont that did not earmark funds for tobacco control activities, were motivated, in part, by the promise that the higher taxes would lead to reductions in youth and adult tobacco use.

Structure of Tobacco Taxes

Different types of taxes are applied to tobacco products. The most basic of these taxes include specific taxes, levied as a fixed amount added to the base price of the product, and ad valorem taxes, levied as a percentage of price. Federal excise taxes and state cigarette excise taxes are specific taxes, whereas most state taxes on other tobacco products and state sales taxes applied to all tobacco products are ad valorem taxes. Some of these taxes, notably state and federal cigarette taxes, are applied per unit of the product (i.e., per cigarette); others, such as federal taxes on chewing tobacco, snuff, and pipe tobacco, are applied based on weight. Other tax structures are possible but are not used in the United States. Some countries, for example, impose differential taxes on imported and domestically produced cigarettes. Similarly, differential taxes may be imposed on the same basic product based on other factors (for example, higher taxes may be imposed on cigarettes that contain more tar and nicotine or are unfiltered). Some of these taxes are imposed at the wholesale level (i.e., federal and state excise taxes on cigarettes and other tobacco products); others are imposed at the retail level (i.e., state sales taxes applied to tobacco products).

Each type of tobacco tax has its own strengths and weaknesses. Ad valorem taxes, for example, have the advantage of increasing with the prices of the products on which they are imposed. That is, the taxes do not need to be continually increased to keep pace with inflation (assuming that the base prices of the products they are applied to rise with inflation). Thus, the real (inflation adjusted) value of revenues generated by these taxes over time is relatively stable. However, this may also be a disadvantage of these taxes because the revenues generated by these taxes can vary as a result of industry price manipulation. Townsend (1998), for example, observed that this has happened in Greece, Spain, and many South American countries where tobacco product prices were kept relatively low, keeping tax revenues low. In addition, many have suggested that ad valorem taxes are likely to lead to reductions in average product quality as producers and consumers switch to lower cost tobacco products (Barzel 1976; British American Tobacco 1994; Sobel and Garrett 1997). Finally, ad valorem taxes are more difficult to administer and more costly to collect.

A major strength of specific taxes is the relative ease and low cost with which they are collected and the relative stability of the nominal revenue stream they generated. In addition, although the tobacco industry may minimize the impact of relatively small unit taxes on the prices of cigarettes and other tobacco products, large specific taxes are almost certain to lead to high prices for these products. At a minimum, they impose a floor on the prices of tobacco products. Nevertheless, the tobacco industry is likely to seek ways to minimize the impact of these taxes. Townsend (1998), for example, describes how the switch to a per-cigarette tax in the United Kingdom (from a weight-based system) led tobacco companies to market "king-sized" and "super king-sized" cigarettes, actually lowering the total tax per amount of tobacco smoked. Similarly, Evans and Farrelly (1998) found that increases in specific cigarette taxes in the United States, while significantly reducing smoking prevalence, led some continuing smokers to switch to longer or higher tar and nicotine cigarettes. This has been interpreted by some as an increase in the quality of the average cigarette consumed (Barzel 1976; British American Tobacco 1994; Sobel and Garrett 1997). In other countries, where the taxes are based on weight, the opposite has occurred. In Australia, for example, tobacco companies have reduced the weight of tobacco per cigarette while increasing the number of cigarettes per pack in an attempt to make cigarettes appear to be a "good value" to consumers.

A major disadvantage of specific taxes is that they need to be increased frequently to prevent their value from being eroded by inflation. If the taxes are not increased often, then their real (inflation adjusted) value will decline over time. Given the importance of tobacco taxes in the prices of tobacco products, stable nominal specific taxes can result in declines in the real prices of tobacco products. Thus, a policy that maintains the nominal value of these taxes over time can offset the impact of other efforts to reduce tobacco use and its consequences. This is clearly seen in the United States through trends in real cigarette prices and taxes over the past 35 years (see figure 3.1). Early in this period, from 1955 through 1971, when states were increasing taxes to both generate revenues and to discourage smoking, both average real cigarette taxes and prices were rising steadily. During this period, the average real state tax doubled from 13.1 cents per pack (1982–1984 dollars) to 26.4 cents per pack, more than enough to offset the decline in the real federal tax (from 29.9 cents to 19.8 cents per pack). As a result, real cigarette prices rose modestly (from 84.7 cents per pack to 96.0 cents per pack).

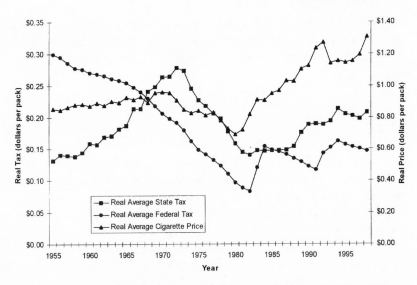

Figure 3.1. Real Cigarette taxes and prices. Prices and taxes are in 1982–1984 dollars. Taxes are for the fiscal year ending June 30th. Average state tax is an average of taxes in all taxing states and D.C. (42 in 1955, 50 and D.C. in 1970 and after) weighted by state tax-paid cigarette sales. Price reflects the median retail price for cigarettes (including generic brands since 1990) in all states, generally as of November 1. Source: Tobacco Institute 1999, and authors' calculations.

During the 1970s, however, states became reluctant to further increase cigarette taxes given that interstate smuggling was perceived to be a significant problem. Consequently, given the stability of both state and federal cigarette taxes and the high inflation of the 1970s, real cigarette taxes and prices fell sharply. The real average state tax declined by nearly 50% from 1971 to 1981, the real federal tax fell by more than 50%, and the average real cigarette price fell by almost 40%.

Since 1981, real cigarette prices have risen significantly, from 69.3 cents per pack in November 1991 to 130.9 cents per pack in November 1998. A tripling of the nominal federal cigarette tax, along with steady increases in average state cigarette taxes, contributed to this increase. However, even with the increases in the real values of federal and state taxes, cigarette taxes as a share of price fell during this period (from 33.1% to 28.2%), implying that the manufacturers' price was rising even more rapidly. Between November 1980 and November 1992, the real value of manufacturers' price rose by more than 70%. This dropped sharply as a result of "Marlboro Friday" in April 1993 when wholesale cigarette prices, first for Marlboro, then followed soon after by other premium brands, were cut by 25%. Over the past two years, however, wholesale cigarette prices have increased sharply as tobacco companies have passed on some of the costs of lawsuit settlements with the states.

International Comparisons

Among high-income countries, the United States has one of the lowest average price and tax on cigarettes. As shown in figure 3.2, cigarette prices, national taxes, and taxes as a share of price are highest in high-income countries and fall as a country's income level falls. Whereas prices in the United States are higher than in most middle-and low-income countries, they are well below average prices in other high-income countries. This is largely the result of the relatively low federal cigarette tax in the United States Moreover, federal taxes as a share of cigarette prices in the United States are well below the average in all of the country groups.

Cigarette Taxes and Cigarette Prices

Increases in cigarette and other tobacco taxes are expected to result in higher prices for these products. In a perfectly competitive market with constant long-run costs of production, an increase in taxes would be fully passed on to consumers in the form of an equivalent price increase. At the opposite extreme, a monopolist would share the burden of cigarette taxes with smokers, with consumers paying a relatively larger share of the tax, as demand was less responsive to price. In the United States, neither extreme characterizes the markets for cigarettes and other tobacco products. Instead, U.S. markets are characterized by a high concentration of production among a small number of firms. In 1996, for example, five firms accounted for 99.9% of all cigarette production, with the two largest firms—Philip Morris and R. J. Reynolds—accounting for nearly three-quarters of this (FTC 1997). Economic theory suggests that each large firm in a highly concentrated market will recognize that its own pricing and marketing strategies will have a significant impact on the sales and profitability of its competitors, as well as on its own sales and profitability. As a result, each understands that any changes in its pricing and marketing strategies will almost certainly be met by changes in the strategies employed by its competitors.

This high concentration and the interdependence among firms in the tobacco industry has important implications for the impact of cigarette taxes and other control policies on the pricing, marketing, and other strategies of cigarette producers. Several early studies of the relationship between cigarette tax increases and price produced generally inconsistent conclusions, with

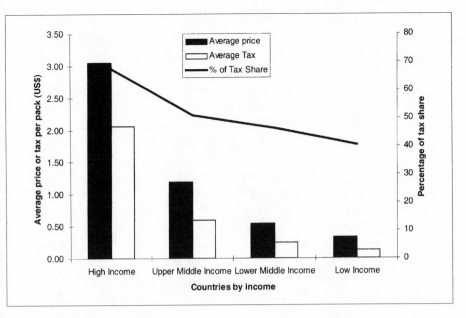

Figure 3.2.   International cigarette prices and taxes. Weighted average price, tax, and share of tax in price per pack by income group countries and the United States, 1996. Source: Unpublished data, World Bank.

some finding that price increased by less than the amount of the tax increase (consistent with monopolistic behavior), whereas others found that the tax was fully passed on to consumers (consistent with relatively competitive behavior) (Barzel 1976; Johnson 1978; Sumner 1981; Sumner and Ward 1981; Bulow and Pfleiderer 1983; Bishop and Yoo 1985; Sullivan 1985; Sumner and Wohlgenant 1985; Ashenfelter and Sullivan 1987). An important limitation of these early studies, however, was that they ignored the dynamic interaction of firms in a highly concentrated industry. That is, these studies typically assumed that the rules for firm behavior were established and then, using data on prices and taxes, the authors worked backward to determine the level of competition in the industry (Harris 1987).

More recent studies have attempted to address this weakness by more formally modeling the dynamic nature of firms in a highly concentrated industry. These recent studies clearly indicate that increases in cigarette taxes lead to significant increases in cigarette prices. The earliest of these studies (Harris 1987), using data on manufacturing costs and state cigarette taxes, concluded that the doubling of the federal cigarette tax in 1983 (an 8 cent tax increase) led to a 17 cent increase in price. Harris argued that U.S. cigarette firms used the scheduled tax increase as a coordinating mechanism for additional industry price increases, noting that the increase in prices began shortly after the tax increase was announced, but well before the tax actually increased.

Subsequent, more rigorous studies by Keeler and his colleagues, however, suggest that this wasn't the case. In a series of articles (Sung, Hu, and Keeler 1994; Barnett, Keeler, and Hu 1995; Keeler, Hu, Barnett, Manning, and Sung 1996), they explored the relationships between state and federal cigarette tax increases and cigarette prices. Their models accounted for the interaction of supply and demand, the highly concentrated, interdependent nature of the cigarette industry, and, in some cases, the addictive nature of cigarette smoking. Using annual state-level data for the period from 1960 through 1990, Keeler and his colleagues (Keeler et al. 1996) estimated that a 1 cent increase in the state cigarette tax would lead to a 1.11 cent increase in cigarette prices, whereas a federal tax increase would lead to an even larger increase in price. They attributed the relatively smaller increase in response to a state tax increase to the potential for cross-border shopping for cigarettes in nearby lower tax and price states. In addition, Keeler and his colleagues concluded that cigarette producers charge relatively low prices in states with stronger tobacco control policies than they do in states with weaker policies. Chaloupka and Slater (1999) provide similar evidence of industry manipulation of price in response to tobacco control efforts. Using data from a 1996 survey of over 700 retail tobacco outlets, they find that prices of branded cigarettes are significantly lower in states with comprehensive tobacco control programs than they are in other states.

Additional evidence on tobacco companies' manipulation of price in response to tobacco tax increases and tobacco control activities comes from internal tobacco company documents made public as a result of state and other lawsuits brought against the tobacco industry. A preliminary examination of these documents highlights the industry's recognition of the impact of tax increases on profitability. A Philip Morris International document from 1985, includes this sentence: "With regard to taxation, it is clear that in the U.S. and in most countries in which we operate, tax is becoming a major threat to our existence." The document goes on: "Of all the concerns, there is one—taxation—that alarms us the most. While marketing restrictions and public and passive smoking (restrictions) do depress volume, in our experience taxation depresses it much more severely. Our concern for taxation is, therefore, central to our thinking" (Moyer 1998).

Similarly, internal documents from R. J. Reynolds and Philip Morris U.S.A. (provided by K. Michael Cummings), discussing a potential 1987 federal cigarette tax increase, illustrate strategies for dealing with these tax increases. In a September 3, 1987, Philip Morris memo on "handling an excise tax increase," Myron Johnston discusses what happened when the federal tax was doubled in 1983 and suggests the following strategy: "take the increase all at once; advertise, blaming it on the feds and encouraging smokers to stockpile; increase prices only to the extent of the tax; and make sure that the cigarettes that the retailers stockpile are *our* brand this time. We might also take the opportunity to again point out the regressive nature of the tax and tell smokers what percent of the price of a pack of cigarettes in their state is due to taxes." Johnston contrasts this with the strategy used in response to the 1983 tax increase when prices were increased five times and by somewhat more than the scheduled tax increase in anticipation of the tax hike, a "fact that was not lost on consumers, who could legitimately blame the manufacturers for the price increases."

R. J. Reynolds considered a somewhat different strategy for responding to the anticipated 1987 federal tax increase that was aimed at softening the impact on smokers and maintaining/gaining market share for its brands. This strategy, outlined in a December 22, 1986, memo from D. W. Shouse, included passing on the full amount of the tax increase to consumers, defending the market share of its core brands and maximizing increases in market share for its discount brands. Losses in core brand market shares were to be minimized by offering a tax rebate/coupon program beginning in July to help offset the short-run impact of the anticipated October tax increase ($2.00 per carton was recommended). In addition, the plan called for including postage-paid reply cards in cartons that would allow smokers to let their congressperson know of their opposition to the tax hike, as well as the creation of a 1-800 number "for smokers to call for additional tax protection if an increase does in fact occur." Smokers participating in the call-in program would have received six $1.00 carton coupons by mail if the tax increase had taken place, a strategy described as "self-selecting, or targeted to price-sensitive franchise smokers." The plan to maximize gains in the discount segment of the market included accelerated introduction of new low-priced brands and national expansion of existing brands (i.e., Doral), along with increased on-carton couponing for discount brands.

Some evidence suggests that price-related marketing strategies of the type suggested in the R. J. Reynolds' memo have become increasingly important in recent years. In the 3 years prior to the most recent federal tax increases in 1991 and 1993, for example, cigarette companies reported expenditures of about $1 million per year on coupons and retail value added. In contrast, average expenditures per year were almost $2.4 million per year from 1991 through 1993, suggesting that cigarette companies expanded discounting in an effort to soften the impact of the tax increase or protect their own market shares. These efforts appear to be short-lived, with average annual expenditures for coupons and retail value added falling to about $1.3 million per year from 194 through 1996 (FTC 1998). Similarly, in the wake of the master settlement agreement, cigarette companies announced an increase of 45 cents per pack in cigarette prices. However, within days, the prices of a number of leading brands were reduced by 45 cents per pack as a result of special promotional discounts; six months later, while somewhat reduced, discounting remained extensive (Chaloupka, Slater, and Wakefield 1999).

2. Tobacco Taxes, Prices, and the Demands for Tobacco Products

One of the most fundamental principles of economics is that of the downward sloping demand curve, implying that as the price of a product rises, the quantity of that product demanded will fall. Several decades ago, many thought that addictive products, including cigarettes and other tobacco products, were exceptions to this principle. However, the large, growing, and increasingly sophisticated economic research on the demands for cigarettes and other tobacco products clearly demonstrates that increases in the prices of these products will lead to reductions in their use. These reductions result not only from reduced use by continuing users but also from increased cessation of use and reduced initiation.

The numerous empirical studies of the past three decades on the effects of tobacco taxes and prices on cigarette smoking and other tobacco use have employed a wide variety of aggregate and individual-level data from the United States and a number of other countries. Similarly, these studies use increasingly sophisticated econometric and other statistical methods. In recent years, several of these studies have attempted to account for the addictive nature of smoking. That is, these studies apply economic models that explicitly recognize the dependence of current consumption decisions on past choices, with some of these models allowing for relatively farsighted behavior. The key implication of these models is that the long-run impact of permanent price increases will exceed the short-run impact, given that demand will adjust gradually over time (see Chaloupka, Tauras, Grossman, and Jha 2000 for a detailed discussion of the economic models of addiction and their applications to tobacco use).

This section highlights the key findings from this body of research, focusing on studies from the United States; more thorough reviews of the literature can be found in Chaloupka and Warner (2000) and Chaloupka, Hu, Warner, Jacobs, and Yurelki (2000). In reviewing these studies, the term "price elasticity of demand" will be used. Economists use this term to define the percent change in the quantity of a good demanded in response to a 1% increase in price. Three basic elasticities will be described. The first is the unconditional, or total price elasticity of demand and reflects the total impact of a change in price on consumption. The second is the prevalence elasticity; this reflects the change in the prevalence of smoking in response to a price increase. The final one is the conditional demand elasticity, reflecting the change in consumption, conditional on use (i.e., the reduction in average daily cigarette consumption among continuing smokers).

Overall Demand Estimates

Numerous studies have examined the impact of changes in cigarette prices on overall cigarette demand. Many of these studies have employed a variety of aggregated data, including national-level cigarette sales and state-level cigarette sales (for a single state over time or for a pooled sample of states over time). Others have used individual-level data taken from large nationally representative surveys. These studies produce a relatively wide range of estimates for the price elasticity of cigarette demand in the United States. However, most estimates fall in the relatively narrow range from −0.25 to −0.50, implying that a 10% increase in cigarette prices would reduce overall cigarette consumption by between 2.5 and 5%. Thus, increases in cigarette taxes, by increasing price, would produce significant reductions in overall cigarette smoking.

Several recent studies have attempted to account for the addictive nature of demand in the context of myopic and farsighted economic models of addiction (i.e., Mullahy 1985; Chaloupka 1991; Keeler, Hu, Barnett, and Manning 1993; Becker, Grossman, and Murphy 1994). As expected, these studies provide strong empirical support for the hypothesis that cigarette smoking is an addictive behavior. In addition, they provide at least some support for the hypothesis that smokers do not behave myopically (implying that smokers would reduce current consumption in response to an increase in the expected future costs of smoking). Finally, as discussed before, these studies consistently estimate that the long-run price elasticity of demand is about double the short-run elasticity. Becker and his colleagues, for example, estimate that the long-run price elasticity is in the range from −0.73 to −0.79. The key policy implication of these studies is that the impact of permanent, inflation-adjusted increases in cigarette taxes and prices will grow over time.

A growing number of studies have used individual level data from nationally representative surveys to separate the impact of price on smoking prevalence from its impact on cigarette consumption among smokers. In general, these studies find that half or more of the effect of price comes from reducing the number of smokers, whereas the remainder is the result of reduced consumption by continuing smokers. For example, a recent study by the Centers for Disease Control and Prevention (CDC 1998) used data from 13 waves of the National Health Interview Survey conducted from 1975 through 1993, estimating an overall demand elasticity of -0.25, and a prevalence elasticity of -0.15. With the epidemiological evidence on the health consequences of smoking and the benefits of cessation, increases in cigarette taxes likely would lead to substantial reductions in the morbidity and mortality resulting from tobacco use.

Smoking Cessation

In general, researchers examining the effects of price on overall smoking prevalence using individual-level data have assumed that the reductions in smoking prevalence resulting from higher prices were largely the result of increased smoking cessation among adults. A few recent studies have attempted to directly examine the impact of prices on smoking cessation. Douglas (1998) used hazard methods applied to retrospective data from the 1987 National Health Interview Survey to estimate the impact of prices on cessation in the context of Becker and Murphy's (1988) economic model of addiction. He found strong evidence that higher cigarette prices reduced the duration of smoking, estimating that a permanent 10% increase in price would reduce the duration of smoking by about 10%.

Tauras (1999) and Tauras and Chaloupka (forthcoming) addressed the same question using longitudinal data on cigarette smoking among young adults taken from the Monitoring the Future Study. Using sophisticated parametric and semi-parametric duration models, Tauras finds consistent evidence that higher cigarette prices significantly raise the probability of smoking cessation. His estimates indicate that a 10% permanent increase in price would raise the probability of cessation among young adults by between 2.4 and 4.7%. Tauras and Chaloupka used these data to explore differences in the effects of price on cessation among young adult men and women, concluding that cessation among both would rise sharply in response to price increases.

Youth and Young Adult Smoking

Grossman and his colleagues (Lewit, Coate, and Grossman 1981; Grossman and Chaloupka 1997) suggest that younger persons would be more sensitive than older persons to changes in cigarette prices for several reasons. First, given the addictive nature of cigarette smoking, they argue that youths who have been smoking for a relatively short time will more likely respond quickly to changes in price than more addicted adult smokers. Second, they argue that peer influences are much more important for young smokers than they are for adult smokers. Thus, increases in price will not only directly reduce youth smoking but will also indirectly reduce it by lowering peer smoking. Third, they note that economic theory implies that the greater the share of income spent on a good, the more price-sensitive demand for that good will be, all else constant. Given that the fraction of disposable income a young smoker spends on cigarettes is likely larger than that spent by an adult smoker, and given the evidence that youths with greater disposable incomes are more likely to smoke, increases in price will likely have a greater impact on youth smoking. Finally, compared to adults, youths are likely to be more present-oriented. In the context of the economic models of addiction, this implies that youths will respond more to changes in the relatively immediate costs of smoking, such as price, whereas adults will be relatively more responsive to changes in the long-term costs of smoking (i.e., increased perceptions of the long-term health consequences of smoking).

Lewit and his colleagues, in the first studies to consider differences in price elasticity by age, produced estimates consistent with the hypothesis that cigarette price increases would have a greater impact on youths and young adults. Lewit and Coate's (1982) estimated price elasticity for young adults (ages 20 through 25 years) was about double the consensus estimate for adults, while Lewit and his colleagues' (1981) estimate for youths (ages 12 through 17) was more than triple that for adults. A decade later, however, two studies based on relatively small samples from the same survey concluded that the price sensitivity of cigarette smoking among youths and young adults was not significantly different from that of adults (Wasserman, Manning, Newhouse, and Winkler 1991; Chaloupka 1991).

Several more recent studies, however, contain strong evidence that the price sensitivity of cigarette smoking is greatest among youths and young adults (Chaloupka and Grossman 1996; Chaloupka and Wechsler 1997; Lewit, Hyland, Kerrelrock, and Cummings 1997; Evans and Huang 1998; CDC 1998; Tauras and Chaloupka 1999). Chaloupka and Grossman, for example, used data on over 110,000 eighth, tenth, and twelfth grade students taken from the 1992, 1993, and 1994 Monitoring the Future Surveys to estimate an overall price elasticity of demand of -1.31 for teenagers. They estimated that just over half of the effect of price was on youth smoking prevalence; the remainder reflected reduced cigarette consumption among young smokers. Similarly, the CDC's 1998 estimate of the price elasticity for young adults was more than double their estimate for the overall population. Most recently, Tauras and Chaloupka, using the longitudinal data from Monitoring the Future, estimated a series of models accounting for unobserved state, time, and individual specific factors that, if ignored, could lead to biased estimates of the effects of prices and other tobacco control policies on demand. Their estimated price elasticity for young adults (−0.79) provides additional support for the hypothesis that price responsiveness is inversely related to age.

Changes in smoking prevalence observed among youths are expected to be largely the result of reduced initiation. A few studies have attempted to directly estimate the impact of price on initiation. Douglas (1998) and Douglas and Hariharan (1994) used retrospective data from the National Health Interview Surveys to address this issue, concluding that cigarette prices had little or no impact on youth smoking initiation. However, as the authors described, errors-in-variables associated with both the retrospective data on age at initiation and the cigarette price data matched to the surveys biased their estimates in the direction of finding no effect. Two recent studies using more appropriate longitudinal data from the National Education Longitudinal Survey produced mixed findings (Dee and Evans 1998; DeCicca, Kenkel, and Mathios 1999); DeCicca and his colleagues present estimates from a variety of models, some suggesting that youth smoking initiation would be reduced by higher cigarette prices and others suggesting that price has no impact on initiation. The authors give greater weight to the latter models, concluding that higher cigarette taxes and prices would not reduce smoking initiation among U.S. teens. Dee and Evans, using a different approach to the treatment of missing data, however, produce estimates for the effects of price on smoking initiation consistent with those from the recent studies based on cross-sectional data described previously. These studies are based on data from a single cohort of youths (eighth grade students in 1988), and some of the models estimated are quite taxing on the limited data employed. Clearly, more research using longitudinal data on multiple cohorts over a longer time period is needed before anyone rejects the consistent findings from studies based on cross-sectional data.

Socioeconomic Status and Price Responsiveness

Economic theory predicts that price sensitivity of demand should be greatest in the lowest income populations and lowest in the highest income populations. This hypothesis is supported by the findings from the relatively few studies that have examined the relationship between the price sensitivity of cigarette demand and socioeconomic status. The CDC (1998), for example, estimated that the price elasticity of demand by persons at or below the median level of family income in their sample was 70% greater than that of persons above the median. Chaloupka (1991) found that cigarette smoking among persons with less than a high school education (a good proxy for income) was much more sensitive to price than smoking among those with at least a high school education.

Similar support is provided from several international studies. Townsend, Roderick, and Cooper (1994), for example, using data from the British General Household Survey, concluded that smoking among people in the highest socioeconomic class was virtually unresponsive to price, while smoking among those in the lowest income groups was highly sensitive to price. The growing number of studies from low- and middle-income countries is also consistent with this hypothesis. Estimates from China (Mao and Xiang 1997; Mao, Xiang, and Kon 1997; Xu, Hu, and Keeler 1998), South Africa (van der Merwe 1998), Zimbabwe (Maranvanyika 1998), Papua New Guinea (Chapman and Richardson 1990), and elsewhere produce estimates of the price elasticity of overall cigarette demand that are consistently higher than those found in studies for high-income countries.

Behavioral Economic Analyses of Cigarette Demand

In a relatively new approach applying the principles of economics to experimental psychology, behavioral psychologists have been examining the impact of prices on cigarette smoking in a laboratory setting. In these experiments, price is reflected by the level of effort that needs to be expended in order to be "rewarded" with a puff on a cigarette. Bickel and Madden (1999) summarize the findings from a number of experiments led by Bickel and other behavioral psychologists. Their research clearly shows that smoking diminishes as price increases. A particularly novel feature of this research is the ability of the researchers to manipulate price over a much wider range than is observed in the real world. For example, the number of responses required to obtain two puffs in their experiments has varied from 100 to 3,200. Based on this, they conclude that the price elasticity of demand rises as price rises, suggesting that the impact of large tax increases on overall cigarette consumption would be disproportionately larger than would be implied by the estimates from the econometric studies based on the much more limited variation in cigarette prices across states and over time.

The Demand for Other Tobacco Products

In contrast to the plentiful literature on the demand for cigarettes, relatively few studies have examined the impact of prices or taxes on the demands for other tobacco products, mainly because of the lack of good data on sales, use, and prices for these other products. Ohsfeldt and his colleagues (Ohsfeldt and Boyle 1994; Ohsfeldt, Boyle, and Capilouto 1997, 1999) used several waves of the Current Population Survey to look at this issue, producing generally consistent evidence that higher smokeless tobacco taxes would lead to reductions in smokeless tobacco use. Chaloupka and his colleagues (1997)

likewise found that smokeless tobacco use among young men would be reduced by higher taxes on smokeless tobacco products. Studies from other
countries for other tobacco products similarly concluded that higher taxes or
prices on various tobacco products would reduce the use of these products
(Thompson and McLeod 1976; Leu 1994; Pekurinen 1989, 1991). In addition, these studies generally provide evidence that cigarettes and other tobacco products are substitutes for one another. That is, an increase in cigarette taxes while holding taxes on other tobacco products constant would
lead to a reduction in smoking but also some increases in the use of other
tobacco products. Evans and Farrelly (1998) provide evidence of a different
type of substitution. Using data on brand choice from the National Health
Interview Survey, they concluded that smokers in high tax states were more
likely to smoke longer cigarettes or cigarettes with higher tar and nicotine
content than were smokers in low tax states. They interpreted this as evidence
that smokers substituted among brands in response to tax changes and that
the health benefits of tax increases would be somewhat reduced by this type
of substitution.

Cigarette Taxes and Other Substance Use

Relatively little is known about the impact of higher cigarette taxes and prices
on other substance use. During the recent debates over national tobacco
legislation, some speculated that the significant increases in cigarette taxes
being considered, while reducing youth smoking, would drive potential
smokers to consume other drugs, particularly marijuana. This speculation is
not consistent with research on patterns of substance use that suggests that
cigarette smoking is a significant predictor of both the probability and frequency of other drug use (i.e., USDHHS 1988; Henningfield, Clayton, and
Pollin 1990). Nor is it consistent with the findings from a few recent econometric analysis of polysubstance use. Chaloupka, Pacula, Farrelly, Johnston,
O'Malley, and Bray (1999), using data from the Monitoring the Future Surveys, found that higher cigarette prices, in addition to reducing youth cigarette smoking, also reduced youth marijuana use. Farrelly and his colleagues
(1999), found similar evidence for adults, using data from the National
Household Surveys on Drug Abuse. In addition, they found that higher cigarette prices reduced alcohol use.

3. Rationales for Tobacco Taxation

Cigarettes and other tobacco taxes have long been taxed by nearly all governments. Historically, as discussed for the United States, these taxes have

been viewed as a relatively easy way to generate revenues. More recently, as the health consequences of tobacco use have become known, many have argued for higher tobacco taxes on public health grounds. Similarly, as the economic costs resulting from tobacco's devastating effects on public health have been quantified, others have argued that higher tobacco taxes would be economically efficient in that the social costs associated with tobacco use could be covered by these taxes. Each of these rationales is reviewed in this section.

Tobacco Taxes and Revenues

The revenue-generating potential of tobacco taxes is by far the most common rationale for tobacco taxation. In the United States, while the nominal amount of revenues generated by tobacco taxes has increased significantly over time, these taxes are now only a minor contributor to overall government revenues. For example, while tobacco taxes accounted for 3.36% of all federal government revenues in 1950, they were only 0.44% of revenues by 1989 (Congressional Budget Office 1990).

Economists have favored cigarette and other tobacco taxes because they have been viewed as consistent with the "Ramsey rule" (Ramsey 1927). This fundamental principle of taxation says that taxes that generate substantial revenues while minimizing the welfare losses associated with the resulting higher prices are preferable to those that cause greater welfare losses. Given the relatively inelastic overall demand for tobacco products, at least in the short run, tobacco taxes appear to satisfy the Ramsey rule. This, in large part, is why institutions such as the International Monetary Fund (Sunley 1998) have favored tobacco taxes.

Given the relatively inelastic demand for cigarettes in the U.S. (overall elasticity of around −0.4) and the relatively low share of taxes in cigarette prices (less than 30%), significant increases in cigarette taxes would not only lead to significant reductions in cigarette smoking but also generate substantial increases in tax revenues. Doubling all federal and state cigarette taxes, for example, would result in about a 12% reduction in overall cigarette sales but would increase cigarette tax revenues by approximately 75%. Although there will almost certainly be some point at which tax revenues fall as taxes rise, Merriman (1994) shows that even in the presence of interstate cigarette smuggling, state cigarette taxes are well below their revenue maximizing levels.

Increases in federal taxes alone, while increasing federal revenues, will have an adverse impact on state revenues. Similarly, some states will be constrained in their ability to raise state cigarette taxes significantly, given the potential for cross-border shopping and smuggling of cigarettes from nearby lower tax states. In general, this is a greater problem the greater the differences in state tax rates and when a larger share of the state population lives near a lower tax state. Nevertheless, all state cigarette tax increases have generated significant increases in state tax revenues.

In some proposals for a national tobacco settlement, cigarette companies would have been required to raise prices, passing on the costs of the settlement to smokers. Many considered this a "tax" on cigarette companies, but it would have had a dramatic impact on state and federal cigarette tax revenues. Given the large price increases that would have resulted from such a pass-through, cigarette sales would have declined significantly, leading to large reductions in state and federal cigarette tax revenues. Similarly, the industry-initiated price increases announced in the wake of the master settlement agreement will have an adverse impact on cigarette tax revenues. Governments, however, can avoid this by raising cigarette taxes, as several have done or are proposing to do.

Cigarette Taxes and Public Health

Given the strong evidence that higher cigarette and other tobacco taxes would reduce tobacco use, particularly among youths and young adults, and given the clear links between tobacco use and a large and growing number of health problems, higher tobacco taxes can be an effective approach to improving public health. Several studies have estimated the potential health benefits of cigarette tax increases based on the estimates of the price elasticity of demand already discussed (i.e., Warner 1986; Harris 1987; General Accounting Office 1989; Chaloupka 1998). Chaloupka, for example, used the estimates from his study with Grossman (Chaloupka and Grossman 1996) to estimate the impact of alternative cigarette tax and price increases contained in several proposals for national tobacco legislation. He estimated, for example, that a $1.50 increase in the federal cigarette tax, phased in quickly and indexed to inflation, would reduce overall cigarette consumption by approximately 30% and cut youth smoking prevalence almost in half. Given CDC's (1996) estimates of the number of youths in the cohort of 0–17-year-olds that would become adult smokers and the number of them that would die prematurely from smoking related diseases, Chaloupka estimated that 2.5 million premature deaths would have been averted by the $1.50 tax increase.

In the only study directly examining the link between cigarette taxes and smoking-related death rates, Moore (1996) provided similar evidence that higher cigarette taxes would be effective in reducing the toll wrought by tobacco use. Using annual state-level death rates from smoking-related diseases (lung cancer, heart disease, cardiovascular disease, and more), he estimated that a 10% increase in cigarette taxes would delay over 5,000 deaths each year.

Tobacco Taxes and Economic Efficiency

Over the past two decades, many of the economic costs associated with cigarette smoking have become clearer. Many of these costs are "internal" costs from the economist's perspective; that is, they are costs that the smoker bears directly. For example, most economists would consider the lost productivity resulting from smoking-related morbidity and mortality to be an internal cost, for it will be reflected in lost income for the smoker. Other costs, however, are "external" or social costs in that they reflect costs imposed by smokers on nonsmokers. Some of these external costs result from nonsmokers' exposure to environmental tobacco smoke. Others include the financial costs associated with nonsmokers' paying for the health care used to treat smoking-related illnesses. In addition, recent arguments suggest that some of the costs traditionally defined as internal that result from decisions made by youths in the presence of imperfect information about the health consequences and addictive nature of smoking could be considered external costs (i.e., Stiglitz 1994; Jha, Musgrove, Chaloupka, and Yurekli 2000).

In the presence of external costs, one notion of economic efficiency implies that individuals should bear the full costs of their consumption. That is, when one person's consumption imposes a cost on another (i.e., cigarette smokers exposing nonsmokers to environmental tobacco smoke), others are bearing part of the cost of that person's consumption. Pigou (1962) suggested that taxes could be used to improve economic efficiency in this situation. According to Pigou, the appropriate tax would raise the tobacco user's marginal cost of tobacco use to the point where it is equal to the marginal social cost (which includes the external costs) of tobacco use.

Estimating the social costs of tobacco use, however, is a complex and highly controversial subject. There is substantial and growing evidence that exposure to environmental tobacco smoke causes a number of health problems, including lung cancer, cardiovascular problems, and more. Similarly, there is strong evidence that maternal smoking during pregnancy and infancy leads to a number of short- and long-term health consequences for exposed children. However, many studies that attempt to estimate the social costs of smoking do not treat the costs resulting from ETS exposure among family members (i.e., nonsmoking spouses and children of smokers) as external costs (i.e., Manning Keeler, Newhouse, Sloss, and Wasserman 1991).

Similarly, there is clear evidence that cigarette smoking has raised total annual health care costs in the United States in recent years by as much as

10% or more (Warner, Hodgson, and Carroll 1999). However, it is also true that nonsmokers live longer than smokers, making it difficult to assess the lifetime impact of smoking on health care costs. Several studies, for example, suggest that lifetime health care costs of smokers are higher than those of nonsmokers (i.e., Manning et al. 1991; Hodgson 1992), yet others have concluded that there are no net cost differences or even that smokers' lifetime costs are lower (i.e, Leu and Schaub 1983; Barendregt, Bonneu, and Van Der Mass 1997). If smokers do impose greater net health care costs over their lifetimes, given that many of these costs are paid for publicly or through group health insurance plans, nonsmokers will bear some of the financial burden of smoking. Some analysts, however, question the appropriateness of counting the reduced health care costs of smokers that result from premature smoking-related death as a "benefit" in these calculations (i.e., Warner 2000). This same objection is raised to studies that count social security and private pension savings as "benefits" in the computation of net social costs.

With these different approaches to counting the costs and benefits of tobacco use, a wide range of estimates of the "optimal" tax on tobacco has been produced. Some estimates suggest that U.S. cigarette taxes are sufficient to or significantly exceed the level necessary to cover net social costs (i.e., Manning et al. 1991; Viscusi 1995). Others suggest that taxes fall well short of what would be needed to cover external costs (i.e., Hay 1991). Clearly, consensus is lacking about the "optimal" or economically efficient level of cigarette and other tobacco taxes. Given the difficult conceptual questions, need for detailed epidemiological and other data, the changing state of knowledge about the health consequences of tobacco use and ETS exposure, and shifting institutional arrangements, more research is clearly needed to determine the economically efficient levels of tobacco taxes.

4. Barriers to Tobacco Taxation

A number of objections are often raised to increases in tobacco taxes, almost always originating from the tobacco industry. As with the pricing and discounting strategies discussed, the internal tobacco industry documents uncovered during recent lawsuits provide interesting insight into the arguments the tobacco industry has used to oppose tax increases. For example, one internal document from the tobacco tax council (provided by K. Michael Cummings) outlines arguments opposing federal cigarette tax increases based on their impact on the macroeconomy, low-income smokers, inflation, and federal and state tax revenues; other documents emphasize the relationship between tax increases, cross-border shopping and smuggling, and tax revenues.

Tobacco Tax Increases and the Macroeconomy

Several tobacco industry–sponsored reports generated over the past two decades have attempted to describe the macroeconomic impact of tobacco growing, manufacturing, retailing, and more (i.e., Price Waterhouse 1992; American Economics Group 1996). These estimates are based on employment in the "core tobacco sector" that includes tobacco growing, manufacturing, and distribution, as well as the "supplier sector," which consists of the industries that produce and distribute intermediate goods used by the core (i.e., the goods and services used in producing tobacco products). In addition, these estimates include "expenditure-induced" effects that arise from incomes generated in the core and supplier sectors being spent on a variety of goods and services. In 1994, for example, the American Economics Group estimated that over 1.8 million jobs generating $53.4 billion in wages and benefits resulted from tobacco. Thus, the objection to tobacco tax increases is that the reduced consumption of tobacco products that would result would lead to significant job losses, reduced incomes, and lower income and other tax revenues.

However, as a number of analysts have pointed out, there is one key flaw in this argument. The argument assumes that the money spent on tobacco products would essentially evaporate. In reality, the money smokers would have otherwise spent on tobacco products will be spent on other goods and services, generating additional employment in the industries that produce and distribute them. In two careful analyses of these issues, Warner and his colleagues (Warner and Fulton 1994; Warner, Fulton, Nicholas, and Grimes 1996) examined the net impact of tobacco under various scenarios about reductions in tobacco use (on the Michigan economy and regional economies, respectively). Their estimates clearly show that, with the exception of the tobacco growing and manufacturing region, the elimination of tobacco products would lead to net increases in employment. The overall impact on the U.S. economy would be similarly positive. Studies from several other countries have reached a similar conclusion (see Jacobs, Gale, Capehart, Zhang, and Zha 2000) for a review of these studies).

The Regressivity of Tobacco Taxes

A second frequently voiced objection to tobacco tax increases is that they will fall disproportionately on the poor. Although U.S. tobacco taxes are relatively regressive (Congressional Budget Office 1990), with smoking prevalence higher among lower income groups, it is not necessarily true that tax increases would fall most heavily on the poor. As described, earlier, recent studies by the CDC (1998) and others indicate that the price responsiveness of cigarette demand will be greater among lower income persons. This implies that a given tax increase will have relatively little impact on cigarette smoking among high-income consumers but will lead to relatively large reductions among low-income consumers. Thus, the burden of the tax increase on high-income smokers will rise significantly, while that on the typical low-income smoker will rise by relatively less. Thus, the overall tax may be regressive, but a tax increase might actually reduce this regressivity.

Moreover, tobacco taxes are only one part of an overall system containing many tax and transfer programs. As the Congressional Budget Office (1990) staff described, increased progressivity of other taxes and increased transfer payments to low-income populations could easily offset the impact of a tobacco tax increase on low-income populations. They considered, for example, three changes that would have offset any regressivity—an increase in food stamp payments, an increase in the earned income tax credit, and a combination of the two (all of which would have cost significantly less than the new revenues generated by a tax increase). More recently, the World Bank (1999) suggested subsidizing nicotine replacement and other cessation therapies as an additional way to both offset any regressivity and further reduce smoking and its health consequences.

Tobacco Taxes and Inflation

The potentially inflationary impact of tobacco tax increases has also been used as an argument against higher tobacco taxes. In the United States, as in most countries, various price indices are based on the prices of a variety of goods and services, including tobacco products. Spending on many government programs and wage and salary increases in many labor contracts are tied to these price indices. Thus, opponents of tobacco tax increases have argued that they will lead to increases in consumer price indices, government spending on social security and other programs, and inflationary wage and salary increases. Although this argument is technically true, relatively modest tax increases would have almost no detectable impact on these indices.

One option that would eliminate any inflationary impact of tobacco tax increases would be the construction of multiple price indices used for different purposes. Existing price indices would continue to be updated for use in historical and international comparisons. Price indices that exclude tobacco products could be developed, however, for use in indexing wages and government spending on various programs tied to a price index. A number of other countries have developed these multiple price indices. France, Luxembourg, and Belgium, for example, exclude tobacco products from the index used for determining government spending on various social programs.

Tobacco Tax Increases, Government Revenues, and Smuggling

As discussed previously, given the low share of cigarette taxes in cigarette prices in the United States and given the relative inelasticity of cigarette demand, increases in cigarette taxes will generate significant increases in tax revenues. The tobacco industry and other opponents of tax increases, however, argue that increases in taxes will not generate substantial new revenues but rather can actually reduce existing revenues as cigarette smuggling increases and a black market in cigarettes develops. Although this is possible, it has not occurred in any state in the United States or in any developed countries where smuggling was perceived to be so problematic that tax rates were reduced (i.e., Canada and Sweden). In Canada, for example, total federal and provincial tax revenues fell by 25% in the year following the tax rollback when compared to the year prior to the tax cuts (when smuggling was at its peak) (Canadian Cancer Society et al. 1999).

Moreover, although it is true that interstate and international differences in cigarette taxes and prices do create incentives for cross-border shopping and smuggling, the actual level of smuggling has been significantly overstated. Several recent studies have examined this issue in the United States and elsewhere. Merriman, Yurekli, and Chaloupka (2000), for example, estimated that somewhere between 6 and 8.5% of cigarettes consumed globally are smuggled. Estimates for the United States, however, are generally lower. Thursby and Thursby (forthcoming), for example, estimate that cross-border shopping and wholesale smuggling account for 3 to 5% of annual U.S. cigarette consumption.

Similarly, although tax and price differentials do contribute to cigarette smuggling, they are far from the only factors and may not even be the most important. Joossens and his colleagues (Joossens and Raw 1995; Joossens and van der Merwe 1997), for example, suggest that the presence of an informal distribution network, nonexistent or weak policies concerning cigarette smuggling and their lack of enforcement, and other factors can be as important as price differences in generating cigarette smuggling. They note, for example, that there is little evidence of cigarette smuggling in high-priced European countries (such as France), yet there is extensive evidence of smuggling in those with relatively low prices (including Spain and Italy). Similarly, in their econometric analysis, Merriman, Yurekli, and Chaloupka (2000) find that the perceived level of transparency (lack of corruption) explains more of the variance in expert estimates of the magnitude of cigarette smuggling than do cigarette prices.

Finally, there is growing evidence that the tobacco companies themselves encourage and participate in cigarette smuggling. In Canada, for example, much of the black market trade was in Canadian cigarettes that had been exported to the United States and then smuggled back into Canada, given Canadian smokers' preferences for the blend of tobacco used in Canadian cigarettes (Sweanor and Martial 1994). Several investigations have led to convictions of tobacco companies and their executives, while other investigations continue (Canadian Cancer Society et al. 1999). Similar investigations and convictions have occurred elsewhere. Likewise, in the empirical application of their sophisticated theoretical model that allows some firms to smuggle a portion of the cigarettes they produce, Thursby and Thursby (forthcoming) estimate that industry-initiated smuggling accounts for a significant and growing portion of cigarette smuggling in the United States.

World Bank officials (1999) suggest that rather than foregoing tax increases because of any fears about smuggling, the more appropriate response is to take firm action against smuggling. They go on to suggest several measures that could be adopted to reduce smuggling, including prominent tax stamps, aggressive enforcement, and consistent application of severe penalties, and more.

Conclusions

Tobacco taxation has long been a key source of revenues for federal, state, and local governments. Given the growing evidence that higher cigarette and other tobacco taxes lead to significant reductions in tobacco use, particularly among younger, less educated, and lower income populations, increased taxes are now viewed as a very effective tool for improving public health. Some object that higher taxes would create more problems than they would address, but, upon closer examination, the arguments on which these objections are based are clearly overstated or inappropriate. The bottom line is that higher cigarette and other tobacco taxes are an effective and appropriate means for reducing the substantial health toll resulting from tobacco use.

REFERENCES

Ashenfelter, O., and D. Sullivan. 1987. Nonparametric tests of market structure: An application to the cigarette industry. *Journal of Industrial Economics* 35(4):483–98.

American Economics Group, Inc. 1996. *The U.S. Tobacco Industry in 1994: Its Economic Impact in the States.* Washington, D.C.: American Economics Group, Inc.

Barendregt, J. J., L. Bonneu, and P. J. Van Der Mass. 1997. The health care costs of smoking. *New England Journal of Medicine* 337:1052–7.

Barnett, P. G., T. E. Keeler, and T-W. Hu. 1995. Oligopoly structure and the incidence of cigarette excise taxes. *Journal of Public Economics* 57(3):457–70.

Barzel, Y. 1976. An alternative approach to the analysis of taxation. *Journal of Political Economy* 84(6):1177–97.

Becker, G. S., M. Grossman, and K. M. Murphy. 1994. An empirical analysis of cigarette addiction. *American Economic Review* 84(3):396–418.

Becker, G. S., and K. M. Murphy. 1988. A theory of rational addiction. *Journal of Political Economy* 96(4):675–700.

Bickel, W. K., and G. J. Madden. 1999. The behavioral economics of smoking. In *The Economic Analysis of Substance Use and Abuse: An Integration of Econometric and Behavioral Economic Research.* Edited by F. J. Chaloupka, M. Grossman, W. K. Bickel, and H. Saffer. Chicago: University of Chicago Press.

Bishop, J. A., and J. H. Yoo. 1985. "Health scare," excise taxes and advertising ban in the cigarette demand and supply. *Southern Economic Journal* 52(2):402–11.

British American Tobacco. 1994. *Tobacco Taxation Guide: A Guide to Alternative Methods of Taxing Cigarettes and Other Tobacco Products.* Woking, England: Optichrome Printing Group.

Bulow, J. I., and P. Pfleiderer. 1983. A note on the effect of cost changes on prices. *Journal of Political Economy* 91(1):182–5.

Canadian Cancer Society, Non-Smokers' Rights Association, Physicians for a Smoke-Free Canada, and Quebec Coalition for Tobacco Control. 1999. *Surveying the Damage: Cut-Rate Tobacco Products and Public Health in the 1990s.* Ottawa: Canadian Cancer Society, the Non-Smokers' Rights Association, and Physicians for a Smoke-Free Canada.

Centers for Disease Control and Prevention (CDC). 1996. Projected smoking related deaths among youth—United States. *Morbidity and Mortality Weekly Report* 45(44): 966–70.

———. 1998. Response to increases in cigarette prices by race/ethnicity, income, and age groups—United States, 1976–1993. *Morbidity and Mortality Weekly Report* 47(29):605–9.

Chaloupka, F. J. 1991. Rational addictive behavior and cigarette smoking. *Journal of Political Economy* 99(4):722–42.

Chaloupka, F. J. 1998. *The Impact of Proposed Cigarette Price Increases.* Policy Analysis No. 9, Health Sciences Analysis Project. Washington, D.C.: Advocacy Institute.

Chaloupka, F. J., and M. Grossman. 1996. *Price, Tobacco Control Policies and Youth Smoking.* National Bureau of Economic Research Working Paper No. 5740.

Chaloupka, F. J., T. W. Hu, K. E. Warner, R. Jacobs, and A. Yurekli. 2000. The taxation of tobacco products. In *Tobacco Control Policies in Developing Countries.* Edited by P. Jha and F. J. Chaloupka. Oxford: Oxford University Press.

Chaloupka, F. J., R. L. Pacula, M. C. Farrelly, L. D. Johnston, P. M. O'Malley, and J. W. Bray. 1999. *Do Higher Cigarette Prices Encourage Youth to Use Marijuana?* National Bureau of Economic Research Working Paper Number 6939.

Chaloupka, F. J., and S. Slater. 1999. *Tobacco Industry Promotions and State Tobacco Control Efforts.* Working Paper. University of Illinois at Chicago Health Research and Policy Centers.

Chaloupka, F. J., S. Slater, and M. Wakefield. 1999. USA: Price cuts and point of sale ads follow tax rise. *Tobacco Control: An International Journal* 8(3):242.

Chaloupka, F. J., J. A. Tauras, M. Grossman, and P. Jha. 2000. The economics of addiction. In *Tobacco Control Policies in Developing Countries*. Edited by P. Jha and F. J. Chaloupka. Oxford: Oxford University Press.

Chaloupka, F. J., and K. E. Warner. 2000. The economics of smoking. In *The Handbook of Health Economics*. Edited by A. J. Culyer and J. P. Newhouse. New York: North-Holland.

Chaloupka, F. J., and H. Wechsler. 1997. Price, tobacco control policies and smoking among young adults. *Journal of Health Economics* 16(3):359–73.

Chapman, S., and J. Richardson. 1990. Tobacco excise and declining consumption: The case of Papua New Guinea. *American Journal of Public Health* 80(5):537–40.

Congressional Budget Office. 1990. *Federal Taxation of Tobacco, Alcoholic Beverages, and Motor Fuels*. Washington, D.C.: U.S. Government Printing Office.

DeCicca, P., D. Kenkel, and A. Mathios. 1999. *Putting out the Fires: Will Higher Cigarette Taxes Reduce Youth Smoking*. Working Paper. Department of Policy Analysis and Management, Cornell University.

Dee, T. S., and W. N. Evans. 1998. *A Comment on DeCicca, Kenkel, and Mathios*. Working Paper. School of Economics, Georgia Institute of Technology.

Douglas, S. 1998. The duration of the smoking habit. *Economic Inquiry* 36(1):49–64.

Douglas, S., and G. Hariharan. 1994. The hazard of starting smoking: Estimates from a split population duration model. *Journal of Health Economics* 13(2):213–30.

Evans, W. N., and M. C. Farrelly. 1998. The compensating behavior of smokers: Taxes, tar and nicotine. *RAND Journal of Economics* 29(3):578–95.

Evans, W. N., and L. X. Huang. 1998. *Cigarette Taxes and Teen Smoking: New Evidence from Panels of Repeated Cross-Sections*. Working Paper. Department of Economics, University of Maryland.

Farrelly, M. C., J. W. Bray, G. A. Zarkin, B. W. Wendling, and R. L. Pacula. 1999. *The Effects of Prices and Policies on the Demand for Marijuana: Evidence from the National Household Surveys on Drug Abuse*. National Bureau of Economic Research Working Paper Number 6940.

Federal Trade Commission (FTC). 1997. *Competition and the Financial Impact of the Proposed Tobacco Industry Settlement*. Washington, D.C.: Federal Trade Commission, Bureaus of Economics, Competition, and Consumer Protection.

———. 1998. *Report to Congress for 1996 Pursuant to the Federal Cigarette Labeling and Advertising Act*. Washington, D.C.: Federal Trade Commission.

General Accounting Office. 1989. *Teenage Smoking: Higher Excise Tax Should Significantly Reduce the Number of Smokers*. Washington, D.C.: General Accounting Office.

Grossman, M., and F. J. Chaloupka. 1997. Cigarette taxes: The straw to break the camel's back. *Public Health Reports* 112(4):290–7.

Harris, J. E. 1987. The 1983 increase in the federal cigarette excise tax. In *Tax Policy and the Economy*. Vol. 1. Edited by L. H. Summers. Cambridge, Mass.: MIT Press.

Hay, J. W. 1991. The harm they do to others: A primer on the external costs of drug abuse. In *Searching for Alternatives: Drug-Control Policy in the United States*. Edited by M. B. Krauss and E. P. Lazear. Stanford: Hoover Institution Press.

Hodgson, T. A. 1992. Cigarette smoking and lifetime medical expenditures. *Millbank Quarterly*70:81–125.

Jacobs, R., H. F. Gale, T. C. Capeheart, P. Zhang, and P. Zha. 2000. The supply-side effects of tobacco-control policies. In *Tobacco Control Policies in Developing Countries*. Edited by P. Jha and F. J. Chaloupka. Oxford: Oxford University Press.

Jha, P., P. Musgrove, F. J. Chaloupka, and A. Yurekli. 2000. The economic rationale for government intervention in tobacco markets. In *Tobacco Control Policies in Developing Countries*. Edited by P. Jha and F. J. Chaloupka. Oxford: Oxford University Press.

Johnson, T. R. 1978. Additional evidence on the effects of alternative taxes on cigarette prices. *Journal of Political Economy* 86:325–8.

Joossens, L., and M. Raw. 1995. Smuggling and cross-border shopping of tobacco in Europe. *British Medical Journal* 310:1393–7.

Joossens, L., and R. van der Merwe. 1997. *Cigarette Trade and Smuggling: Project Update #7*. The Economics of Tobacco Control Project, Cape Town, South Africa.

Keeler, T. E., T-W. Hu, P. G. Barnett, and W. G. Manning. 1993. Taxation, regulation and addiction: A demand function for cigarettes based on time-series evidence. *Journal of Health Economics* 12(1):1–18.

Keeler, T. E., T. W. Hu, P. G. Barnett, W. G. Manning, and H. Y. Sung. 1996. Do cigarette producers price-discriminate by state? An empirical analysis of local cigarette pricing and taxation. *Journal of Health Economics* 15:499–512.

Leu, R. E. 1984. Anti-smoking publicity, taxation, and the demand for cigarettes. *Journal of Health Economics* 3(2):101–16.

Leu, R. E., and T. Schaub. 1983. Does smoking increase medical expenditures? *Social Science and Medicine* 17:1907–14.

Lewit, E. M., and D. Coate. 1982. The potential for using excise taxes to reduce smoking. *Journal of Health Economics* 1(2):121–45.

Lewit, E. M., D. Coate, and M. Grossman. 1981. The effects of government regulation on teenage smoking. *Journal of Law and Economics* 24(3):545–69.

Lewit, E. M., A. Hyland, N. Kerrebrock, and K. M. Cummings. 1997. Price, public policy and smoking in young people. *Tobacco Control* 6(S2):17–24.

Manning, W. G., E. B. Keeler, J. P. Newhouse, E. M. Sloss, and J. Wasserman. 1991. *The Costs of Poor Health Habits*. Cambridge, Mass.: Harvard University Press.

Mao, Z. Z., and J. L. Xiang. 1997. Demand for cigarettes and factors affecting the demand: A cross-sectional survey. *Chinese Health Care Industry Management* (in Chinese) 5:227–9.

Mao, Z. Z., J. L. Xiang, and Z. P. Kon. 1997. Demand for cigarette and pricing policy. *Chinese Health Economics* (in Chinese) 16(6):50–2.

Maranvanyika, E. 1998. The search for an optimal tobacco control policy in Zimbabwe. In *The Economics of Tobacco Control: Towards an Optimal Policy Mix*. Edited by I. Abedian, R. van der Merwe, N. Wilkins, and P. Jha. Cape Town, South Africa: Applied Fiscal Reseach Centre, University of Cape Town.

Merriman, D. 1994. Do cigarette excise tax rates maximize revenue? *Economic Inquiry* 32(3):419–28.

Merriman, D., A. Yurekli, and F. J. Chaloupka. 2000. How big is the worldwide smuggling problem? In *Tobacco Control Policies in Developing Countries*. Edited by P. Jha and F. J. Chaloupka. Oxford: Oxford University Press.

Moore, M. J. 1996. Death and tobacco taxes. *RAND Journal of Economics* 27(2):415–28.

Moyer, D. B. 1998. *The Tobacco Almanac: A Reference Book of Facts, Figures and Quotations About Tobacco.* Washington, D.C.: U.S. Government Printing Office.

Mullahy, J. 1985. Cigarette smoking: Habits, health concerns, and heterogeneous unobservables in a micro-econometric analysis of consumer demand. Ph.D. diss., University of Virginia.

Ohsfeldt, R. L., and R. G. Boyle. 1994. Tobacco excise taxes and rates of smokeless tobacco use in the US: An exploratory ecological analysis. *Tobacco Control* 3(4): 316–23.

Ohsfeldt, R. L., R. G. Boyle, and E. I. Capilouto. 1997. Effects of tobacco excise taxes on the use of smokeless tobacco products. *Health Economics* 6(5):525–32.

———. 1999. Tobacco taxes, smoking restrictions, and tobacco use. In *The Economic Analysis of Substance Use and Abuse: An Integration of Econometric and Behavioral Economic Research.* Edited by F. J. Chaloupka, M. Grossman, W. K. Bickel, and H. Saffer. Chicago: University of Chicago Press.

Pekurinen, M. 1989. The demand for tobacco products in Finland. *British Journal of Addiction* 84:1183–92.

Pekurinen, M. 1991. *Economic Aspects of Smoking: Is There a Case for Government Intervention in Finland?* Helsinki: Vapk-Publishing.

Pigou, A. C. 1962. *A Study in Public Finance.* 3d rev. ed. London: Macmillan.

Price Waterhouse. 1992. *The Economic Impact of the Tobacco Industry in the United States in 1990.* Arlington: Price Waterhouse.

Ramsey, F. P. 1927. A contribution to the theory of taxation. *Economic Journal* 37:47–61.

Sobel, R. S., and T. A. Garrett. 1997. Taxation and product quality: New evidence from generic cigarettes. *Journal of Political Economy* 105(4):880–7.

Stiglitz, J. E. 1994. *Wither Socialism?* Cambridge, Mass.: MIT Press.

Sullivan, D. 1985. Testing hypotheses about firm behavior in the cigarette industry. *Journal of Political Economy* 93(3):586–98.

Sumner, D. A. 1981. Measurement of monopoly behavior: An application to the cigarette industry. *Journal of Political Economy* 89(5):1010–9.

Sumner, D. A., and M. K. Wohlgenant. 1985. Effects of an increase in the federal excise tax on cigarettes. *American Journal of Agricultural Economics* 67(2):235–42.

Sumner, M. T., and R. Ward. 1981. Tax changes and cigarette prices. *Journal of Political Economy* 89(6):1261–5.

Sung, H-Y., T-W. Hu, and T. E. Keeler. 1994. Cigarette taxation and demand: An empirical model. *Contemporary Economic Policy* 12(3):91–100.

Sunley, E. M. 1998. *The Design and Administration of Alcohol, Tobacco and Petroleum Excises: A Guide for Developing and Transition Countries.* Working Paper. Fiscal Affairs Department, International Monetary Fund.

Sweanor, D. T., and L. R. Martial. 1994. *Smuggling of Tobacco Products: Lessons from Canada.* Ottawa: Non-Smokers' Rights Association/Smoking and Health Action Foundation.

Tauras, J. A. 1999. *The Transition to Smoking Cessation: Evidence from Multiple Failure Duration Analysis.* Working Paper. Department of Health Management and Policy, University of Michigan.

Tauras, J. A., and F. J. Chaloupka. Forthcoming. Determinants of smoking cessation: An analysis of young adult men and women. In *The Economic Analysis of Substance*

Use and Abuse: The Experiences of Developed Countries and Lessons for Developing Countries. Edited by M. Grossman and C. R. Hsieh. United Kingdom: Edward Elgar Limited.

————. 1999. *Price, Clean Indoor Air Laws, and Cigarette Smoking: Evidence from Longitudinal Data for Young Adults.* National Bureau of Economic Research Working Paper Number 6937.

Thompson, M. E., and I. McLeod. 1976. The effects of economic variables upon the demand for cigarettes in Canada. *Mathematical Scientist* 1:121–32.

Thursby, J. G., and M. C. Thursby. Forthcoming. Interstate cigarette bootlegging: Extent, revenue losses, and effects of federal intervention. *National Tax Journal.*

Tobacco Institute. 1999. *The Tax Burden on Tobacco.* Washington, D.C.: The Tobacco Institute.

Townsend, J. L. 1998. The role of taxation policy in tobacco control. In *The Economics of Tobacco Control: Towards an Optimal Policy Mix.* Edited by I. Abedian, R. van der Merwe, N. Wilkins, and P. Jha. Cape Town, South Africa: Applied Fiscal Reseach Centre, University of Cape Town.

Townsend, J. L., P. Roderick, and J. Cooper. 1994. Cigarette smoking by socioeconomic group, sex, and age: Effects of price, income, and health publicity. *British Medical Journal* 309(6959):923–6.

van der Merwe, R. 1998. The economics of tobacco control in South Africa. In *The Economics of Tobacco Control: Towards an Optimal Policy Mix.* Edited by I. Abedian, R. van der Merwe, N. Wilkins, and P. Jha. Cape Town, South Africa: Applied Fiscal Reseach Centre, University of Cape Town.

Viscusi, W. K. 1995. Cigarette taxation and the social consequences of smoking. In *Tax Policy and the Economy.* Edited by J. M. Poterba. Cambridge, Mass.: MIT Press.

Warner, K. E. 1986. Smoking and health implications of a change in the federal cigarette excise tax. *Journal of the American Medical Association* 255(8):1028–32.

————. 2000. *The Economics of Tobacco: Myths and Realities.* Working Paper. Department of Health Management and Policy, University of Michigan.

Warner, K. E., and G. A. Fulton. 1994. The economic implications of tobacco product sales in a nontobacco state. *JAMA* 271(10):771–6.

Warner, K. E., G. A. Fulton, P. Nicolas, and D. R. Grimes. 1996. Employment implications of decline tobacco product sales for the regional economies of the United States. *JAMA* 275:1241–6.

Warner, K. E., T. A. Hodgson, and C. E. Carroll. 1999. Medical costs of smoking in the United States: Estimates, their validity, and their implications. *Tobacco Control* 8(3):290–300.

Wasserman, J., W. G. Manning, J. P. Newhouse, and J. D. Winkler. 1991. The effects of excise taxes and regulations on cigarette smoking. *Journal of Health Economics* 10(1):43–64.

World Bank. 1999. *Curbing the Epidemic: Governments and the Economics of Tobacco Control.* Washington, D.C.: The World Bank.

Xu, X., T-W. Hu, and T. E. Keeler. 1998. *Optimal Cigarette Taxation: Theory and Estimation.* Working Paper. Department of Economics, University of California, Berkeley.

4

Marketing Policies

John Slade

The subject of this chapter is tobacco product marketing. Public health efforts seek to reduce illness and death through prevention and treatment (USDHHS 2000). The intermediate goals for accomplishing this include reducing new use of tobacco products, reducing use among current users, and, perhaps, helping those who use tobacco to continue in less dangerous ways (Warner, Slade, and Sweanor 1997; Bolliger et al. 2000). Controlling the industry's marketing of tobacco products and sponsoring public health messages (countermarketing) have become two important tools in this effort.

This chapter uses the term "marketing" to mean advertising and promotion, which is a large part of the tobacco enterprise. The five largest U.S. cigarette makers spent $8.24 billion for these purposes in 1999 (FTC 2001). A pack of Marlboro costs $0.16 to make (half of this is for the tobacco), yet marketing costs for that pack in the United States are $0.55 (Newman 1999).

The chapter is organized into five main sections. The first explores some of the perspectives from which discussions of tobacco product marketing take place. The second examines the question of whether advertising and promotion for tobacco products actually work. There is a brief review of the history of tobacco advertising and promotion over the past 50 years in the United States and then a summary of current advertising practices. The final main section describes a range of opportunities for public health advances in this area.

1. Perspectives

At Philip Morris International, we are committed to marketing cigarettes responsibly. We do not market cigarettes to minors, and we firmly believe that cigarettes should be consumed only by informed adults who have chosen to smoke.

(Philip Morris International 2000a)

The cigarette makers often talk about people making a "decision" to smoke and about needing to be able to provide continued service to "adults who choose to smoke." For an activity that is so often an addiction (USDHHS 1988; Royal College of Physicians 2000), these are very peculiar words.[1]

The R. J. Reynolds (RJR) Tobacco Company used to publish a glossy "smokers-rights" newsletter titled *Choice*. A cover photo on one issue showed people outside an office building in what appeared to be sleet and freezing rain (R. J. Reynolds 1991). They were miserably huddled together against the cold and wet, smoking. Although the photo was intended as a comment on the discourtesy shown by the building owner toward some office workers, it was not, of course, a picture of social smoking. Instead, it was a powerful illustration of drug addiction.

The essence of addiction is a loss of choice, an undermining of free will, a loss of control over use.[2] Although this loss of control is not absolute and unchanging, it is a powerful force. Nearly three-quarters of people who smoke do not want to do so (USDHHS 2000). They want to quit but find this difficult to do. The tobacco manufacturers face the unpleasant reality that most of their customers do not want to be their customers. The language of choice creates a veneer of autonomy and helps hide the underlying, unpleasant reality of addiction. The individual smoker might overcome the addiction, but this complex and highly uncertain phenomenon is not clearly communicated by the unadorned word "choice."

Initiation to tobacco use results from a complex interaction of forces, including tobacco product marketing and design. Speaking of initiation as a matter of choice and of personal decision making puts the spotlight on the individual and markedly diminishes the roles of other players. It especially leaves the tobacco product maker with no assigned role in the drama. This is a false image. A more apt image is that the process of initiation to tobacco is a seduction, one that usually occurs during late childhood or adolescence. Even though this process is similar to that which leads people to try out a wide variety of consumer goods, rarely are those goods addictive and even more rarely are they as hazardous as cigarettes are. Similarly, continuing to smoke is poorly characterized as simply a matter of choice. Tobacco manufacturers actively entice their (usually addicted) customers to keep smoking by skillful manipulation.

As discussed in the following sections, communication between tobacco product makers and the public is almost entirely conducted at an emotional level through brand imagery. This communication is contrary to basic principles of informed consent and consumer protection.

Perceptions of Risk

Viscusi (1992) has observed that when smokers are asked about how many cancers cigarettes will eventually cause in 100 smokers, they overestimate the actual risks. He has developed this observation into an elaborate rationale that leads him to conclude that smokers know the risks and that they continue to smoke anyway, although fully informed.

Although Viscusi's theory is superficially appealing, other data lead to different conclusions. Among current adult smokers, only 29% believed that they had a higher-than-average risk of having a heart attack, and only 40% believed that their risk of getting cancer was higher than average (Ayanian and Cleary 1999). Even if a person believes in the abstract that smoking is a cause of serious illness, it is quite another thing to feel personally vulnerable to this risk.

Slovic (2000a, 2000b) has presented a cogent critique of Viscusi's argument. First, Viscusi's analysis overlooks the need for the individual to know about the nature and severity of the consequences and not merely the chance that they will occur. For instance, in Ontario, only 43% of smokers thought that the risk of death from lung cancer was as high as 50% (it is actually over 80%) (Sweanor 2000).

Second, optimism bias overshadows a person's general understanding of risk. People do not see themselves at as great a risk as others are. Slovic points out that the risks from cigarettes are cumulative over a relatively long period of time. A person might understand an individual cigarette to confer no discernable risk whatsoever and privately believe that he or she will quit smoking in a few months or years. This means that a person's day-to-day smoking can easily be privately regarded as of little or no harm, as virtually safe when, in fact, the exposure will be longer than anticipated because of addiction. Adolescents markedly overestimate their ability to stop smoking. Among high school seniors who were smoking one or more cigarettes per day when asked, as high school seniors, whether they would not be smoking in five years, the actual rate of not smoking was half that which had been predicted (USDHHS 1994).

Furthermore, nearly 80% of people who smoke recall considering health issues "not at all" when they began to smoke (Slovic, in press), and people who smoke rank cigarettes much lower on a list of hazards than do people who do not smoke (e.g., BATCo 1988).

In short, whereas Viscusi paints a picture of people making careful decisions about smoking as a rational economist might, Slovic (in press) shows that people do not, in the main, function this way. Most who smoke regret having started and want to quit (USDHHS 2000).

Informed Consent

Beginning in October 1999, Philip Morris USA, the leading domestic cigarette maker, began promoting a Website that set forth the company's perspective on a wide range of issues (Philip Morris USA 1999). Among other things, Philip Morris said:

> *Cigarette Smoking and Disease in Smokers*: There is an overwhelming medical and scientific consensus that cigarette smoking causes lung cancer, heart disease, emphysema and other serious diseases in smokers. Smokers are far more likely to develop serious diseases, like lung cancer, than non-smokers. There is no "safe" cigarette. These are and have been the messages of public health authorities worldwide. Smokers and potential smokers should rely on these messages in making all smoking-related decisions.

A number of influential observers, including *The New York Times* (2000), regarded these sentences as an admission on the part of Philip Morris that cigarettes caused disease. This perception was understandable, yet it was incorrect.

The company's 10-K filing with the Securities and Exchange Commission for 1999 noted:

> On the issues of the role played by cigarette smoking in the development of lung cancer and other diseases in smokers, and whether nicotine, as found in cigarette smoke, is addictive, the Company [has] stated that despite the differences that may exist between its views and those of the public health community, it would, in order to ensure that there will be a single, consistent public health message on these issues, refrain from debating the issues other than as necessary to defend itself and its opinions in the courts and other forums in which it is required to do so. (Philip Morris Companies 2000, 6)[3]

In short, the Philip Morris Website merely conveyed the views of scientists and public health officials, not the views of the company. Moreover, even though the company said that consumers should "rely" on this scientific consensus, the company made no comment about whether Philip Morris would rely on this consensus in advertising and promoting its tobacco products.[4] But from an examination of the character and the content of the marketing programs of the major U.S. tobacco companies, it is obvious that none of them relies on the scientific consensus about smoking and disease in designing these campaigns.

In connection with a presentation in 2000 to the World Health Organization on the Framework Convention on Tobacco Control, the company modified its position a bit. The Website now says that the company agrees with the scientific consensus. This supposed agreement has not, however, led to any change in its marketing practices.

The companies take no responsibility for helping consumers understand the dangers of cigarette use beyond what governments require them to do. This behavior stands in contrast to what one higher court has laid out as an appropriate standard for informed consent:

> A manufacturer of a product has a duty to warn consumers of the dangers inherent in the use of its product, of which it knows or has reason to know. The warning must be adequate. It should be communicated clearly and understandably in a manner calculated to inform the user of the nature of the risk and the extent of the danger; it should be in terms commensurate with the gravity of the potential hazard, and *it should not be neutralized or negated by collateral efforts on the part of the manufacturer.*[5] (emphasis added)

To the contrary: the tobacco companies engage in an $8.2 billion annual effort designed to neutralize or negate the warnings issued by others or required on their packaging and advertising by government. Moreover, the tobacco companies have sought to neutralize public concerns about cigarettes with products that have the appearance of safety, such as filtered cigarettes and so-called low tar brands (Slade 1989).

The Nature of Tobacco Product Advertising

Tobacco presents such great difficulties for public health largely because its use became embedded in the culture long before the full extent of its danger was clearly recognized. Although it is inconceivable that government would permit the new introduction of a product known beforehand to be as addictive and deadly as the cigarette, it is also unlikely that the cigarette will ever be banned. Despite its enormous hazard, tobacco is still treated in the marketplace more like candy or soda pop than like cyanide or morphine. Advertising for tobacco products resembles that for many consumer goods, and this contributes to the harm these products cause.

Tobacco product advertising is largely about brands. As Pollay (1998) has pointed out, the products themselves are nearly identical. Not only does branding permit differentiation, it lets marketers infuse products with characteristics they can talk about besides the unpleasant, intrinsic ones of addiction, illness, and death.

A key part of branding is the association of each brand with specific images and fantasies, which in turn are keyed to be appealing at an emotional level to the targeted consumers. Mere familiarity through repetition (Bornstein 1989) and associations of products with positive images (Winkielman, Zajonc, and Schwarz 1997) are two techniques that work at the affective level to condition responses to products. Far from being the rational offering of product information that the tobacco marketers would have us believe it to be, tobacco product marketing is designed to be manipulative, seductive, and enticing.

Brand images are often presented with enough richness that fantasies can be created about the characters in the ads: The Marlboro man, Virginia Slims women, Joe Camel. Stories, images, and fragments of real life are each more powerful influences on people than statistics (Hendickx, Vlek, and Oppewal 1989), so such presentations can directly undermine the impact of dry numbers (or dry words in the boxed warning) about harm from tobacco.

The importance of the brand, and the interaction of advertising with product development, is illustrated by the impact of Virginia Slims when it was introduced in 1967. This newly created brand gave Philip Morris an opportunity to fashion advertising aimed at women with a product whose very name and design (each cigarette has a relatively small circumference) allude to the weight-control properties of cigarettes (USDHHS 1988).[6]

Pierce and his colleagues used the National Health Interview Surveys to examine age of initiation to smoking for men and women (Pierce, Lee, and Gilpin 1994). They constructed time series by gender and age group from 1944 through 1988 and calculated sex-age-year initiation rates. There were marked downward trends for smoking initiation among males over this time period. Among females, smoking initiation surged abruptly beginning in 1967 among girls younger than 18 years, whereas there were no large changes for older women. This effect was much more pronounced among girls who later did not attend college. This study provides strong evidence that the introduction of Virginia Slims (and its imitators, such as Eve and Silva Thins) led to a marked increase in the uptake of smoking by adolescent girls.

In this example, Philip Morris did not even need to recruit the new customers to use Virginia Slims itself for the product to be a success. Because Philip Morris also sells Marlboro, the leading brand among novice smokers, the company is likely to be indifferent about whether the person who learns about the weight-control properties of smoking from Virginia Slims advertising uses that brand or Marlboro. The main advantage of the Virginia Slims campaign, then, could be that it provides a way for Philip Morris to communicate with girls about specific attributes of cigarettes that it cannot fit into the Marlboro brand image and so cannot talk about in advertising for Marlboro.

Initiation   Peer influence is an important predisposing factor for the uptake of tobacco use (USDHHS 1994). This is frequently talked about in terms of "peer pressure," but this term falsely colors what takes place. The term "peer pressure" has a pejorative, pathological quality about it, as though a person's friends were responsible for his or her taking up smoking. Peer influences are normal processes that occur around thousands of aspects of daily life. In marketing terms, they are referred to as "word of mouth." Marketers regularly seek to influence word of mouth, to help their products catch the buzz (Ellison 2000). The marketing of tobacco products frequently features that seem focused on facilitating word of mouth.

Continuation, Relapse   For people who already smoke, tobacco product makers try to create an inviting and diversionary environment. They offer innumerable rewards for smoking, including discount coupons, merchandise, sweepstakes, and opportunities to participate in sporting events. Thus, much of the marketing activity, especially that which occurs via direct mail, has the character of relationship marketing. The product itself is perhaps secondary to the emotional bond, the interaction between the consumer and the image that the company projects about the brand. The products themselves are more widely distributed than milk, bread, or gasoline, making it easy to forget one's promise to oneself about not buying another pack.

2. Tobacco Product Advertising and Promotion Are Effective

Advertising for tobacco products increases consumption (Saffer and Chaloupka 1999). A comprehensive advertising ban lowers consumption, but limits on advertising, short of a ban across numerous media, have little or no effect. For the most part, studies concluding that advertising for these products does not affect consumption (e.g., Duffy 1996) approach the issue from a perspective that cannot find the effect that exists.[7]

Most of the negative studies measure advertising by annual or quarterly national expenditures (Saffer and Chaloupka 1999). At this gross level of analysis, the data are so highly aggregated that the variations resulting from advertising activity average out and cannot be readily distinguished. Studies that measure advertising in a more fine-grained fashion, on a regional basis and utilizing shorter periods for measurement, more likely identify positive effects of advertising.[8]

An alternative approach is to examine the effects of national advertising bans on tobacco use. A study by Hamilton (1975) of advertising restrictions in 11 countries in the Organization for Economic Cooperation and Development (OECD) from 1948 to 1973 found no reduction in tobacco use in association with advertising bans. In contrast, Laugesen and Meads (1991) found an effect when the data set examined was expanded to 22 OECD countries and the time frame shifted to the 1960–1986 period.

Saffer and Chaloupka (1999) built on these prior studies. They examined the pattern of tobacco consumption in comparison with the number of media from which cigarette advertising had been banned in 22 OECD countries for the 1970–1992 period. They found that if tobacco advertising had been banned from only a few types of media (for instance, from television and radio), there was no measurable benefit, yet if the ban extended to additional media (such as newspapers, magazines, outdoor and transit advertising), there was a significant relationship between the ban and reduced tobacco consumption. In their analysis, an extensive advertising ban, one that markedly reduced the availability of alternative media in which advertising could continue, reduced consumption by 6.3% over a period of 6 years. This is a potent intervention, for the effect would continue to influence consumption over time because it alters the dynamic of entry into and exit from the market.

Just as it is possible to increase tobacco use by promoting tobacco products, it is also possible to reduce tobacco use by employing media messages that encourage quitting or not starting. Counteradvertising, efforts by government or voluntary health agencies to reduce tobacco product use through advertising, can be effective at reducing consumption (Saffer and Chaloupka 1999). This effect has been observed in the United States in the late 1960s in association with counteradvertising on television under the "Fairness Doctrine," as well as in connection with advertising sponsored by tobacco control programs in California and Massachusetts in recent years. It has also been observed in a number of European countries and in Australia and Israel.

What Advertising Does

Tobacco product advertising is mainly about product image, its potential role in a person's lifestyle, its "personality" (Pollay 1998; Saffer and Chaloupka 1999).[9]

> Cigarette advertising is primarily designed to create various fantasies of sophistication, pleasure, social success, independence or ruggedness. These attributes become the product personality which advertisers expect will appeal to specific consumers. For a relatively small expenditure on tobacco, the consumer psychologically connects to the fantasy lifestyle and personality characteristics portrayed in the advertising. This process can induce individuals, who are not smokers, to try the product, for those who are smokers, to smoke more, for those who might have quit, to continue and for those who have quit, to start again. (Saffer and Chaloupka 1999, 2)

Branding is an essential part of tobacco product marketing. With the creation of brands, it is possible to segment the market and so increase sales by making appeals to particular subgroups within the entire market (Simonich 1991). These segments can be defined by region, demographics, behavior, psychographics, or combinations of these factors. Branding is the process of creating products that are distinguishable and appealing to different target groups by their product design, packaging, and marketing. There may be individual brands or, as is common in the tobacco business, brand families with a dozen or more variations on the core brand (e.g., Marlboro). More than 1,200 distinct varieties of cigarette brands were sold in the United States in 1997 (FTC 1999).[10]

The marketing of tobacco products features "images and art, not logic and copy" (Pollay 1998). Speaking of the images in an advertisement for Marlboro shortly after the brand had been repositioned from an unfiltered cigarette for women to a filtered cigarette for men, Martineau (1957) commented, "They [the visuals] are emotional supports which . . . make smoking seem reasonable, justifiable, and highly desirable. They obviously cannot be thrown in people's faces in their bare essence: but when they are implied, when they are communicated, they are understandable and satisfying" (18).

An analysis of internal advertising agency documents in the United Kingdom has shown that advertising agencies working for cigarette companies behave as though they believe that advertising increases consumption (Hastings and MacFadyen 2000). Internal agency documents occasionally voice concern that people might give up smoking and point to low tar cigarettes as an alternative to quitting. Moreover, the agencies realize that image is the key to promoting smoking among young people: they view smoking as a "rite of passage" and recognize that the young are seeking "an identity." Similarly, an examination of internal tobacco industry documents in Canada has shown that tobacco product marketing frequently involves appeals to "starters" (young people) and to "concerned smokers" (those with health concerns who want to quit) (Pollay 2000).

Even though the use of image-based advertising that contains little specific information is not unusual in advertising for other consumer goods, tobacco products are not ordinary consumer goods. Tobacco products are unreasonably dangerous, and they are unregulated. Moreover, the consumers of these products are usually addicted, concerned about their health, and desirous of quitting.

A number of specific direct and indirect effects of tobacco product marketing have been proposed as mechanisms by which this activity produces its beneficial effects for this singular industry (USDHHS 1989). The direct effects are these:

- Facilitating initial experimentation and uptake of tobacco use by young people
- Serving as a cue for consumption among current users by reinforcing the desirability of smoking and providing an economic incentive to smoke through promotions
- Reducing motivation to quit by allaying health concerns and, through such mechanisms as couponing, reducing the monetary cost of smoking
- Encouraging those who have stopped to resume

The indirect effects are these:

- Discouraging criticism of the tobacco industry in the media by creating financial dependence through the purchase of advertising space for tobacco products and for products other corporate divisions may produce, such as foodstuffs
- Fostering active support for the company through good works in philanthropy
- Creating and sustaining a general environment that is favorable to tobacco products and their makers, promoting the general acceptability of these products despite their capacity to injure and kill both users and nonusers

The evidence supporting the validity of these effects has grown stronger since these were catalogued in 1989, both with empirical studies and with the recent availability of inside information from tobacco company documents (Glantz, Slade, Bero, Hanaver, and Barnes 1996; Hurt and Robertson 1998).[11] However, the bulk of work in this area has focused on the effect of marketing tobacco products on novices and on the appeal of so-called light cigarettes to smokers concerned about their health.

Tobacco Marketing Helps Recruit New Smokers

The Food and Drug Administration documented an intent and effect of advertising for cigarettes in its proposed assertion of jurisdiction over these products and its proposed rule.[12] In a summary statement, the agency commented:

[T]he preponderance of quantitative and qualitative studies of cigarette advertising suggests: (1) A causal relationship between advertising and youth smoking behavior, and (2) a positive effect of stringent advertising measures on smoking rates and on youth smoking. Moreover, industry statements indicate the importance of the youth market segment to the industry's continued success. Actions taken by industry members to attract young smokers have also resulted in attracting children and adolescents. Finally, examples of specific campaigns directed at young people support the hypothesis that cigarette advertising and promotion play an important role in encouraging young people to start smoking, to sustain their smoking habit, and to increase consumption. Therefore, the agency finds that stringent restrictions on advertising are essential if smoking by adolescents is to be reduced.[13]

The proposed rule generated more than 300,000 comments to the agency, more than the agency has ever received for any other regulatory action. The agency's analysis of these comments only confirmed its earlier conclusions about tobacco product advertising and the young.[14]

Among the more recent studies of cigarette advertising and young people, several have documented that young people, to a far greater extent than adults, smoke the most heavily advertised brands (Pollay et al. 1996), and there is an especially strong relationship between brand advertising in magazines with high youth readership and the use of these brands preferentially by young people (King, Siegel, Celebrucki, and Connolly 1998; King and Siegel 1999). This relationship also holds for advertising patterns in magazines read by African American youths and the choice of brands in this market segment (King, Siegel, and Pucci 2000).

Sports sponsorship, to which the cigarette companies turned in a major way following the broadcast ad ban (Kluger 1996), influences children's experimentation with cigarettes (Vaidya, Naik, and Vaidya 1996).

Promotional activities have always been part of tobacco product marketing, but there was a marked increase in the distribution of promotional items for tobacco products in the late 1980s and early 1990s. The effects of this phenomenon on the uptake of cigarettes by the young could be readily measured by survey techniques, for it is relatively easy to ascertain, for instance, whether a respondent has or does not have any of these items. Several studies have documented the association of promotional items and tobacco use by young people (Coeytaux, Altman, and Slade 1995; Pierce, Choi, Gilpin, Farkas, and Berry 1998; Sargent, Dalton, and Beach 2000) and have shown that participation in promotional activities by nonsmoking youths is highly associated with a person's susceptibility to smoke (Altman, Levine, Coeytaux, Slade, and Jaffe 1996; Pierce et al. 1998). Biener and Siegel have shown that involvement with tobacco product promotions and advertising "precedes, and is likely to facilitate, progression to established smoking" (Biener and Siegel 2000).

Evidence reviewed by Emery and her colleagues indicates that about a third (34%) of new experimentation with tobacco products in the early 1990s would not have occurred but for the marketing activities of tobacco companies (Emery, Choi, and Pierce 1999). Because tobacco consumption by young people is only a small fraction of the overall market at any one time (perhaps 3% of the market), this figure is not in conflict with the overall assessment that advertising accounts for 6.3% of consumption (Saffer and Chaloupka 1999).

Light Cigarettes Are Falsely Presented as Reasonable Alternatives to Quitting

In late 1963, a few weeks before the release of the first surgeon general's report, the American Tobacco Company introduced Carlton, the first ventilated brand, in a classic public relations effort to steal a march on the report (Kluger 1996). Carlton was introduced as the company's solution to the smoking and health problem. The company managed to observe the letter of the FTC prohibition at the time against advertising "tar" yields by simply printing them on the pack itself.

The saga of so-called light or low tar cigarettes has played out in recent decades at the intersection of the FTC test, cigarette design, and advertising as one of the ways manufacturers addressed the health concerns on the minds of most of their customers (NCI 1996; Warner et al. 1997; Hurt and Robertson 1998; Slade and Henningfield 1998; Leavell 1999; Slade 1999; Pollay 2000; Wilkenfeld, Henningfield, Slade, Burns, and Pinney 2000).[15]

The manufacturers have used "Lights" as a way to falsely reassure smokers and keep them in the franchise.[16] Although there is no health benefit of lower tar smokes (NCI 1996; Burns 2000; Wilkenfeld et al. 2000), and the cigarette makers realize this (e.g., Glantz et al. 1996, 89, 129), in recent decades, the cigarette makers have successfully promoted "low tar" brands with thinly veiled promises of lower health risk. By 1998, brands with an FTC tar yield of 12 mg or less accounted for 57% of the market (FTC 2000). There is little doubt that, had it not been possible for cigarette makers to provide this false reassurance, more people would have quit smoking, and the burden of illness and death that we face today from tobacco products would be far less.

Consumers have been misled by advertising for light cigarettes (Cohen 1996; Kozlowski et al. 1998; Kozlowski, Pillitteri, and Ahern 1998; Pillitteri, Shiffman, Gitchell, Burton, and Shimer 2000), and advertising messages that counter the results of this deception are effective (Kozlowski et al. 1999). The European Union (EU) has banned the terms "light," "mild," and the like for tobacco products because of this deception.

3. Past Attempts to Control Tobacco Product Marketing

Sequence of Events

In the 1930s, 1940s and early 1950s, cigarette advertising frequently included claims that drew the attention of the Federal Trade Commission (e.g., "No worry about throat irritation even when you inhale!") (USDHHS 1989; Kluger 1996). The commission's efforts to police these claims had little effect, however, for it was unable to stop the misleading claims until after the lengthy hearing and appeal processes had been exhausted.

In 1955, the commission issued a set of advertising guidelines that served to quiet the most blatant health claims. At the time, filters were taking over the market, and health claims for one brand against another were common. By the late 1950s, claims about tar yields had become prominent and the pressure on the commission's guidelines increased following the 1964 report of the Surgeon General's Advisory Committee (Public Health Service [PHS] 1964).

One of the responses of the cigarette manufacturers to the 1964 report was the establishment of a voluntary advertising code (Richards, Tye, and Fischer 1996). Introduced with great fanfare in 1964, it initially featured an enforcement office headed by a former governor of New Jersey. The enforcement provisions were dismantled in 1967. No enforcement actions had ever been taken. Accountable to no one, the companies regularly engaged in practices outside of the code (Richards et al. 1996).

The FTC began a rule-making proceeding that would have led to warning labels on cigarette packs, but Congress supervened in 1965 with a law that dictated the wording of the warning label ("Caution: cigarette smoking may be hazardous to your health"). In 1969, when the warning label legislation was renewed, Congress gave the cigarette makers liability protection for having the required warning label on their packs (USDHHS 1989; Kluger 1996). In 1972, warnings began to be required on cigarette advertisements. Congress again revised the warnings on cigarette packs, and the FTC revised those on advertising in 1985 to the present set of four rotating warnings, none of which mentions either addiction or death.

The FTC test was established and implemented in 1967 as a way to bring order to the claims in cigarette advertising. The test set a machine smoking standard for "tar" and nicotine that used parameters developed in the labs of the American Tobacco Company in the 1930s (NCI 1996). The smoking machine took a 35 ml draw over 2 seconds once a minute until the cigarette being tested was smoked down to a specific length. The amount of nicotine trapped in the machine's filter and the amount of particulate matter on the filter that was neither water nor nicotine ("tar") were reported in milligrams per cigarette. A requirement to report carbon monoxide yields was added in the early 1980s, but only "tar" and nicotine yields are required in cigarette advertising from the major companies. There is no requirement that yields be included on packaging, and there is no testing or disclosure requirement for cigarettes produced by the small cigarette makers, for these requirements are contained only in an agreement between the FTC and the major manufacturers.

The Federal Communications Commission (FCC), in response to a petition filed by John Banzhaf, required broadcasters to provide free air time under the Fairness Doctrine for counterads if broadcasters also carried cigarette commercials. Between 1967 and 1970, counteradvertising from the voluntary health agencies appeared on television in a volume of about a quarter that of cigarette commercials (USDHHS 1989; Kluger 1996; Saffer and Chaloupka 1999). While the counterads ran, cigarette consumption declined. The counterads left the air, following the broadcast ad ban on January 2, 1971. The money that had been spent on television ads was now poured into billboards, magazines, and sports sponsorship, venues beyond the reach of the Fairness Doctrine. Cigarette consumption rose.

Beginning in the late 1980s, R. J. Reynolds successfully revived the Camel brand on the back of a cartoon character, Joe (DeSmith 1998). By late 1991, it was becoming clear that the Camel campaign was succeeding with kids more than with adults (DiFranza et al. 1991; Fischer, Schwartz, Richards, Goldstein, and Rojas 1991; Pierce et al. 1991). Part of the successful marketing effort for Camel was a remarkably aggressive effort to distribute promotional items. Catalogs for "Camel Cash" premiums appeared in magazines such as *Rolling Stone*, in convenience stores across the country, and in mailboxes of people on the company's mailing lists. Camel Cash was distributed as a coupon inserted between the cellophane and the back of the package of filtered Camel packs. Philip Morris soon imitated this with its Marlboro Miles promotion, its own catalog blaring, "Get the Miles, Get the Gear." The universal product code (UPC) on each pack of Marlboros was designated as worth 5 "Miles."

In California, Mangini filed a lawsuit against the R. J. Reynolds Tobacco Company for targeting kids with the Joe Camel campaign. The lawsuit was settled in December 1997 with the withdrawal of the Joe Camel cartoon character from brand advertising and with the public disclosure of 80,000 pages of documents related to the campaign (available at www.library.ucsf.edu/tobacco/mangini).

The FDA issued regulations[17] that would have limited the reach of the Joe Camel campaign, but its authority was successfully challenged by the cigarette makers.[18]

In the meantime, lawsuits brought by state attorneys general beginning in 1994 against the major tobacco manufacturers for Medicaid cost recovery led to a Master Settlement Agreement (MSA) involving 46 states, 6 territories, and the major tobacco companies in November 1998 (MSA 1998). This agreement has resulted in a number of changes in tobacco product marketing in the settling states and, effectively, throughout the country (table 4.1) (USDHHS 2000).

Results

What have been the results of all these shifts and changes in tobacco product marketing over the past 50 years?

From the perspective of public health, not much. The PHS has concluded, "Since 1964, numerous attempts to regulate advertising and promotion of tobacco products have had only modest success in restricting such activity" (USDHHS 2000, 260). Limited restrictions are known not to affect consumption (Saffer and Chaloupka 1999).

There have been marked shifts in the form and character of tobacco product advertising over the years in response to various factors, including those regulatory controls already listed. The broadcast ad ban led to shifts of advertising to magazines, billboards, and sports sponsorships. The billboard ban under the MSA has been associated with a marked increase in point-of-sale cigarette advertising at retail locations (Wakefield et al. 2000), and cigarette advertising actually *increased* in magazines with high youth readership comparing pre-MSA with the MSA era (Turner-Bowker and Hamilton 2000; Campaign for Tobacco-Free Kids 2000).

Auto racing sponsorship, a source of enormous visibility and brand identification (Blum 1991; Philip Morris 1993), remains intact for Marlboro and Winston following the MSA, and, as discussed later, concerts sponsored by tobacco brands have proliferated in night clubs. Marketing in such "adults-only" venues has markedly increased, and much of the marketing for these products in general is still not without appeal to the young.

4. The Current Scene

In 1999, the major cigarette makers in the United States spent $8.2 billion on domestic cigarette advertising and promotions (table 4.2) (FTC 2001). Notwithstanding the gentle restrictions subsequently imposed by the MSA, tobacco product marketing remains robust in 2001.

Adults who do not smoke usually are only minimally aware of tobacco product marketing. The following brief catalog of current tobacco marketing

Table 4.1. Summary of the Marketing Provisions of the
Master Settlement Agreement

Provision	Description
Prohibition of youth targeting	Participating manufacturers may not target youth in the advertising, promotion, or marketing of tobacco products or take any action the primary purpose of which is to initiate, maintain, or increase youth smoking.
Ban on use of cartoons	Participating manufacturers may not use any cartoon in the advertising, promoting, packaging or labeling of tobacco products.
	"Cartoon" is taken to mean a depiction of an object, person, animal, creature, or similar caricature that uses comically exaggerated features, attributes human characteristics to animals, plants or other objects, or attributes unnatural or extrahuman abilities to the character.
Limitation of tobacco brand name sponsorships	Participating manufacturers may not engage in brand name sponsorship of concerts, of events with an audience comprised of a significant percentage of youth, of events in which any paid participants or contestants are youth, or of any athletic event between opposing teams in any football, basketball, baseball, soccer, or hockey league.
	Participating manufacturers may engage in one brand name sponsorship per company per year, and Brown & Williamson is exempt from the ban on sponsorship of concerts with respect to its GPC Country Music Festival and its Kool Jazz Festival.
	Specific rules for sponsored events permit brand name advertising of the sponsored brand in connection with the events being sponsored but no mention of the sponsorship in the advertising for the brand itself. In addition, media can be paid to mention brand name sponsorships, and brand name merchandise can be sold if it deals with the sponsored event. Finally, outdoor advertising with brand name sponsorship is permitted despite the fact that such advertising of tobacco products is itself not permitted.
	The company name, as long as it is not also a tobacco product brand name, can be used in sponsorship without restriction. A brand name may not be used to name a stadium. Brand sponsorship of football, basketball, baseball, soccer, or hockey teams is not permitted.
Outdoor and transit advertising	Billboards advertising tobacco brands are not permitted, and neither are placards placed in arenas, stadiums, shopping malls, or video arcades, and in public transportation.
Adult-only facilities	There are no prohibitions on advertising within any facility in which the operator ensures or has a reasonable basis to believe that no underage person is present.
Payments related to tobacco products in media	Participating manufacturers may not pay to have tobacco products, packaging, or advertising used or referred to in entertainment media except for media that is to be displayed in an adult-only facility, that is not intended for public distribution, or that consists of instructions in the use of "nonconventional cigarettes" and is provided only to adults.
Brand name merchandise	Participating manufacturers may not employ products bearing the brand name of a tobacco product other than the product itself and advertisements for it except for use within an adult-only facility for products not distributed to the general public.
Miscellaneous restrictions	Free sampling permitted only in adult-only facilities; no gifts to underage persons based on proof of purchase; minimum pack size of 20 cigarettes and 0.60 ounces of tobacco for roll your own packages

Source: MSA 1998.

Table 4.2. Domestic Cigarette Advertising and Promotional
              Expenditures for the Year 1999

Type of advertising	Millions of dollars	% of total
Newspapers	50.9	0.6
Magazines	377.4	4.6
Outdoor	53.8	0.7
Transit	5.6	0.1
Point of sale	329.4	4.0
Promotional allowances	3,543.0	43.0
Sampling distribution	33.7	0.4
Specialty item distribution	335.7	4.1
Public entertainment	267.4	3.3
Direct mail	94.6	1.2
Endorsements/testimonials	—	—
Internet	0.7	0.0
Coupons	531.0	6.5
Retail value added	2,560.0	31.1
All others	54.7	0.7
Total	8,237.6	100.0

Source: FTC 2001.

Promotional allowances. The largest category of expenditure includes payments to retailers for shelf space.

Specialty item distribution. This category includes distribution of brand-related merchandise through the mail or at promotional events.

Direct mail. The top three companies each maintain and regularly use mailing lists
containing tens of millions of names. The amount in this line may represent only direct
mail expenses (such as database management) that are not attributable to other lines such
as the coupon line, which may include expenses for the distribution of coupons as well
as the value of the coupons that are redeemed.

Retail value added. This category includes both multiple-pack promotions such as buy
one, get one free and free promotional items with cigarette purchase ("trinkets and trash").

in the United States at this time is presented to heighten the reader's awareness of the breadth and depth of this activity.

Conventional Advertising: Magazines

Display advertising is common in magazines that have high youth readership
(Campaign for Tobacco-Free Kids 2000; Turner-Bowker and Hamilton
2000). Ads have featured drawings reminiscent of Varga girls and of James
Dean for Camel (RJR), spacious Western vistas for Marlboro (Philip Morris),
and hip bar scenes with a threatening undertone of sexual tension between
a man and a woman for Kool (Brown & Williamson). In magazines more
likely to be read by adults with an interest in quitting, ads whose layout and
message ("You can do it") resemble advertising for a nicotine replacement
product have appeared for Merit (Philip Morris), and a picture of a slim,

reflective young woman "Thinking about number one" refers to both being good to yourself and using the 1 mg "tar" cigarette from Brown & Williamson, Carlton.

Marketing at Retail

Display Space   The market leader, Philip Morris, is making an effort to move its cigarette displays behind the counter (but remaining in highly visible locations) while the smaller major companies seek to continue to have their packs within a hand's reach of desire. The companies pay retailers for display space, and this has become a major expenditure (table 4.2). There is fierce competition between the companies for this space (Ress 1999), perhaps in anticipation of additional limits on other forms of marketing. Regarding retail space in the post-MSA environment, a Brown & Williamson executive commented, "Increasingly, the store will be treated not just as an outlet for volume but as a targeted communication channel" (Pollack 1999). The importance the manufacturers assign to optimizing their retail presence is indicated by the amount of money that goes to retailers in the form of promotional allowances. This category was 43% of total advertising and promotional expense in 1999. This represents a substantial portion of the total income retailers receive for offering cigarettes to their customers.

Signage   Signs advertising tobacco products and special offers have become more prominent following the MSA (Wakefield et al. 2000).

Matches   R. J. Reynolds supplies matches advertising Camel, Salem, or Winston in profuse designs to many retailers. Series of matches with as many as 36 different designs circulate for a few months, to be replaced by another series for the same or a different RJR brand. In many cities, discarded matchbooks on the street are usually from the RJR effort. Philip Morris will occasionally distribute matches for Marlboro or Parliament. These have graphically striking designs and are made with higher quality materials and have a more polished finish and appearance than those from RJR, but they appear only in limited quantities and only for a limited period of time. The message Philip Morris seems to send with this strategy is that the Camel matches may be OK for everyday use, but Marlboro matches are special.

Promotions

Items at Retail   Although not as common as 10 years ago, promotional items are still given away from time to time with the purchase of cigarette packs. For instance, during summer 2000, Brown & Williamson offered an FM radio free with the purchase of one pack of Kool. The radio was smaller than a pack of cigarettes and was stylishly shaped like a computer mouse with a headset for its tail. The in-store display for this promotion carried the headline, "KBOOM: BUY 1 PACK GET THE BOOM FREE."

Items by Mail Order   Catalog redemption of Camel Cash, Marlboro Miles, and UPC codes for a range of other brands (Newport, Basic, Virginia Slims) for merchandise is practiced, but the goods on offer are of higher quality and no longer carry the tobacco brand logo, as compared to pre-MSA practices. The catalogs continue to be crafted as extensions of the specific brand images and fantasies. They are available at retail, by calling toll-free numbers, and through mailing lists.

Sweepstakes and Contests   Sweepstakes for Marlboro ("Cowboy Place"), Winston ("Want to Win a Million?" geared to the NASCAR Winston Cup series), and Basic ("The Best Things in Life are Basic") offer alluring rewards with chances to win. Newport ("Rhythm and Sound Dance Contest") offers a dancing competition in which contestants send in videotapes of themselves dancing. Semi-final winners travel to Miami for a live final round contest. Persons too young to enter these games can still be drawn into the fantasies portrayed in the promotional literature. Entry forms are distributed at retail, in magazines, and through the mail.

Event Sponsorships and Tie-ins   Auto races (Marlboro, Winston, Kool) and concerts (Salem, Kool, Lucky Strike) are the main sponsorships on offer at this time. Special VIP clubs with membership cards and racing event tie-ins are created and sustained through direct mail as part of the relationship marketing that the sponsorships so readily facilitate among people dedicated to the sports.

Direct Mail

Overview   Each of the major companies has a huge database of consumers. Brown & Williamson, the smallest of the three major companies, has more than 25 million names in its national database (S. Rosenblatt, personal communication, May 9, 2000), and RJR has more than 800,000 names in Florida alone (Blackmer 1996). Despite representations to the contrary by the companies, it is not uncommon for young people to receive mail from tobacco companies. An October 1999 survey of middle and high school students in New Jersey revealed that 11.3% of nonsmoking students and 24.3% of students who reported smoking in the last 30 days had received mail addressed to them from a tobacco company (Adler and Slade 2000).

Typical Mail Pieces   Mail pieces are used to distribute coupons and catalogs and to help launch new variations on a brand family. Coupons are coded so they can be tracked to the individual to whom they were mailed when they are redeemed. Questionnaires that permit further refinement of company databases are frequently employed and often include extra copies that recipients are asked to pass along to friends.

Controlled Circulation Tobacco Brand Magazines   Each major company now publishes full-fledged magazines that portray key brand attributes through both advertising and editorial content (table 4.3). These magazines are distributed only through the mail to persons on the respective company mailing lists. Although the magazines contain advertising for other products, the entire environment of each magazine is carefully tailored to fit the selling message of the featured brand.

"Adults-Only" Marketing

Concerts   Both Brown & Williamson and R. J. Reynolds sponsor concerts in adults-only environments, but the promotion for these concerts includes conventional advertising channels in the alternative newspapers of the larger cities (Applebome 1999; Brown & Williamson 2000). The sponsorships associate the brands (Lucky Strike and Salem) with entertainment, a communication mode that is completely devoid of any informational content about the products.

Table 4.3. Tobacco Product Brand Magazines

Magazine title	Sponsor	Featured brand(s)	Editorial themes
Real Edge	Brown & Williamson	Lucky Strike, Kool	Adventure, sports, sex, music
Flair	Brown & Williamson	Capri, Kool, Lucky Strike, Misty	Fashion, romance, health and beauty, starlets
The Art of Simple Living	Brown & Williamson	Misty, Capri, Carlton	Friends, family, home, Self
Unlimited	Philip Morris	Marlboro	Action, adventure, good times
CML	RJ Reynolds	Camel	The hip, good life
Heartland USA	UST	Skoal, Copenhagen	Rodeo, fishing, hunting, drag Racing, kayaking

Sources: Respective magazines.

Bars and Clubs   Marlboro, Camel, and Kool are featured in the entertainment pages of alternative newspapers as sponsors of bars and nightclubs and often of the entertainment there. The brands provide promotion and entertainment guides to establishments under contract with them, and in turn, the night spots feature the sponsored brand in various ways (Gellene 1997; Naymik 1997; Solomon 1997; Hwang 1999). A product representative may also be there to be friendly with customers and to give away product.

The Pack

Trading Cards   Beginning in the 1880s, cigarette cards were used as a means of generating interest in and loyalty to particular brands (Howsden 1995). These well-designed miniature cards featured subjects such as flags, actresses, flowers, and soldiers in sets of up to 50 or more different cards on a given theme. With the rise of mass advertising techniques in the first quarter of the twentieth century, cigarette cards disappeared from the marketing mix. Cards have recently returned here and there as specialty items, perhaps in recognition by marketers that a new mix of communication devices will be needed for tobacco products to successfully convey the brand image to consumers in the current environment. Brands such as Salem, Doral, and Natural American Spirit have featured these engaging cards. Salem has included cards on the backs of selected packs as features for a limited period of time as part of a concert series promotion. Doral has offered cards celebrating each of the fifty states, similar to the U.S. Mint's offerings on quarter dollars. Natural American Spirit has put cards with various themes on its cigarette packs, available both by mail order and at retail, in sets of up to 36 cards, putting a series out for a limited period of time and then replacing it with another series. People on the company's mailing list have received posters depicting each card in a given series.

Novel Brands and Formulations   Unusual formulations (Camel "exotic blends"), cigarette brands boasting that they contain no additives ("No Bull" Winston, Natural American Spirit, among others) or that their menthol is from "natural" sources (Salem and Kool) have appeared in the marketplace in recent years. These products trade off of novelty and associations with health food fads. The appearance of such products underlines the fact that cigarette makers have no obligations to a regulator to justify and to obtain pre-market approval for changes in product composition (Slade and Henningfield 1998). Claims are sometimes modified after the fact, as occurred with the toning down of the "additive free" claims for Winston and Natural American Spirit following settlements with the FTC (FTC 2000).

The Cigarette Pack as Advertisement   Before mass marketing was the norm, the cigarette pack was the main direct link between the manufacturer and the consumer (Mullen 1979). It remains a key element in the relationship, and its importance can only grow if other means of communication are limited by regulation. Package design is a key part of the brand image and is an ever-present element of the product.

Collectors' Packs   The cigarette pack itself provides an intimate space for advertising and promotion. The UPC codes and Camel Cash provide the connection to promotions. However, the pack design itself can be readily modified (Slade 1997; Rossel 2000). As Rossel comments,

> Who needs a large canvas when you have a cigarette pack to apply imaginative design? With special editions, smokers always carry a little piece of art in their pockets. Some of the colourful and diverse boxes have even gained cult status among consumers. And manufacturers' experience with special editions is unanimously positive. (48).

In Switzerland, a Philip Morris brand, Star, has for years featured a multitude of novel, artsy pack designs all circulating simultaneously. In recent years, both Philip Morris and R. J. Reynolds in the United States have sold limited edition special packs for a range of brands including Marlboro, Parliament, Camel, and Salem. Most often, these have been conventional hard packs with advertising-linked pictures or graphics, but, occasionally, Brown & Williamson (Kool) and R. J. Reynolds (Camel) have issued packs of 20 sticks in flat tins with special graphics. A tin for Kool, for instance, featured an embossed image of an Indy-style race car, providing a link with the company's racing sponsorship. Sometimes, these special packs are explicitly called "collectors' packs" and each one of a series is numbered, like the trading cards.

Word of Mouth

Some marketing activities can best be understood as attempts to promote good word of mouth. Here are several examples.

Brown & Williamson   A toll-free customer service number for Brown and Williamson has had a series of highly unusual messages. The first one told the caller, "Brown & Williamson loves you," while indicating that its competitors do not.

The second one in the series features a quartet of male voices serenading the caller with this song:

> Ohhhhh, the tobacco plant is a lovely plant
> Its leaves so broad and green,
> But you shouldn't think about the tobacco plant
> If you're still a teen.
>
> 'Cause tobacco is a big person's plant,
> And that's the way it should be,
> So if you're under 21, go and climb a tree.
>
> Ohhhhh, the tobacco plant is a lovely plant
> ([*spoken solo voice*] and that, my friends, is no yarn!)
> We let it ripen in the fields and hang it in the barn.

A female voice invites the caller to write a better song before providing instructions for which buttons on the phone to press for service and for information.

The third one depicts a rap artist talking with an announcer. Throughout the schtick, the rap artist's words are repeatedly bleeped out.

All three recorded messages are irreverent and unexpected. The series coincides with the decidedly more aggressive advertising that Brown and Williamson has been doing for Kool and Lucky Strike. These telephone recordings are likely intended to have such novelty that their message will travel from person to person, generating positive word of mouth.

Salem   A new packing of Salem, the slide pack, has come to feature a novelty inside. On Salem, the tipping paper, the paper that holds the filter onto the tobacco rod, has always been white. In the slide pack, this paper is a striking dark green on one (and only one) of the twenty cigarettes. This special cigarette is always in the same location in the pack, where it is seen when the pack is first opened. It may be a silly point of difference, but it exemplifies one of the brand's slogans, "It's not what you expect." Again, the intent of going to this trouble with one special stick among twenty may be to generate positive word of mouth for the product.

Eclipse and Accord

R. J. Reynolds and Philip Morris have each developed and tested a novel nicotine delivery device resembling a cigarette that the respective companies believe represents a "reduced risk" product (Slade 2000). Both companies would like to make health claims for their version of this class of product, Eclipse for Reynolds and Accord for Philip Morris. Philip Morris, with its deep pockets, has taken a gradual, evolutionary approach to this, trying to shape the regulatory environment and waiting for the process to evolve before making its move with health claims. Reynolds, in contrast, has jumped in with health claims for Eclipse, as well as sales of the product by phone and over the Internet beginning in the spring of 2000 (Stephenson 2000).

Advertising for Eclipse has featured claims that, among smokers, the product may reduce the risk of cancer, that it may reduce bronchial inflammation, and that it may lessen heart disease risk if the person does not have preexisting heart disease. The claims are based on studies that, for the most part, compare Eclipse with middle-range delivery cigarettes when it may well be that the market for Eclipse is those who already smoke the lowest delivery brands. When Eclipse is compared to the lowest delivery brands, its deliveries are similar to, or actually greater than, these products, even ones from Reynolds (Slade, Connolly, and Lymperis in press). Thus, there is substantial doubt whether this product offers any actual benefit to those who will actually use it.

In the 1950s, filtered cigarettes were promoted as a solution to health concerns (Slade 1989). A generation later, low tar filled this role. The companies that have developed these products hope that Eclipse and Accord will serve this function in the new century. It is looking more and more like these products stand in the same tradition of public relations substituting for public health. The marketing of these products is, then, a serious concern for public health, and any health claims made for products like this should be approached with the utmost caution.

5. Opportunities for Control

Limits on Marketing

Setting Limits on Marketing   As discussed previously, setting limits on tobacco product marketing in only a few venues without banning the activity from multiple media does little or nothing to reduce tobacco product use because advertising simply migrates to the still permitted outlets. Voluntary agreements with industry, as well as industry-generated advertising codes, have been window dressing, providing this peculiar industry with the appearance of being responsive to public health concerns without providing substance.

Banning Advertising   Saffer and Chaloupka (1999) have demonstrated that advertising bans work. A ban must be thoroughgoing so that the effects of alluring imagery and enticements inherent in tobacco product marketing are all but stifled. In the United States, such an approach raises concerns about abridging a company's free speech rights. However, commercial speech is not accorded the same protection that other forms of speech enjoy. Curtailing tobacco product marketing is a reasonably limited response to the enormous damage that tobacco products do to the public health[19] (USDHHS 2000). Nonetheless, any proposed limits on tobacco product marketing in the United States are certain to face strong legal challenges. At the end of the day, it is possible that the Supreme Court will not permit an approach that protects the public to the greatest extent possible from these uniquely hazardous products. That possibility should not, though, limit the description of an approach that is reasonably designed to protect the public.

The industry will test the limits of any ban that is enacted, and governmental resolve in enforcement will be key to its success. In the early 1990s, a group representing religious investors had a dinner meeting in New York City with a group of Philip Morris executives to discuss the investors' concerns about the company's behavior. One of these concerns involved "brand stretching," the practice of using a cigarette brand name and image to promote other products. The practice promotes a product's brand image apart from the product and has been used to skirt ad bans. The French government had recently implemented a ban on advertising cigarettes in magazines. A member of the investor group passed around the table an ad in a French magazine for a travel agency called "Marlboro Travel." The ad depicted a Western scene typical of cigarette advertising for the namesake brand. As the ad passed around the table, nearly all the Philip Morris executives commented that the ad was not, actually, a cigarette ad but was simply an ad for another, albeit similarly positioned, business. When the magazine got to Charles Wall, the most senior company attorney at the table, he voiced disagreement with his colleagues. "This is a cigarette ad," he flatly declared, "but it is up to the French government to say so."

A comprehensive ban on tobacco product advertising and promotion in the United States would eliminate numerous practices. Advertising promoting brands, promotions, or tobacco use would not be permitted, whether in media, at point of sale, in "adult-only" venues, or through the mails. There would be no sweepstakes offers and no promotional item catalogs or promotional items offered at retail. There would be no free samples.[20] There would be no sponsorships (e.g., sporting events, concerts). There would be no "brand stretching," the introduction, for instance, of Camel brand boots, or of Marlboro travel agencies (as in the French example) or Marlboro clothing stores (such as actually exist in many locations in Asia, Europe, and South America). In addition, tobacco products would be placed out of sight at retail, and brand imagery would be removed from tobacco product packages. Retailers would not be permitted to advertise or promote products that could not be advertised by manufacturers other than to indicate, in the driest possible manner, that the products were available and at what price.

Limiting Product Displays   The pack is itself an advertisement (Mullen 1979; Slade 1997; Rossel 2000). When in-store ads for tobacco products were banned in Canada in the late 1980s, the companies responded by creating massive displays of packs stacked like wallpaper behind the sales counter. In the United States, there is a growing effort to remove self-service displays of tobacco products to reduce opportunities for shoplifting. These efforts have resulted in tobacco products placed behind the counter in plain view or placed in containers on the counter open to the clerk but not the consumer. Display space for product at retail has become an intensely competitive arena among the cigarette makers (Ress 1999). To blunt the advertising message transmitted by the pack, an advertising ban should require that tobacco products not be on open display. Rather, they should be *under* the counter at retail.

Promotional allowances were the greatest single expenditure for cigarette marketing in 1999 (table 4.2). This money, more than $3.5 billion, was spent largely to assure prime product placement at retail. Moving the product under the counter, out of sight, would sharply reduce the value of what the manufacturers get from these slotting fees. Were product displays to be eliminated, expenditures on promotional allowances would decline markedly.

Plain Packaging   In the hands of a consumer, the pack is a small, decorative work of art, designed to be appealing, a badge for the brand (Mullen 1979; Slade 1997; Rossel 2000). It links the consumer to the brand image, the fantasy creation of the marketing staff at the company and the advertising agency. The pack design is not essential to the product inside except as part of the selling message for the product.

Were cigarette packaging to become standardized, that is, to be the same from brand to brand but for the brand name and brand-specific disclosures, the degree to which the pack conveyed the brand image would be limited (Expert Panel Report 1995). A review of the empiric literature on plain packaging has concluded that "generic packaging of cigarettes *could* be an important component of a comprehensive program designed to reduce cigarette smoking, and particularly by young people" (Swanson and Donavan 1996, 7). The report indicates that the studies it reviewed provided only indirect measures and called for "studies that more directly assess the link between generic packaging and likely impact on smoking behavior" (Swanson and Donovan 1996, 7).

Because the package is part of the marketing effort, and the pack becomes a billboard in retail displays (a factor not assessed in any of the studies reviewed), a move to plain or standard packaging would likely be an important complement to an advertising ban. Furthermore, it is difficult to see how this suggestion can be properly tested apart from actually trying it out.

Countermarketing

Paid Advertising   Counteradvertising can reduce tobacco use (Popham et al. 1994; Saffer and Chaloupka 1999; McVey and Stapleton 2000). It can be effective at preventing tobacco use from becoming established among the young (Siegel and Biener 2000), it can reduce the use of tobacco products by adults, as seems to have happened in the United States during the late 1960s fairness doctrine period (USDHHS 1989), and it can promote quitting by adults (Popham et al. 1993).

Not every campaign is necessarily effective, and the best public health efforts, like those generated by persons with a vested interest in promoting tobacco use, rely on a thoughtful understanding of marketing (Rust 1999) and on careful market research (e.g., Massachusetts Department of Public Health 2000). Media campaigns are more likely to be successful if they are relatively large, strategically focused, and linked to community public health activities (USDHHS 2000). Themes especially helpful in these efforts include emphasizing industry manipulation, environmental tobacco smoke, addiction, and quitting (Goldman and Glantz 1998). At the same time, ads that have themes of underage access, short-term effects of smoking, dry presentations of long-term health effects, and romantic rejection because of tobacco use do not seem promising approaches. A highly personalized, emotionally involving exploration of how tobacco has devastated a person's life and a family can be very powerful, and Massachusetts has used this approach in several ad series (Connolly 2000).

Balbach and Glantz have discussed the political environment in which countermarketing takes place (1998). Based on the experience in California, where marketing and public health decisions about the media campaign have been subject to political interference, we know that effective media efforts can be compromised. The problem requires continual monitoring of a government's program by voluntary public health and medical groups and active intervention in the political process by these groups if the campaign is compromised.

Labeling (Warnings, Messages, and Disclosures)   Package warnings, since their introduction in the 1960s, have mainly served as shields for tobacco companies facing product liability claims (Kluger 1996; USDHHS 2000). The present warnings on U.S. cigarette packs don't even use the words "death" or "addiction," and they are inconspicuous by current international standards.

Large, graphic warnings are feasible (Mahood 1995, 1999) and are, in fact being implemented in Canada (Health Canada 2000). The warning system in Canada features color pictures of children, of diseased lungs, of a limp cigarette (symbolizing impotence) along with pointed comments endorsed by the government about problems caused by cigarettes. The warnings cover the top half of the major faces of the packs. The Canadian Cancer Society (Informa Market Research Co. 1999) and Health Canada, after testing the approach these warnings take, have found it effective at conveying the desired information to consumers. An indirect indication of their expected effectiveness has been hinted at by Philip Morris. The company has indicated to WHO that it opposes the use of graphic messages in cigarette package warnings (Philip Morris International 2000b),[21] perhaps because these images undermine the brand image otherwise conveyed by the package design.

In addition to large, graphic health warnings, the Canadian system includes package inserts that provide quit-smoking advice to consumers. This feature is especially reasonable because most cigarette consumers would like to stop (USDHHS 2000). Tips on quitting, especially if linked with referral numbers for stop smoking clinics, quit lines, or the universal resource locators (URLs) for Internet quit-smoking services, might prove to be an especially helpful way to magnify the cognitive dissonance many smokers feel each time they take a cigarette from their pack. A health warning is incomplete without an indication of how to stop, and the package insert can point the way.

In addition to health warnings and assistance with quitting, packages can also provide ingredient and toxic constituent disclosures (NCI 1996). The amount of publicly available information about cigarettes and their smoke constituents has increased as a result of governmental requirements (especially by the governments of Massachusetts, British Columbia, and Canada).[22] Disclosure about what is in a tobacco product, and what it delivers to the consumer, are reasonable things for consumers to expect from the makers of their cigarettes, cigars and smokeless tobacco products.[23]

Becoming Accountable

The major tobacco companies are presently seeking respect and respectability (France 1996), but the companies might take steps to earn respect before simply declaring that they have changed and are somehow doing business in a new manner.

The multinational tobacco companies have worked long and hard to avoid being held accountable to government regulators for their addictive, deadly product[24] (Glantz et al. 1996; Kluger 1996; Hurt and Robertson 1998; Francey and Chapman 2000). If the companies ever become subject to appropriate regulation, they would still likely retain the fruits of decades of past fraud, misrepresentation, and deceit. As juries come to award punitive damages for the ongoing bad faith behavior of these companies (e.g., *Engle v. R. J. Reynolds Tobacco Co.*[25]), a question arises about what behavior on the part of the companies would be necessary not only for them to stop engaging in the deceitful conduct but also what would be necessary for them to undo the fraud. Although the misbehavior may largely have occurred in the past, elements of it continue, and the companies continue to benefit enormously from past misdeeds.

Systematically Reducing "Unwanted" Sales   In June 1997, a proposed settlement of the Medicaid lawsuits was put forward by the major tobacco companies and most of the suing attorneys general. That proposed agreement included a "lookback" provision. Under its terms, companies would have been obligated to pay what amounted to fines if their respective shares of the underage market for cigarettes or smokeless tobacco did not decline to a certain degree over time. Not only did the overall agreement eventually fall apart, this particular provision came to be a source of conflict over the degree to which it would be enforceable and the degree to which large market shares of the underaged market would be penalized.

Despite this inauspicious initial airing, the fundamental idea is sound. If the companies actually do not want to have underaged customers, then, to the degree that they do, they should be glad to at least forego any income made from products used by those customers. This market is about $1 billion per year, so the profit made on underaged use is substantial. A larger incentive against the underaged consumers using a company's product would be provided by making the penalty an even larger amount (Glantz 1993). Such economic incentives would help companies focus on effective means to reduce tobacco product usage by the underaged by making it in their economic self-interest.

Child-Proofing Advertising   The major companies have declared that they will not "target" young people with their marketing. However, the companies view marketing "targeted" at folks just a bit older as completely fair and important for them to pursue. If it happens that an ad directed at a 20-year-old also has appeal for someone at age 15, that is accidental, incidental, and not of concern to the company. This self-serving standard is clearly neither child-friendly nor child-centered.

A child-centered standard would be that tobacco product marketing, to the extent that it continues to exist at all, should be *child-proof*: advertising and promotion should be actively tested on young people and demonstrated to have little to no appeal to those for whom tobacco product purchase is forbidden.

Helping Customers Quit   Most who smoke want to stop (USDHHS 2000). Even though the Web sites for both Philip Morris and RJR sanctimoniously declare that their customers should "rely" on the scientific evidence that cigarettes kill, neither company uses this conclusion as the basis for its marketing and promotion. Were this to happen, all the marketing efforts for Marlboro, Camel, Virginia Slims, Salem, and Benson & Hedges would urge customers to quit and actively help novices not start.

Conclusion

The present situation is inside out. An ordinary consumer products company, faced with the reality of the damage it was doing to customers, would be taking extraordinary steps to save lives. Instead, members of this peculiar industry wait for government to force them to take ordinary steps to improve consumer protection, and even then actively oppose effective measures.

There may be no alternative for the tobacco product makers. Unlike ordinary consumer products, tobacco products are inherently poisonous and addictive. Because the companies' first obligation is to enhance shareholder value and not to protect public health, the only way the public health will be protected is for governmental requirements to be imposed, over the opposition of the peculiar industry.

NOTES

1. Nicotine interacts with specific receptors in the brain, both stimulating them and stimulating their further synthesis. The repeated ingestion of nicotine is reinforcing, and tobacco use meets standard clinical criteria for drug addiction. Tobacco use controls behavior in a manner that is clinically recognized as addiction more frequently than does the use of alcohol, heroin, or cocaine (Anthony, Warner, and Kessler 1994). Whereas the term "addiction" is often applied colloquially and imprecisely to a wide range of activities, its use in this chapter is in the technical sense of drug dependence. The definition of drug addiction used by Kalant (2000, 127) captures this meaning:

> Drug addiction is a strongly established pattern of behavior characterized by 1) the repeated self-administration of a drug in amounts which reliably produce reinforcing psychoactive effects, and 2) great difficulty in achieving voluntary long-term cessation of such use, even when the user is strongly motivated to stop.

The 1988 Surgeon General's Report on nicotine addiction (UDSHHS 1988) and the Royal College of Physician's report on nicotine addiction in Britain (2000) develop this topic more fully.

2. In unguarded moments, tobacco industry insiders understand this very well. In 1980, a Tobacco Institute staffer wrote, "Shook, Hardy reminds us, I'm told, that the entire matter of addiction is the most potent weapon a prosecuting attorney can have in a lung cancer/cigarette case. We can't defend continued smoking as 'free choice' if the person was 'addicted' " (Knopick 1980, 2).

3. A provision of the Master Settlement Agreement (MSA 1998, Section III[r]) states,

> No Participating Manufacturer may make any material misrepresentation of fact regarding the health consequences of using any Tobacco Product, including any tobacco additives, filters, paper or other ingredients. Nothing in this sub-section shall limit the exercise of any First Amendment right or the assertion of any defense or position in any judicial, legislative or regulatory forum.

The company seems to have relied on this proviso in at least one judicial proceeding since posting its "overwhelming . . . consensus" comment on the corporate website. In a filing in New York just a month later, the company took the following position: "Philip Morris admits that smoking is a risk factor for, and may in fact cause, certain kinds of diseases in humans, but states that *it has not been scientifically established whether cigarette smoking causes any of these diseases in humans*" Simon et al. v. Philip Morris et al., No. 99 Civ. 1988 (E.D.N.Y. Nov. 29, 1999).

4. The R. J. Reynolds Tobacco Company makes a similar comment that consumers should "rely" on information about smoking and health on its website (R. J. Reynolds 2000).

5. *Buchan v. Ortho Pharmaceutical* [1986] 54 O.R.2d 92.

6. See Kilbourne (1999) for an insightful discussion of how this and other advertising that targets women are constructed.

7. The explanation usually offered by supporters of the industry position for the lack of effect of advertising on consumption is that tobacco represents a "mature market" (e.g., Waterson 1996). Pollay has pointed out that the cigarette market has none of the characteristics of a mature market and that senior researchers at the J. Walter Thompson ad agency concluded in 1976 that this concept does not apply to cigarettes (Pollay 1998). In tacit agreement with this conclusion, internal documents from the tobacco industry that discuss advertising never use this concept. Rather, this notion seems reserved for the industry's public relations efforts.

8. A similar analysis has also been done with regard to advertising for alcoholic beverages with the same result (Saffer 1996).

9. A particularly readable account of advertising, especially related to women and both alcoholic beverages and tobacco products, has recently been presented by Kilbourne (1999).

10. Branding sells tobacco use to particular target groups. Although this is often paired with the use of the particular brand advertised by the particular target group, it also can happen, as in the example of Virginia Slims mentioned earlier, that a brand can communicate strong ideas about smoking in general that lead to a general increase in tobacco use by a target group.

11. The relationship between cigar consumption and the marketing practices of the industry has not received detailed study, but the rise in cigar consumption in the 1990s among both adults and teens occurred in the setting of renewed, intense promotion for these products (NCI 1998).

12. 60 Fed.Reg. 41,314–41,787 (1995).

13. 60 Fed.Reg. at 41,334.

14. 61 Fed.Reg. 44,396–45,318 (1996). In the United States, the marketing of moist snuff, in conjunction with the design of these products, follows the same pattern of youth appeal (Connolly 1995; Slade 1995), with a resulting pattern of use by the young that follows the marketing plan of the major manufacturer (Tomar, Giovino, and Eriksen 1995).

15. The other major way the companies have provided false reassurance to customers is through public relations techniques, for instance by claiming that there remained a "controversy" about whether smoking was a cause of any human illness and by supporting a public relations–driven research effort, the Tobacco Industry Research Committee in the 1950s which became the Council for Tobacco Research (CTR) (Kluger 1996). Although CTR was dismantled as part of the Master Settlement Agreement, Philip Morris has recently launched its own program to support the work of academic scientists through a call for proposals (Philip Morris Incorporated 2000). This program, by cultivating relationships with academic scientists, may permit the company to continue to reap the public relations benefits of sponsoring scientific research in carefully delimited areas. At the same time, the company shows no signs of actually relying on what science has already learned about addiction and illness from cigarettes in how it markets its products.

16. Some advertisements for these brands in the 1970s showed that these brands were in competition with abstinence. For instance, an ad for True showed an earnest woman saying, "All the fuss about smoking got me thinking I'd either quit or smoke True. I smoke True."

17. 61 Fed.Reg. 44,396–45,318 (1996).

18. *FDA v. Brown & Williamson et al.*, No. 98–1152 (Sup.Ct. decided March 21, 2000).

19. 60 Fed.Reg. 41,314–41,787 (1995); 61 Fed.Reg. 44,396–45,318 (1996).

20. Coupons and buy-one-get-one free promotions have the effect of lowering the price consumers pay for tobacco products. It may be possible to curtail these practices through the state's minimum price laws. Even though these laws are designed to limit price competition among retailers, it may be possible to put them to a public health purpose in this way.

21. The company's precise wording is worth noting: it opposes "proposals to use 'shock' images in health warnings designed to disparage cigarette consumers" (Phillip Morris International 2000b, 4).

22. This is still an evolving and unsettled area of regulatory law. Exactly what authority state and federal governments will eventually have in this area is uncertain. Although the companies claim that many proposed disclosures are "trade secrets," it seems more likely than not that the particulars being sought are already known within the large companies, in part from analysis and reverse engineering of the products of competitors. The only groups not already in on the key secrets are, probably, the government and the public.

23. Governmentally required messages on packaging, assistance with quitting, and disclosures about ingredients and poisons need not constitute the universe of governmental labeling requirements for tobacco products (E. LeGresley and H. Selin, personal communication 1996). The pack might also carry messages that provide consumers with facts that inform them about the product they are using. For instance, a Marlboro pack might include the message, "More children smoke Marlboro than any other brand on the US market." A pack of Eve might have a boxed message saying, "Eve can give you facial wrinkles." Any pack might convey this message: "Half of all parents killed by smoking die in middle age. Isn't that too soon to lose yours?"

The idea would be to provide food for thought, additional prompts to stop smoking with messages that are appropriate extensions of health warnings, messages that incidentally counter the selling message of the product in other ways than straightforward health warnings do. These suggestions about an expanded view of health messages for tobacco product packages should be explored with appropriate consumer research.

24. 60 Fed.Reg. 41,314–41,787 (1995); 61 Fed.Reg. 44,396–45,318 (1996).

25. *Engle v. R. J. Reynolds Tobacco Co.*, No. 94-08273 CA 22 (Dade County Circuit Court, Florida).

REFERENCES

Adler, R. K., and J. Slade. 2000. *Direct mail marketing of tobacco products in the United States*. Eleventh World Conference on Tobacco or Health, Chicago, Illinois.

Altman, D. G., D. W. Levine, R. Coeytaux, J. Slade, and R. Jaffe. 1996. Tobacco promotion and susceptibility to tobacco use among adolescents aged 12 through 17 in a nationally representative sample. *American Journal of Public Health* 86:1590–3.

Anthony, J. C., L. A. Warner, and R. C. Kessler. 1994. Comparative epidemiology of dependence on tobacco, alcohol, controlled substances, and inhalants: Basic findings from the National Comorbidity Survey. *Experimental and Clinical Psychopharmacology* 2:244–68.

Applebome, P. 1999. Tobacco's imprimatur is less bold, but still on cultural events. *New York Times*, 21 June, B1.

Ayanian, J. Z., and P. D. Cleary. 1999. Perceived risks of heart disease and cancer among cigarette smokers. *JAMA* 281:1019–1021.

Balbach, E. D., and S. A. Glantz. 1998. Tobacco control advocates must demand high-quality media campaigns: The California experience. *Tobacco Control* 7:397–408.

BATCo. 1988. Smoking and health: German smokers' attitudes, perceptions and preferences. BAT document number 400170334–400170344 in the BAT archives at Guildford, UK. Montreal: BATCo.

Biener, L., and M. Siegel. 2000. Tobacco marketing and adolescent smoking: More support for a causal inference. *American Journal of Public Health* 90(3):407–11.

Blackmer, E. M. 1996. Affidavit. In *Engle et al. v. RJ Reynolds Tobacco Company et al.*, No. 94–08273 CA 20 (Dade County Circuit Court, Florida), 30 April.

Blum, A. 1991. The Marlboro Grand Prix. Circumvention of the television ban on tobacco advertising. *New England Journal of Medicine* 324(13):913–7.

Bolliger, C. T., J-P. Zellweger, T. Danielsson, X. van Biljon, A. Robidou, A. Westin, A. P. Perruchoud, and U. Sawe. 2000. Smoking reduction with oral nicotine inhalers: Double blind, randomised clinical trial of efficacy and safety. *British Medical Journal* 321:329–33.

Bornstein, R. F. 1989. Exposure and affect: Overview and meta-analysis of research, 1968–1987. *Psychological Bulletin* 106:265–89.

Brown & Williamson. 2000. Lucky Strike's band to band 2000 music competition kicks off round three: Over $100,000 in cash and prizes. PR Newswire, 29 August.

Burns, D. 2000. *Are low tar and nicotine cigarettes less hazardous?* Paper presented at Eleventh World Conference on Tobacco or Health, 7 August, in Chicago, Illinois.

Campaign for Tobacco-Free Kids. 2000. *Big tobacco: Still addicting kids.* Online. Available: http://tobaccofreekids.org/reports/addicting/legacy.shtml.

Coeytaux, R. R., D. G. Altman, and J. Slade. 1995. Tobacco promotions in the hands of youth. *Tobacco Control* 4(3):253–7.

Cohen, J. B. 1996. Smokers' knowledge and understanding of advertised tar numbers: Health policy implications. *American Journal of Public Health* 86(1):18–24.

Connolly, G. N. 1995. The marketing of nicotine addiction by one oral snuff manufacturer. *Tobacco Control* 4(1):73–9.

———. 2000. Letter regarding Massachusetts media campaign. Boston, 28 June.

DeSmith, D. 1998. *A Camel Named Joe: The Illustrated History of an American Pop Icon.* Boston: duCap Books.

DiFranza, J. R., J. W. Richards, P. M. Paulman, N. Wolf-Gillespie, C. Fletcher, R. D. Jaffe, et al. 1991. RJR Nabisco's cartoon camel promotes Camel cigarettes to children. *JAMA* 266(22):3149–52.

Duffy, M. 1996. Econometric studies of advertising, advertising restrictions, and cigarette demand: A survey. *International Journal of Advertising* 15:1–23.

Ellison, S. 2000. Motorola's "silent Bill" arrives via e-mail. *The Wall Street Journal,* 3 August, B13.

Emery, S., W. S. Choi, and J. P. Pierce. 1999. The social costs of tobacco advertising and promotions. *Nicotine & Tobacco Research* 1(supp. 2):S83–91.

Expert Panel Report. 1995. *When packages can't speak: Possible impacts of plain and generic packaging of tobacco products.* Ottawa: Health Canada.

Federal Trade Commission (FTC). 1999. *"Tar," Nicotine, and Carbon Monoxide of the Smoke of 1252 Varieties of Domestic Cigarettes for the Year 1997.* Washington, DC: Federal Trade Commission.

———. 2001. *Report to Congress for 1999 Pursuant to the Federal Cigarette Labeling and Advertising Act.* Washington, DC: Federal Trade Commission.

Fischer, P. M., M. P. Schwartz, J. Richards, Jr., A. O. Goldstein, and T. H. Rojas. 1991. Brand logo recognition by children aged 3 to 6 years. Mickey Mouse and Old Joe the camel. *JAMA* 266(22):3145–48.

France, M. 1996 Is Big Tobacco ready to deal? *Business Week.* December 23, 1996, 32.

Francey, N., and S. Chapman. 2000. "Operation Berkshire": The international tobacco companies' conspiracy. *British Medical Journal* 321:371–4.

Gellene, D. 1997. Joining the clubs: Tobacco firms find a venue in bars. *Los Angeles Times*, 25 September, D-1 (Home Edition).

Glantz, S. A. 1993. Removing the incentive to sell kids tobacco—a proposal. *JAMA* 269(6):793–4.

Glantz, S. A., J. Slade, L. A. Bero, P. Hanauer, and D. E. Barnes. 1996. *The Cigarette Papers*. Berkeley: University of California.

Goldman, L. K., and S. A. Glantz. 1998. Evaluation of antismoking advertising campaigns. *JAMA* 279(10):772–7.

Hamilton, J. L. 1975. The effect of cigarette advertising bans on cigarette consumption. In *Proceedings of the Third World Conference on Smoking and Health*. Washington, DC: U.S. Department of Health, Education, and Welfare.

Hastings, G., and L. MacFadyen. 2000. A day in the life of an advertising man: Review of internal documents from the UK tobacco industry's principal advertising agencies. *British Medical Journal* 321:366–71.

Health Canada. 2000. *New tobacco regulations become law*. Press release. Ottawa: Health Canada, 28 June.

Hendickx, L., C. Vlek, and H. Oppewal. 1989. Relative importance of scenario information and frequency information in the judgment of risk. *Acta Psychologica* 72: 41–63.

Howsden, G. 1995. *Collecting Cigarette & Trade Cards*. Tampa: Pincushion Press.

Hurt, R. D., and C. R. Robertson. 1998. Prying open the door to the cigarette industry's secrets about nicotine. *JAMA* 280:1173–81.

Hwang, S. L. 1999. Tobacco companies enlist the bar owner to push their goods. *The Wall Street Journal*, 21 April, A-1.

Informa Market Research Co., Ltd. 1999. *Focus group research on new health warnings on tobacco packages*. Toronto: Informa, for the Canadian Cancer Society.

Kalant, H. 2000. Nicotine as an addictive substance. In *Nicotine and Public Health*. Edited by R. Ferrence, J. Slade, R. Room, and M. Pope. Washington DC: American Public Health Association.

Kilbourne, J. 1999. *Deadly Persuasion*. New York: Free Press.

King, C., III, and M. Siegel. 1999. Brand-specific cigarette advertising in magazines in relation to youth and young adult readership, 1986–1994. *Nicotine & Tobacco Research* 1:331–40.

King, C., III, M. Siegel, C. Celebucki, and G. N. Connolly. 1998. Adolescent exposure to cigarette advertising in magazines: An evaluation of brand-specific advertising in relation to youth readership. *JAMA* 279(7):516–20.

King, C., III, M. Siegel, and L. G. Pucci. 2000. Exposure of black youths to cigarette advertising in magazines. *Tobacco Control* 9:64–70.

Kluger, R. 1996. *Ashes to Ashes: America's Hundred-Year Cigarette War, the Public Health, and the Unabashed Triumph of Philip Morris*. New York: Knopf.

Knopick, P. 1980. Memorandum to W. Kloepfer. Dated September 9. Minnesota trial exhibit # 14,303. Tobacco Institute Bates No. TIMN0107822/7823.

Kozlowski, L. T., M. E. Goldberg, C. T. Sweeney, R. F. Palmer, J. L. Pillitteri, B. A. Yost, E. L. White, and M. M. Stine. 1999. Smoker reactions to a "radio message" that light cigarettes are as dangerous as regular cigarettes. *Nicotine & Tobacco Research* 1:67–76.

Kozlowski, L. T., M. E. Goldberg, B. A. Yost, E. L. White, C. T. Sweeney, and J. L.

Pillitteri. 1998. Smokers' misperceptions of light and ultra-light cigarettes may keep them smoking. *American Journal of Prevention Medicine* 15:9–16.

Kozlowski, L. T., J. L. Pillitteri, and F. M. Ahern. 1998. Advertising fails to inform smokers of official tar yields of cigarettes. *Journal of Applied Biobehavioral Research* 3(1):55–64.

Laugesen, M., and C. Meads. 1991. Tobacco advertising restrictions, price, income, and tobacco consumption in OECD countries 1960–1986. *British Journal of Addiction* 86:1343–54.

Leavell, N-R. 1999. The low tar lie. *Tobacco Control* 8(4):433–6.

Mahood, G. 1995. Canadian tobacco package warning system. *Tobacco Control* 4(1): 10–4.

Mahood, G. 1999. Warnings that tell the truth: Breaking new ground in Canada. *Tobacco Control* 8(4):356–61.

Martineau, P. 1957. *Motivation in Advertising: Motives that Make People Buy*. New York: McGraw-Hill.

Massachusetts Department of Public Health. 2000. *Summary of 1998 Advertising Campaign Assessments*. Boston: Massachusetts Department of Public Health, Tobacco Control Program.

Master Settlement Agreement. 1998. Online. Available through the National Association of Attorneys General (www.naag.org), November.

McVey, D., and J. Stapleton. 2000. Can anti-smoking television advertising affect smoking behaviour? Controlled trial of the Health Education Authority for England's anti-smoking TV campaign. *Tobacco Control* 9:273–82.

Mullen, C. 1979. *Cigarette Pack Art*. London: Galley Press.

National Cancer Institute (NCI). 1996. *The FTC Cigarette Test Method for Determining Tar, Nicotine, and Carbon Monoxide Yields of U.S. Cigarettes*. Washington, DC: U.S. Department of Health and Human Services, Public Health Service, National Institutes of Health, National Cancer Institute.

———. 1998. *Cigars: Health effects and trends*. 1998. Washington, DC: U. S. Department of Health and Human Services, Public Health Service, National Institutes of Health, National Cancer Institute.

Naymik, M. 1997. Camel clubbing. *The Cleveland Free Times,* 28 May–3 June, 9–12.

New York Times. 2000. New strategy at Philip Morris. Editorial. *New York Times,* 4 March, A-14.

Newman, A. 1999. Smoke one for the tax man. *The New York Times Magazine,* 28 February, 21.

Pierce, J. P., W. S. Choi, E. A. Gilpin, A. J. Farkas, and C. C. Berry. 1998. Tobacco industry promotion of cigarettes and adolescent smoking. *JAMA* 279:511–515.

Pierce, J. P., E. Gilpin, D. M. Burns, E. Whalen, B. Rosbrook, D. Shopland, et al. 1991. Does tobacco advertising target young people to start smoking? Evidence from California. *JAMA* 266(22):3154–3158.

Pierce, J. P., L. Lee, and E. A. Gilpin. 1994. Smoking initiation by adolescent girls, 1944 through 1988: An association with targeted advertising. *JAMA* 271(8):608–11.

Philip Morris. 1993. *Formula 1: Worldwide Evaluation*. Minnesota litigation document, Bates numbers 2500156422–2500156476. Online. Available: http://www.pmdocs.com.

Philip Morris Companies Inc. 2000. *Form 10-K, Annual Report to the Securities and Exchange Commission for the Year Ended December 31, 1999*. New York: Philip Morris Companies.

Philip Morris Incorporated. 2000. *Request for Applications: 2000 Research Focus, Philip Morris External Research Program*. Linthicum Heights, MD: Research Management Group.

Philip Morris International. 2000a. Online. Available: http://www.pmintl.com/tobacco_bus/PMI/corp_resp/market.html. Site last accessed August 2000.

————. 2000b. *Comments to WHO on the Framework Convention for Tobacco Control*. 30 August.

Philip Morris USA. 1999. Online Available: http://www.philipmorris.com. Site last accessed August 2000.

Pillitteri, J. L., S. Shiffman, J. G. Gitchell, S. L. Burton, and A. G. Shimer. 2000. *Smokers who switched to "light" cigarettes: Misperceptions, motivations, and messages to promote quitting*. Paper presented at the Society for Research on Nicotine and Tobacco.

Pollack, J. 1999. B & W's Carlton relaunch first since new ad rules. *Advertising Age* March 1, 1999, 12.

Pollay, R. W. 1998. How cigarette advertising works: Rich imagery and poor information. Expert report for *Imperial Tobacco Ltd et al. v. Attorney General of Canada*, Public Version.

Pollay, R. W. 2000. Targeting youth and concerned smokers: Evidence from Canadian tobacco industry documents. *Tobacco Control* 9(2):136–47.

Pollay, R. W., S. Siddarth, M. Siegel, A. Haddix, R. K. Merritt, G. A. Giovino, and M. P. Eriksen. 1996. The last straw? Cigarette advertising and realized market shares among youth and adults, 1979–1993. *Journal of Marketing* 60(2):1–16.

Popham, W. J., L. D. Potter, D. G. Bal, M. D. Johnson, J. M. Duerr, and V. Quinn. 1993. Do anti-smoking media campaigns help smokers quit? *Public Health Reports* 108(4):510–3.

Popham, W. J., L. D. Potter, M. A. Hetrick, L. K. Muthen, J. M. Duerr, and M. D. Johnson. 1994. Effectiveness of the California 1990–1991 tobacco education media campaign. *American Journal of Preventive Medicine* 10(6):319–26.

Public Health Service (PHS). 1964. *Smoking and Health. Report of the Advisory Committee to the Surgeon General of the Public Health Service*. U.S. Department of Health, Education, and Welfare, Public Health Service, Center for Disease Control. Washington, D.C.

R. J. Reyolds Tobacco Company. 1991. Give your workplace a *reasonable* smoking policy. *Choice* 5(28), cover.

————. 2000. Online. Available: http://www.rjrt.com. Site last accessed August 2000.

Ress, D. 1999. Fighting for more shelf space: New rules haven't cooled cigarette wars. *Richmond Times-Dispatch,* 28 June.

Richards, J. W., Jr, J. Tye, and P. M. Fischer. 1996. The tobacco industry's code of advertising in the United States: Myth and reality. *Tobacco Control* 5(4):295–311.

Rossel, S. 2000. Special editions: The art of smoking. *Tobacco Journal International* May/June, 48–50.

Royal College of Physicians. 2000. *Nicotine Addiction in Britain*. London: Royal College of Physicians.

Rust, L. 1999. Tobacco prevention advertising: Lessons from the commercial world. *Nicotine & Tobacco Research* 1(suppl. 1): S81–9.

Saffer, H. 1996. Studying the effects of alcohol advertising on consumption. *Alcohol and Health Research World* 20(4):266–72.

Saffer, H., and F. Chaloupka. 1999. Tobacco advertising: Economic theory and international evidence. Cambridge, MA: National Bureau of Economic Research, Working Paper 6958. Online. Available: http://www.nber.org/papers/w6958.

Sargent, J. D., M. Dalton, and M. Beach. 2000. Exposure to cigarette promotions and smoking uptake in adolexcents: Evidence of a dose-response relation. *Tobacco Control* 9(2):163–8.

Siegel, M., and L. Biener. 2000. The impact of an antismoking media campaign on proression to established smoking: Results of a longitudinal youth study. *American Journal of Public Health* 90(3):380–6.

Simonich, W. L. 1991. *Government antismoking policies*. New York: P. Lang.

Slade, J. 1989. The tobacco epidemic: Lessons from history. *Journal of Psychoactive Drugs* 21(3):281–91.

———. 1995. Are tobacco products drugs? Evidence from US Tobacco. *Tobacco Control* 4(1):1–2.

———. 1997. The pack as advertisement. *Tobacco Control* 6(3):169–70.

———. 1999. Introductory notes on the tobacco problem. *Nicotine & Tobacco Research* 1(suppl. 2):S27–30.

———. 2000. Innovative nicotine delivery devices from tobacco companies. In *Nicotine and Public Health*. Edited by R. Ferrence, J. Slade, R. Room, and M. Pope. Washington DC: American Public Health Association.

Slade, J., and J. E. Henningfield. 1998. Tobacco product regulation: Context and issues. *Food and Drug Law Journal* 53(suppl.):43–74.

Slade, J., G. N. Connolly, and D. Lymperis. Eclipse: Is there really no cigarette like it? *Tobacco Control* in press.

Slovic, P. 2000a. Rejoinder: The perils of Viscusi's analyses of smoking risk perceptions. Journal of Behavioral Decision Making 13:273–6.

———. 2000b. What does it mean to know a cumulative risk? Adolescents' perceptions of short-term and long-term consequences of smoking. *Journal of Behavorial Decision Making* 13:259–66.

———. In press. Rational actors and rational fools: The influence of affect on judgment and decision making. *Roger Williams Law Review*.

Solomon, C. 1997. Tobacco companies bankroll their own. *Seattle Times,* 10 December. Online. Available: www.seattletimes.com.

Stephenson, J. 2000. A "safer" cigarette? Prove it, say critics. *JAMA* 283(19):2507–08.

Swanson, M., and R. Donovan. 1996. *Generic packaging of cigarettes: A literature review*. Report to Tobacco Working Group, 23 May, Western Australia.

Sweanor, D. 2000. Informed consent: What smokers know and what they need to know. In *Tobakksindustriens erstatningsansvar, Vedlegg 2*. Edited by E. Bjerkestrand. Oslo: Norwegian Council on Smoking and Health.

Tomar, S. L., G. A. Giovino, and M. P. Eriksen. 1995. Smokeless tobacco brand preference and brand switching among US adolescents and young adults. *Tobacco Control* 4(1):67–72.

Turner-Bowker, D., and W. L. Hamilton. 2000. *Cigarette Advertising Expenditures before and after the Master Settlement Agreement: Preliminary Findings*. Boston: Massachusetts Department of Public Health, 15 May.

U.S. Department of Health and Human Services (USDHHS). 1988. *Nicotine Addiction: A Report of the Surgeon General*. Rockville, MD: U.S. Department of Health and Human Services, Public Health Service, Centers for Disease Control, Center for Health Promotion and Education, Office on Smoking and Health.

———. 1989. *Reducing the Health Consequences of Smoking: 25 Years of Progress: A Report of the Surgeon General*. Rockville, MD: U.S. Department of Health and Human Services, Public Health Service, Centers for Disease Control, Center for Chronic Disease Prevention and Health Promotion, Office on Smoking and Health.

———. 1994. *Preventing Tobacco Use among Young People: A Report of the Surgeon General*. Atlanta, GA: U.S. Department of Health and Human Services, Centers for Disease Control and Prevention, National Center for Chronic Disease Prevention and Health Promotion, Office on Smoking and Health.

———. 2000. *Reducing Tobacco Use: A Report of the Surgeon General*. Atlanta, GA: U.S. Department of Health and Human Services, Centers for Disease Control and Prevention, National Center for Chronic Disease Prevention and Health Promotion, Office on Smoking and Health.

Vaidya, S. G., U. D. Naik, and J. S. Vaidya. 1996. Effect of sports sponsorship by tobacco companies on children's experimentation with tobacco. *British Medical Journal* 313:400.

Viscusi, W. K. 1992. *Smoking: Making the Risky Decision*. New York: Oxford University Press.

Wakefield, M. A., Y. M. Terry, F. J. Chaloupka, D. C. Barker, S. J. Slater, P. I. Clark, and G. A. Giovino. 2000. *Changes at the Point-of-Sale for Tobacco Following the 1999 Tobacco Billboard Ban*. Chicago: ImpacTeen Research Paper No. 4. Online. Available: http://www.uic.edu/orgs/impacteen.

Warner, K. E., J. Slade, and D. T. Sweanor. 1997. The emerging market for long-term nicotine maintenance. *JAMA* 278(13):1087–92.

Waterson, M. 1996. Advertising, brands and markets. In *Advertising and Markets*. Edited by J. C. Luik and M. J. Waterson. Oxfordshire, UK: NTC Publications Ltd.

Wilkenfeld, J., J. Henningfield, J. Slade, D. Burns, and J. Pinney. 2000. It's time for a change: Cigarette smokers deserve meaningful information about their cigarettes. *Journal of the National Cancer Institute* 92(2):90–2.

Winkielman, P., R. B. Zajonc, and N. Schwarz. 1997. Subliminal affective priming resists attributional interventions. *Cognition and Emotion* 11(4):433–65.

5

Reducing Harm to Smokers:
Methods, Their Effectiveness,
and the Role of Policy

Kenneth E. Warner

Historically, efforts at tobacco control have focused on three strategies to diminish the toll of smoking: preventing the initiation of smoking by children, reducing nonsmokers' involuntary exposure to environmental tobacco smoke (ETS), and encouraging adults who smoke to stop. The first of these is necessary to avoid future smoking-produced illness in the youngest generation and to break the seemingly endless cycle of childhood addiction followed by premature adult death. The second is essential to protect the innocent, nonsmoking victims of ETS. The last is crucial to minimize the near-future damage on smoking adults caught in the cycle of addiction and disease decades ago.

In general, tobacco control *policy* has focused on the first two objectives, with relatively little policy directed at adult cessation, at least little explicitly identified as motivated, even in part, by the objective of encouraging adults to quit smoking.[1]

More than 45 million American adults are smokers; more than 70% say that they would like to quit; in a given year approximately a third make a serious cessation attempt; fewer than 3% of smokers actually succeed in quitting each year; and the vast majority of these—more than 90%—quit on their own, without using formal cessation programs or devices (USDHHS 1989). Would-be quitters confront a growing array of smoking cessation pharmaceuticals, as well as novel cigarettes and innovative nicotine-delivery devices created by the tobacco industry, many designed with an exterior appearance similar to that of cigarettes (Warner, Slade, and Sweanor 1997). Any reduction in tobacco-produced mortality over the next three decades necessarily must come from reductions in the risks current smokers face. Even 100% success in preventing children from starting to smoke would have no discernible impact on the mortality toll of smoking until the fourth decade of the next century.[2]

As a result of these facts, interest in expanding access to smoking cessation services and in exploring nontraditional means of reducing smokers' risks has burgeoned in recent years. Armed with effective new pharmaceuticals, members of the smoking cessation community—physicians, nurses, psychologists, and other professionals who work with smokers desiring to quit—evince a rejuvenated optimism that they can and must make a difference in the disease burden of smoking. At the same time, cessation professionals know that even the most effective treatments succeed with only a minority of patients. They know, too, that many smokers perceive barriers to the receipt of treatment (financial and otherwise) and that others are not ready or willing to try to quit, though wanting to reduce their risk of experiencing tobacco-produced disease. As a consequence, smoking cessation professionals are calling for expanded access to services and products, primarily in the form of insurance and health plan coverage of cessation treatment.

A subset of the cessation community is also calling for open-minded consideration of additional means of reducing risk. The most commonly mentioned means involve encouraging continuing smokers to reduce the number of cigarettes they consume and spurring the development of more consumer-attractive nicotine-delivery systems devoid of the tars and carbon monoxide that make cigarettes so dangerous. More controversial are recommendations that smokers should switch to less hazardous forms of tobacco consumption, such as smokeless tobacco (Tilashalski, Rodu, and Cole 1998; Rodu and Cole 1999), and that cigarette manufacturers should be encouraged to develop and market genuinely less hazardous cigarette-like products.

This chapter examines the options available to smokers to reduce the dangers they confront from smoking and explores the role of policy in enhancing harm reduction for smokers. Following this introductory section, the chapter includes a brief treatise on the uses and abuses of the term "harm reduction" and an explanation of how the term is used here. The next section describes the principal methods available to current smokers to reduce harms, both those well established as efficacious and those recently hypothesized as necessary additions to the harm-reduction armamentarium. The fourth section compares the cost-effectiveness of smoking cessation techniques, the only category of harm reduction thus far evaluated for cost-effectiveness. The fifth section explores how policy can influence smoker's use of existing harm-reduction techniques and encourage (or discourage) the development of new ones. This section reviews the questions and challenges posed by a contemporary environment characterized by rapid and creative technological innovation and pervasive uncertainty about desirable directions for future policy. The last section offers concluding observations about the potential of harm reduction in tobacco control.

A caveat: because of the broad scope of the chapter, many issues and much evidence germane to the topic of harm reduction for smokers will receive relatively cursory treatment. In particular, with the breadth and depth of coverage elsewhere, this is not a definitive detailed treatise on the efficacy of smoking cessation therapies (USDHHS 1996). Rather, the objective of the chapter is to draw together the essential components of harm reduction for smokers, to elucidate the social and policy issues that confront the tobacco control community. Readers will be provided numerous citations for more thorough discussions of each of the components.

1. Harm Reduction

Proponents of tobacco control have borrowed the term "harm reduction" from the debate concerning society's response to illicit drug use. Harm reduction regarding illicit drugs is posited as a more humane and realistic alternative to the conventional "just-say-no" approach to dealing with drugs. The just-say-no approach relies heavily on the expectation that law enforcement—interdiction of drugs at the nation's borders, arrest and prosecution of users and sellers—can diminish the amount of drug use and its toll. Further, the approach pays optimistic lip service to the notion that education can avert drug abuse in the next generation.

In contrast, harm reduction advocates insist that much drug use is unavoidable. They argue that much of the toll of illegal drug use results from its illegality, rather than inherent characteristics of the substances in question or of their effects on human behavior (Nadelmann 1989). In lieu of the futile and expensive effort of trying to stem the flow of drugs (Reuter, Crawford, and Cave 1988), and the inhumane and expensive measure of imprisoning users, they call for greater investment in treatment. As one option, they recommend less harmful alternatives, such as methadone for heroin addicts. In general, they call for the decriminalization, if not necessarily legalization, of currently illicit drugs (Bayer and Oppenheimer 1993).

At first, the relevance to smoking may seem tenuous, for the simple reason that smoking is legal (subject to age and place restrictions). But the connection is actually quite logical and close: for decades now, the public health community's approach to smoking has been an unambiguous "just say no." The message to children is never to start; to adult smokers, the message is to quit. Intentionally or not, the nation's tobacco control campaign has ostracized and marginalized smokers, marking their compulsive behavior as pathetic and antisocial (Schaler and Schaler 1998). Indeed, today's smoker is made to feel like a degenerate drug user. And like that drug user, the smoker is the victim of a powerful addiction (USDHHS 1988).

Enter tobacco control's version of harm reduction. Due to awareness of the harmful effects of tobacco, millions of Americans want to end their addiction to nicotine but believe themselves unable to do so. As noted earlier, nearly three-quarters of smokers identify themselves as would-be quitters, yet barely 3% succeed in quitting in any given year. Until recently the entire effort to help addicted smokers has rested on encouraging them to quit, to sever their ties to nicotine completely. Sweanor (1997) argues that this approach condemns millions of them to an early and avoidable grave. Among the alternatives to quitting smoking for those who cannot quit, as well as for those who do not want to quit but do wish to reduce risk, are reductions in the daily consumption of cigarettes and substitution of less harmful nicotine-delivery systems for cigarettes. Additional, more controversial possibilities include substitution of less dangerous tobacco products for cigarette smoking (e.g., smokeless tobacco or cigarettes modified to be less toxic) and the use of novel cigarette-like products developed by the cigarette manufacturers that are marketed as reducing risk. In each case, compared to the dangers posed by the unaltered smoking pattern, the alternative holds the potential of reducing the smoker's risk. The notion of encouraging such alternatives to the just-say-no philosophy is itself quite controversial, however. As discussed later in the chapter, effective promotion of such alternatives could conceivably increase *population* risk, even while it reduces risk for many individual smokers.

In the context of the illicit drug debate, harm reduction has clearly come to connote alternatives to the strict law enforcement model of dealing with the purveyors and consumers of drugs. By extension, harm reduction has been used, loosely, in the tobacco control field to refer to alternatives to quitting, in recognition of the just-say-no strategy's failure to vanquish the enormous disease burden resulting from widespread addiction to nicotine.

Logically, however, this connotation of harm reduction is inappropriate, or at least incomplete. Clearly, the most successful method to reduce harm is complete abstinence: quitting smoking altogether. Alternatives such as less intensive smoking or substitution of less dangerous nicotine-yielding products can also reduce harm if the smokers would have continued their established smoking behaviors otherwise. Thus, logically, harm reduction should encompass all means of reducing the risks posed by smoking and nicotine use, both the old standard (cessation) and the more novel approaches that stop short of complete abstinence. This is how I use the term throughout this chapter.

2. Harm Reduction Methods

Smoking Cessation

Techniques employed to encourage smoking cessation run the gamut from simple exhortations to quit by individual or institutional authority figures, such as the surgeon general or the American Lung Association, to elaborate physician-directed treatments incorporating cessation and maintenance counseling, complemented by nicotine replacement therapy (NRT) products or buproprion (an antidepressant that assists in smoking cessation). In between lie diverse interventions such as voluntary association self-help cessation manuals, broadcast media cessation campaigns, hypnotherapy, group behavioral counseling, and acupuncture. Of course, as noted earlier, historically, unassisted quitting (typically "cold turkey") has dominated all assisted techniques by a large margin.

Each of the common methods may increase the odds of quitting for some group of smokers, by means of a genuine treatment effect or, at minimum, a placebo effect. Treatment effects have been established for many of the techniques, including media campaigns (Flay 1987), self-help manuals, group behavioral counseling, NRT and buproprion, and physician-directed counseling interventions ranging from two minutes of cessation counseling to more formal counseling on cessation and maintenance combined with pharmaceutical treatment. Treatment effects for hypnotherapy and acupuncture are not well established (USDHHS 1996; Hughes, Goldstein, Hurt, and Shiffman 1999).

As noted earlier, of the fewer than 3% of smokers who quit each year, the vast majority do so without the aid of formal cessation materials, programs, or pharmaceuticals. These cold turkey quitters have a success rate of less than 10% (reflecting the fact that about a third of smokers make a serious cessation attempt in any given year). Low-intensity interventions, such as printed self-help materials and media campaigns, increase the cessation rate modestly. Behavioral counseling, by physicians or others, can double the cessation rate, as can pharmacotherapy (NRT or buproprion). Even just two minutes of counseling by a physician can increase a patient's "background" (unaided) rate of quitting. The combination of serious physician counseling with patient follow-up and use of pharmacotherapy can produce cessation rates in the vicinity of 30% (Flay 1987; USDHHS 1996; Hughes et al. 1999). However, achieving permanent cessation is a difficult endeavor with any intervention technique. According to one major federal government study, nearly 40% of people who quit for a year relapsed thereafter (USDHHS 1990).

Introduction of the NRT products in the mid-1980s revolutionized smoking cessation treatment, instilling an energetic creative force and a newfound optimism in treatment professionals. Somewhat stagnant until then, tinkering with different modes of counseling patients, those in the field aggressively pursued the new avenues NRT opened. From one product initially (nicotine polacrilex, or "gum"), the nicotine pharmaceutical family rapidly expanded to two (patch), with the nasal spray and inhaler following a decade later. Other pharmaceutical forms of nicotine delivery are under consideration as well, including a nicotine lozenge. The institutional mode of delivery changed along with the technology, with over-the-counter availability of gum and patch replacing their prescription-only status. The medical community is experimenting with combinations of products, for example, concurrent use of patch and gum. The pharmaceutical approach to treating nicotine addiction experienced a sea change with the introduction of an effective nonnicotine drug treatment, buproprion (Hughes et al. 1999).

The advent of NRT medicalized the treatment of smoking (Warner 1994). Prior to its availability, neither physicians nor patients exhibited much interest in treatment of nicotine addiction. Physicians felt ill prepared to counsel patients on their health behaviors (with counseling never a forte of medical education, and rarely a reimbursable event); patients sought a "magic bullet," a prescription, in their physician encounters (Warner and Warner 1993). The availability of NRT gave both physicians and patients a reason to discuss smoking, thereby significantly increasing the prospects for patients to quit (along with, of course, the independent pharmacological effect of NRT). For physicians strongly committed to helping their smoking patients quit, more sophisticated knowledge of counseling needs and techniques has increased the cessation rate substantially.

As pharmacological innovation was revolutionizing the treatment of nicotine addiction, experts on behavioral counseling were developing innovative approaches to counseling patients. Taking advantage of increasingly accessible computer technology to provide instant feedback, behavioral scientists have developed financially feasible means of tailoring cessation messages and strategies to the needs and desires of specific individuals. Whether in doctors' offices or shopping malls, tailoring personalizes the cessation process, providing participants with individually relevant suggestions for enhancing the prospects for quitting. Evidence suggests that tailoring can greatly increase sustained quitting (Strecher 1999).

With new pharmaceuticals and new counseling strategies, smoking cessation professionals have more powerful weapons to combat tenacious nicotine addictions. However, a heady optimism that the new armamentarium would conquer smoking has yielded to a frustration that, despite the availability of these innovations, national cessation rates have not increased substantially. Even with the new techniques, smokers who quit permanently remain the exception rather than the rule. Further, for a variety of reasons—financial, knowledge, prior negative experience, and otherwise—significant proportions of the smoking population do not avail themselves of the new opportunities to try to quit. This is itself a phenomenon worthy of substantial study.

Alternatives to Cessation

Recognition that neither NRT nor improved counseling will be the salvation of America's 45 million smokers has led a subset of the smoking cessation community to contemplate, and in some instances actively pursue, alternatives to quitting as methods of reducing smokers' risks. Some of these approaches really will constitute alternatives; others, however, will serve (or be intended to serve) as complements for more conventional cessation strategies. Much of the interest in alternatives derives from unwillingness to simply "forget" smokers not ready to quit. Thus, one desirable, often self-conscious, function of alternative approaches is to move smokers along the continuum of readiness to change (Prochaska, DiClemente, Velicer, and Rossi 1993). As such, smokers may migrate over time from an alternative to cessation. Professionals hope most will.

Less Intensive Smoking   Emerging interest in the harm reduction potential of less intensive smoking, typically through consumption of fewer cigarettes per day, must evoke an ironic déjà vu among many tobacco control veterans. In the middle of the century, when widespread public concern about the health consequences of smoking first arose, the popular view was that "excessive" smoking was dangerous. Many perceived "moderate" smoking as harmless. Physicians advised many patients to cut back the number of cigarettes they smoked, rather than encouraging them to quit.

Today, a group of smoking cessation experts is contemplating the same strategy for smokers who believe they cannot or do not want to quit. Drawing on the widely accepted belief that fewer cigarettes are less harmful than more cigarettes—there is a clear dose-response relationship between number of cigarettes smoked and risk of disease (USDHHS 1989)—these professionals believe that reduced smoking may be the only viable alternative for an important subset of smokers. They believe, too, that reductions in daily consumption may eventually increase the probability that such smokers will quit altogether. In this view, the conventional wisdom that quitting cold turkey is the most successful method may represent an unfortunate generalization.

There may well be a group of smokers who fail when attempting to quit cold turkey but might succeed through a strategy of gradually phasing out smoking, even including smokers who view reduced consumption (not cessation) as their ultimate goal. Although some research supports the value of reduced smoking (Glasgow, Klesges, Lesges, et al. 1985), other research finds it ineffective (Hughes, Cummings, and Hyland 1999).

Even if reduced smoking could reduce exposure to tar and carbon monoxide, promotion of this alternative is not without risks. Clearly, smokers will find it easier to cut back on their daily consumption than to quit altogether. So encouraging reduced smoking could conceivably convert potential quitters into less intensive smokers. Continued smoking, even at significantly reduced quantities, does not reduce harm when quitting would have occurred otherwise. Thus, the effectiveness of encouraging less intensive smoking, for smokers who say they cannot or will not quit, rests on the balance achieved between reducing consumption among otherwise ongoing smokers and reducing consumption in lieu of quitting. The less intensive smoking strategy also assumes that smokers consuming fewer cigarettes will not compensate completely or largely by smoking those fewer cigarettes more intensively (e.g., inhaling more deeply, puffing more frequently, or smoking the cigarette closer to the butt end). How much compensation occurs when smokers intentionally try to cut back is unclear, although there is widespread agreement that compensation does occur, at least partially (Kozlowski and Pillitteri 1996; Shiffman, Mason, and Henningfield 1998).

Experts contemplating the reduced smoking strategy are fully cognizant of its risks. To them, important questions must be answered empirically before reduced smoking becomes a widely advocated practice: does reduction in the number of daily cigarettes, among confirmed smokers, increase the likelihood of eventual cessation? Does reduction in the number of cigarettes typically reduce the ingestion of tar, nicotine, and carbon monoxide by a proportionate (or nearly proportionate) amount? Does encouraging less intensive smoking decrease the aggregate extent of quitting in a smoking population?

There is an additional route to reducing smokers' risks through reductions in the number of cigarettes smoked: combining reduced smoking with use of NRT. Shiffman and colleagues (1998) note the potential of this approach in their discussion of "exposure reduction therapy," but they conclude that the evidence on its effectiveness is, to date, sparse. Some of that evidence, however, is definitely promising (Fagerstrom, Tejding, Westin, and Lunell 1997).

Substitution of Less Dangerous Tobacco Products   For the nicotine addict who cannot find satisfaction in NRT products, switching from smoking cigarettes to less hazardous forms of tobacco consumption could conceivably reduce risk considerably. In recent years, Rodu (1995), an oral pathologist at the University of Alabama, and his colleagues (Tilashalski, Rodu, and Cole 1998; Rodu and Cole 1999) have argued in favor of converting "inveterate smokers" to smokeless tobacco use. His argument is straightforward, though not without its detractors (Tomar 1996): many confirmed smokers, he believes, can find smokeless tobacco an acceptable substitute for cigarettes, recognizing the risk-reduction benefits it confers in contrast to continued smoking. And smokeless tobacco use, although definitely not without disease risks of its own, is unarguably less risky than smoking.

Rodu's proposal has not met with much enthusiasm in the public health community, in part because there are far less dangerous alternatives to smokeless tobacco for smokers willing to part with their cigarettes but not nicotine. In addition to their health advantage over smokeless tobacco, those alternatives—NRT products—have the advantage of helping many smokers to renounce not only smoking but also nicotine altogether.

One intermediate alternative has received little attention in the United States. Large numbers of Swedish men use *snus*, a smokeless tobacco product (moist snuff) that has low levels of nitrosamines. To date, the evidence suggests that long-term consumers of *snus* do not have noticeably elevated risks of disease, with oral cancer risk greatly diminished compared to that posed by conventional oral tobacco use (Ahlbom, Olsson, and Pershagen 1997).

Less Hazardous Cigarettes and Pseudo-Cigarettes   The notion of providing smokers with less hazardous cigarettes has a long, if thus far futile, history. Filtered cigarettes were advertised aggressively by the cigarette industry in the 1950s as a means of reducing, presumably avoiding, the risk of lung cancer that scientists had strongly associated with smoking. The impact of the advertising campaign was sudden and dramatic: filtered cigarettes went from being virtually nonexistent in 1950 to become the dominant product on the market a decade later. An unprecedented two-year decline in adult per capita cigarette consumption in the early 1950s, the result of the public's concern about smoking and lung cancer, was quickly reversed, and per capita consumption resumed its otherwise uninterrupted upward trend over the next decade (USDHHS 1989).

A similar phenomenon occurred in the late 1960s and early 1970s, when public attention focused on cigarette tar and nicotine yields, with the presumption that high tar and nicotine cigarettes were more dangerous. The industry responded by introducing low tar and nicotine cigarettes, advertised, sometimes explicitly, as a risk-reduction alternative to quitting smoking. The smoking public again leaped at the presumed technological fix: just like filtered cigarettes, low tar and nicotine brands grew to become the dominant product in a decade (USDHHS 1989).

With hindsight, we now appreciate that the tobacco industry always perceived both filtered and low tar and nicotine cigarettes as public relations devices intended to limit the economic damage from smokers' health concerns (Slade 1993; Glantz, Slade, Bers, et al. 1996). The industry never conceived of them as true risk-reduction technologies. As the evidence suggests, however, the public did perceive these innovations as risk-reducing alternatives to quitting. Even much of the medical profession endorsed the new products. In the early 1980s, for example, leading textbooks of internal medicine recommended that doctors counsel their smoking patients to switch to low tar and nicotine cigarettes (Holbrook 1983; Willner 1983).

There has never been any evidence of heart disease risk reduction from "reduced-yield" cigarettes. Early evidence suggested, however, that for smokers who did not otherwise alter their smoking behavior, switching to reduced-yield cigarettes may have conferred a modest reduction in the risk of lung cancer (USDHHS 1981; Samet 1996). Recent diagnostic and autopsy evidence, however, shows that smokers of low tar and nicotine cigarettes have been developing new histologic types of cancers further down into the lungs, indicative of the deeper inhalation used by many "low-yield" cigarette smokers to compensate for reductions in the ease of ingesting accustomed doses of nicotine (Levi, Franceschi, La Vecehia, Randimbison, and Te 1997).

Most smokers who switch engage in such compensating behaviors, some conscious, others not (e.g., smoking reduced-yield cigarettes further down the butt, puffing harder, and occluding the microscopic holes, or air vents, in the filters designed to reduce yields by diluting the smoke), thereby diminishing any potential health benefits (Kozlowski and Pillitteri 1996; Shiffman, Mason, and Henningfield 1998). Finally, some smokers, perhaps many, certainly have substituted filtered and low tar and nicotine cigarettes for smoking cessation (USDHHS 1989; Giovino, Tomar, Reddy, et al. 1996). Without any doubt, they have *increased* their smoking-attributable disease risk. To the extent that this response dominates actual ingestion of lower levels of cigarette smoke toxins, the advent of filtered and low tar nicotine and cigarettes may well have increased the population risk of smoking (USDHHS 1989).

The idea of tinkering with the composition of the cigarette was broached by a prominent member of the smoking cessation community in the 1970s. Russell (1976) proposed that cigarettes be manufactured to yield a moderate dose of nicotine but a diminished quantity of tar. His notion was that a lower tar-nicotine ratio would satisfy smokers' nicotine needs while reducing their exposure to toxins.

Russell's proposal did not find a sizeable receptive audience. It has been resurrected in the late 1980s and 1990s, however, in the form of new industry-produced pseudo-cigarettes that greatly reduce tar deliveries, while providing nicotine and carbon monoxide. The first two such products, Premiere and Eclipse, were developed and test marketed by the R. J. Reynolds Tobacco Co. Neither product burns tobacco; indeed, according to its patent, Premier did not even require tobacco as a raw ingredient. Rather, the device produced an aerosol from glycerin and a tobacco extract adsorbed onto alumina beads close to a carbon fuel element (R. J. Reynolds Tobacco Company 1988; Slade 1993). Premier included processed tobacco papers allegedly to serve a legal purpose: by producing a product that looked externally like a cigarette, contained tobacco, and was called a cigarette, the company hoped that the FDA would deem the product a cigarette and therefore off limits for regulation; the agency had never regulated tobacco products. Although the agency was considering attempting to regulate Premier as a drug-delivery system, its consideration was rendered irrelevant when RJR withdrew the product, having concluded it was failing its market tests (Slade 1993).

There is evidence that RJR expected, or at least hoped, to receive the public health community's endorsement of Premier. At a meeting with the surgeon general and several other government officials, an attorney for the company allegedly explained that the product reduced the risk of cancer associated with smoking. In notes written following the meeting, the director of the Office on Smoking and Health interpreted the presentation as soliciting the Public Health Service's endorsement of Premier, or at least its neutral reaction (Mintz 1987). It is a measure of the public health community's fervent distrust of the tobacco company that introduction of Premier was strongly opposed by all involved in tobacco control.

Premier has been replaced by Eclipse, a somewhat more cigarette-like device that releases nicotine (and glycerin) from reconstituted tobacco in the course of heating, not burning, the tobacco. As with Premier, Eclipse yields nicotine and carbon monoxide but little tar. Eclipse has been test-marketed in several countries and, as of this writing, is still in test markets in America.

Smoking cessation professionals have approached Eclipse with a deep-seated skepticism but with not entirely closed minds. Like its technological predecessors, Eclipse might well reduce disease risk, possibly substantially, for smokers who would use it instead of continuing to smoke regular cigarettes. (But see the caveat in the next paragraph.) However, it raises the prospect of sustaining smoking in smokers who otherwise would quit. It is plausible (although far from certain) that Eclipse, or a product like it, might be deemed acceptable in some places in which smoking is not permitted, because it emits little sidestream smoke into the environment. Many smokers who are not currently permitted to smoke cigarettes in the workplace would likely supplement their before and after work cigarette smoking by consuming Eclipse at work. This would clearly represent an increase in risk for such smokers by exposing them to additional carbon monoxide, one of the major constituents of smoke associated with acute toxicity and, more generally, with development of heart disease (USDHHS 1989). The risk is that on-the-job consumption of Eclipse might reduce the quitting that accompanies workplace smoking bans (Brownson, Eriksen, Davis, and Warner 1997).

Even the health consequences for the individual who merely substitutes Eclipse for conventional smoking remain unclear. Indeed, the product illustrates the complexity of assessing likely risks and benefits in new nicotine-delivery technologies (Stratton et al. 2001). Eclipse clearly reduces total tar yield substantially. According to its manufacturer, it reduces carcinogens in smoke by 64 to 87%. However, an analysis from a state laboratory in Massachusetts found dramatically higher levels of two carcinogens, acetaldehyde and acrolein, in Eclipse compared with conventional ultralight cigarettes (Associated Press 2000). Further, Eclipse poses a risk not associated with conventional cigarettes. Because its carbon heating element burns at temperatures that could injure consumers, the tip is surrounded by a fiberglass shield. Fiberglass particles break loose during the process of packaging and shipping the product. As a consequence, Eclipse smokers inhale some of these fibers (Pauly et al. 1998). Whether this creates a serious danger for users of the product is unknown; but it demonstrates that the very process of modifying products in an attempt to reduce smoking-related risks may inadvertently introduce new hazardous exposures (Stratton et al. 2001).

An intriguing recent development concerns the patenting of a process for removing the nitrosamines from cigarette smoke. In 1999, the Brown & Williamson cigarette company purchased 1.2 million pounds of tobacco cured with this process, with the intent of introducing a cigarette with little or no nitrosamine (Hwang 1999). In 2000, under a contractual arrangement with Brown & Williamson, a company named Star Scientific began test-marketing the low-nitrosamine cigarette under the brand name Advance (Fairclough 2000). The questions posed by this innovation are complex: will the advertising of a low-nitrosamine cigarette produce a net increase in smoking by giving smokers the illusion of a safe cigarette (which, of course, it would not be; it would produce several carcinogens in its conventional tar, carbon monoxide, and nicotine)? Should advertising of such a feature of cigarettes be prohibited precisely for this reason? Could it be prohibited, given the prospect of political opposition and the likelihood of a constitutional challenge on grounds of violating free speech? How could the regulatory process ensure that technological risk-reducing innovations such as this one would be adopted in the production of all cigarettes, assuming that its risk reduction potential could be scientifically established? From a purely public health standpoint, the ideal likely would be required adoption of the innovation, with advertising of it to the public not permitted. If it is even possible, achieving such an outcome is a regulatory challenge of the first order. Both the public health ideal and the difficulty of achieving it appear later in the chapter in the section on policy.

The position of the mainstream public health community on the issue of the development of less hazardous cigarettes and pseudo-cigarettes seems clear. In general, that community appears to believe that there is no such thing as a safe cigarette and that all attempts to create one are either naïve (the scientific community) or disingenuous (the tobacco industry). A just-say-no philosophy prevails in much of the public health community. That attitude notwithstanding, the sheer pace of technological innovation, and the pot of gold at the end of the rainbow for the successful entrepreneur, virtually ensures that this approach to smoking risk reduction will not go away soon. Philip Morris has joined the fray, test-marketing its own new device, Accord. Other companies have announced development of a cigarette with no nicotine and another cigarette modified to reduce the yield of polynuclear aromatic hydrocarbons (PAHs), a highly carcinogenic class of substances. Scores of additional patents for alternative nicotine delivery systems have been filed by the major tobacco manufacturers and others.

Long-Term Nicotine Maintenance   NRT products have been approved by the FDA and marketed by the pharmaceutical companies as short-term substitutes for the nicotine in cigarettes while smokers are attempting to quit. To date, the first two of the products brought to market—nicotine polacrilex, commonly called nicotine "gum," and nicotine transdermal patches—have been authorized by FDA as over-the-counter products. Two more recent innovations, a nicotine inhaler and a nicotine nasal spray, are now available by prescription only. Other products, including a nicotine lozenge, are in various stages of development and regulatory review.

Although the extent of the phenomenon remains unknown, it is clear that some proportion of NRT users have used these products well beyond the medically indicated short-term trial for smoking cessation, often a year or more. Further, perceiving themselves seriously addicted to nicotine and better off with NRT than cigarettes, a subset of these users has no intention of ever quitting NRT. Their physicians often endorse this position, a position that prominent researchers support as well (Shiffman et al. 1998).

It is a small step, but an important one, for physicians to move from tolerating such use of NRT to advocating it for individuals most addicted to nicotine and most likely to relapse to smoking should they be deprived of NRT. The notion of using NRT on a long-term basis has been broached in the literature (Warner et al. 1997) and is receiving serious consideration in policy-oriented health groups around the world (e.g., Scollo 1998).

Although no knowledgeable scientist considers nicotine use "risk free," the best evidence to date finds no obvious major health risks from consuming nicotine in the doses people typically self-administer it (Benowitz 1998). If this becomes the conventional wisdom within the medical community, and doctors begin to encourage patients to use NRT on a sustained basis, a now skeptical public might eventually view nicotine per se as relatively benign, perhaps analogous to caffeine, itself an addictive stimulant widely regarded as minimally (if at all) dangerous. Should such a day arrive, the notion that smokers would switch permanently to NRT products (which then might be called NMPs, for nicotine maintenance products) would be considered unremarkable. Indeed, the use of NMPs by nonsmokers might be deemed largely unobjectionable as well.

Such a day is well in the future, because of considerable skepticism in the medical community about the safety of long-term nicotine use and the widely held belief in the general public that nicotine itself is dangerous. The development of NMPs that would be sufficiently attractive to smokers to serve as adequate substitutes for cigarettes is likely years into the future as well. Nevertheless, this mode of tobacco harm reduction may well gain acceptance for a subgroup of NRT consumers who are there already, with physicians willing to support their decisions, as well as a flurry of innovation in nicotine delivery technology from both the tobacco and pharmaceutical industries. This assumes continued over-the-counter availability of NRT products, of course.

Proponents point out that long-term nicotine maintenance has existed for centuries, in the form of tobacco product use. The tobacco industry is seeking its share of the harm reduction, long-term nicotine maintenance market through its development of products like Eclipse. Clearly, however, maximal harm reduction will be achieved if consumers who otherwise would have continued to smoke switched to nicotine-only products, the current generation of NRT products as well as nicotine-only products still to be developed. From a therapeutic point of view, hope lies with this strategy. Of course, risks and other concerns persist, even if nicotine-only products come to dominate the market (Warner et al. 1997).

Conclusion   Smoking cessation remains the ideal form of tobacco harm reduction. With the new generation of NRT products now available to smokers and more to come, and sophisticated individually tailored behavioral approaches to cessation emerging, more, not less, attention should be devoted to encouraging cessation in the future. As this survey of tobacco harm reduction techniques indicates, however, a wide variety of strategies is, or soon will be, supplementing or competing with cessation and with continued smoking. The hope of all tobacco control professionals, of course, is that the alternative methods will be employed only by smokers who cannot or will not renounce nicotine entirely. If the alternative approaches substitute for effective cessation, they may not prove to be harm reducing at all. Indeed, to the contrary, they would risk increasing harm from tobacco (and nicotine) to the public as a whole.

With filtered and low tar and nicotine cigarettes fresh in their minds, tobacco control professionals are rightly skeptical that a new "easy" alternative to quitting will serve the interests of public health. Nevertheless, the limited success to date of the just-say-no route to reduce tobacco harm recommends a cautious and creative open-mindedness to the array of new possibilities. The challenges will be not only to assess how safe, effective, and cost-effective the various approaches to harm reduction are, and for whom each technique is appropriate, but also to determine how the entire field of harm reduction strategies can and should be regulated, if at all.

3. Cost-Effectiveness of Harm Reduction Interventions

Economists and other interested parties have assessed the cost-effectiveness of smoking cessation interventions ranging from the distribution of how-to-quit booklets to formal behavioral modification programs supplemented with NRT. As discussed later, although recent contributions to the literature differ in the specifics of their conclusions (Cromwell, Bartosch, Fiore 1997; Warner 1997), all analysts familiar with the literature endorse one finding: effective smoking cessation interventions are also cost-effective. Indeed, smoking cessation interventions compare favorably with a wide range of health care interventions (Tengs, Adams, Pliskin, et al. 1995). In fact, cost-effectiveness expert David Eddy (1992) has labeled smoking cessation "the gold standard of healthcare cost-effectiveness."

Cost-effectiveness has not been evaluated for any of the alternative smoking harm reduction interventions discussed in section three; in fact, the essential precursor of cost-effectiveness analysis (CEA), determination of effectiveness, has not occurred for any of these approaches. The fact that all of the alternatives are considered second-best approaches to cessation per se points to an important conclusion about attempts to evaluate their cost-effectiveness: their cost-effectiveness should not be compared to general estimates of the cost-effectiveness of cessation, because cessation presumably will be completely ineffective (hence, cost-ineffective) for people using these techniques. However, some individuals who reduce their risks through alternative methods likely would have quit entirely had they not availed themselves of the alternatives. This complicates analysis of the cost-effectiveness of the alternatives considerably.

The CEA of smoking cessation typically evaluates either the cost per cessation, a behavioral measure of success, or the cost per life-year saved (LYS), a health outcome. Tables 5.1 and 5.2 present illustrative findings from the literature for each type of outcome measure. Behavioral outcomes CEAs (table 5.1), although of inherent interest, offer little by way of comparison with other health behavior change interventions for the obvious reason that quitting smoking has different health implications than, for example, reducing weight. In contrast, analysis of the cost per LYS by smoking cessation (table 5.2) can be compared with health and health care interventions sharing the same health endpoint.

For perspective concerning the health outcome studies, the literature on health and health care CEA finds a few lifesaving interventions considered costless (because they save more money than they cost), several interventions that save life-years for a few hundreds or thousands of dollars, and many that cost from $20,000 to $150,000 per LYS or more. According to Tengs et al. (1995), examples of lifesaving interventions that also reduce costs include mandatory motorcycle helmet laws, a number of childhood immunizations, methadone maintenance for heroin addicts, and prenatal care programs. Inexpensive, but not costless, interventions include beta blockers for survivors of myocardial infarctions, cervical cancer screening, and pneumonia vacci-

Table 5.1. Cost per Cessation—Illustrative Studies

Authors	Type of intervention	Cost per quitter (1995 dollars)[a]
Altman et al. 1987	Self-help	$240 at 1 yr., $84 at 5 yrs.
	Cessation contest	$500 at 1 yr., $260 at 5 yrs.
	Cessation class	$670 at 1 yr., $470 at 5 yrs.
Windsor, Warner, and Cutter 1988	1. Standard information and advice	$190
	2. 1+ standard self-help manual	$220
	3. 1+ pregnancy self-help manual	$92
Tillgren et al. 1995	1. Mass media	$290
	2. 1 + County organization	$250
Fiscella and Franks 1996	Nicotine patch as adjunct to physician counseling	$7,300
Warner et al. 1996	Work site smoking cessation program	$1,500
Cromwell et al. 1997	Implementation of the AHCPR smoking cessation guideline	$3,779

[a]See Warner 1997.

Table 5.2. Cost per Life-Year Saved—Illustrative Studies

Authors	Type of intervention	Cost per life-year saved (1995 dollars)[a]
Oster et al. 1986	Nicotine gum as adjunct to physician counseling	Men: $8,500–13,000 Women: $14,000–20,000
Cummings, Rubin, and Oster 1989	Physician counseling	Men: $1,500–2,100 Women: $2,500–4,300
Krumholz et al. 1993	Nurse-managed cessation counseling	$300
Tillgren et al. 1993	Mass media quit contest + county-level organization	$1,400–1,600
Fiscella and Franks 1996	Nicotine patch as adjunct to physician counseling	$7,300
Cromwell et al. 1997	Implementation of the AHCPR smoking cessation guideline	$2,587

[a]See Warner 1997.

nation for the elderly. Interventions such as hypertension screening in an asymptomatic population cost in the few tens of thousands of dollars per LYS, as does home dialysis for end-stage renal disease patients. Many cholesterol treatments are estimated to cost over $100,000 per LYS, as is intensive care for seriously ill patients with complications. Some government toxin exposure control regulations, intended to reduce cancer risk, are estimated to cost in the tens or hundreds of millions of dollars per LYS.

By comparison with other health care interventions (and, indeed, with common sense), virtually all the smoking cessation interventions appear to represent "good buys"—health care value for the dollar spent. This is likely the most important "take home" message from the cessation CEA literature. In all instances, smoking cessation interventions save life-years at a cost of only hundreds or a few thousands of dollars, far less than such well-established medical procedures as treatment of hypertension, cholesterol screening and treatment, coronary artery bypass, and so on.[3]

It is tempting to interpret the results presented in table 5.2 as implying that certain specific smoking cessation interventions—those with low cost per LYS—are clearly preferable to the high-cost interventions and hence that cessation resources should be devoted almost exclusively to the former. This would be a misinterpretation, however, for at least two reasons. First, differences in variables studied, analytical methods, and data make the various studies not strictly comparable. The safest comparisons are "order of magnitude" comparisons. Thus, it is likely safe to conclude that a "low-tech" educational campaign, saving life-years for a few hundred dollars each, is more cost-effective than a "high-tech" physician-directed counseling program supplemented with NRT, which costs several thousands of dollars per LYS.

Second, thus far, few CEAs have addressed the question of for whom a particular intervention is effective and cost-effective. Although a media smoking cessation campaign is almost certainly a cost-effective intervention, reflecting its ability to reach a large audience of smokers at a low cost per viewer or reader (Flay 1987), the fact is that the vast majority of "participants" in such campaigns fail to quit smoking. Among these will be some smokers so heavily addicted to nicotine that they may need NRT to quit. For them, the media campaign is completely cost-*in*effective, whereas NRT, possibly with professional counseling, may be highly cost-effective.[4] Until CEAs involve interventions tailored to specific types of smokers most likely to benefit from them, any smoking cessation intervention that compares favorably with other health and health care measures on grounds of cost-effectiveness should be considered a desirable intervention, including all of the effective smoking cessation methods evaluated to date.

It is easy to miss this point. For example, a prominent tobacco control scholar observed that individual smoking cessation treatment should be abandoned in favor of public health campaigns against smoking, because the former cost far more per quitter than the latter (Chapman 1985). If resources are severely limited, one might make this argument on the grounds of maximizing social welfare under conditions of constrained optimization. When one considers that resources devoted to these different tobacco control interventions are not perfectly (or even modestly) substitutable, and that the smoking cessation clinic is still cost-effective compared to other health care interventions, the argument for supporting *both* activities seems stronger than that placing them in competition with one another (Warner 1997).

Comparison of the cost-effectiveness ratios in table 5.2 with findings concerning the effectiveness of smoking cessation interventions offers an intriguing insight into the relationship between health care effectiveness and cost-effectiveness. As described earlier, the literature indicates that, in general, the more intensive the intervention, the more effective it is. This has an obvious intuitive appeal. Far less intuitive is the conclusion suggested in table 5.2 that, again in general, the more resource-intensive interventions are *less* cost-effective than those that demand fewer resources (at least when one can compare cost-effectiveness based on cost-effectiveness ratios alone, as discussed before) (Warner 1997). The explanation lies in the relative increase in cost and effectiveness as one moves from the least to the most resource-intensive intervention. Comparing broad categories of interventions by their resource intensity, one finds that the cost of the interventions escalates more rapidly than does their effectiveness. Hence, as intervention effectiveness increases, the cost per LYS rises as well.[5]

There may be subtleties in the literature, but there is no subtlety in the bottom-line conclusion resulting from this review: on the basis of cost-effectiveness, smoking cessation in its myriad forms is a highly worthwhile public health and health care investment. Even so, the national investment in smoking cessation is modest, and many health care organizations that have never hesitated to finance coronary bypass operations do not cover the smoking cessation intervention that might prevent them. The lack of investment in cessation reflects the interaction of a number of factors, including skepticism on the part of many providers and smokers that cessation treatment will work, the absence of emphasis on behavioral counseling in medical education, and the fact that providers not reimbursed for the service will either devote uncompensated time to it or charge their (often ambivalent) patients out-of-pocket fees (Warner and Warner 1993). Another consideration is that health care providers may perceive, quite possibly accurately, that membership turnover might translate into competing organizations realizing the later health benefits of ex-members who quit at the first organization's expense.

The next section addresses the issue of what can be done from a policy perspective about the relative dearth of health care organizations' provision of smoking cessation services, as well as how policy can (or should) address the availability and use of alternative nicotine-delivery technologies. The lack of evidence on the effectiveness of harm reduction strategies other than smoking cessation has precluded CEA of any of the alternatives. The literature currently offers no guidance as to the relative desirability of the various harm reduction strategies, a problem that will not be resolved easily.

4. The Role of Policy in Harm Reduction

Smoking Cessation Treatment

According to one estimate, in 1997 approximately 75% of managed care organizations (MCOs) provided some form of smoking cessation benefit, although the principal form, provided by more than half of survey respondents, was distribution of self-help materials. Only a little over a third provided full coverage for smoking cessation classes (with an additional fifth providing partial coverage). Coverage of pharmaceutical therapy was rare (McPhillips-Tangum 1998).

Coverage of smoking cessation appears to have grown in recent years. With health care organization "report cards" like HEDIS (the Health Plan Employer Data and Information Set) grading MCOs in part on the availability of covered smoking cessation treatment, continued spread of coverage seems likely. To many public health professionals, however, there should be no need to await the vagaries of the market place to ensure that smokers who want to quit do not confront a financial barrier against doing so (Koplan 1998). Advocates of coverage argue that reluctant MCOs should be required to pay for cessation treatment.

What is "right" to do here is not unambiguously clear. Although cessation treatment is certainly socially cost-effective, it is not obviously financially remunerative for health care providers (Warner 1998). In addition, providers who offer coverage face the risk of adverse selection—attracting to their plans customers who, by virtue of their smoking, are at higher than average risk of experiencing an expensive disease. One can argue, too, that most smokers can readily afford treatment; some forms of treatment are not substantially more expensive than continuing to smoke in lieu of the treatment. Further, if the members of an MCO really wanted coverage of cessation, presumably they would indicate their desire for coverage and their willingness to pay for any modest increase in premiums to cover it. But, then, why should non-smokers, the majority of the population, want to subsidize smokers' efforts to quit? There may be reasons—notably, for example, smokers' quitting could eventually reduce nonsmokers' health care insurance premiums—but short-sighted, self-interested nonsmokers are not likely to jump to this conclusion.

The failure of MCOs to cover cessation treatment acts as a barrier to treatment in two ways. The first is the obvious one: smokers desiring treatment will have to pay out of their own pockets. Lacking confidence in their ability to quit, they may be reluctant to sink money into this particular black hole. The widely recognized phenomenon that the demand for preventive services is inversely related to the price of the services holds for smoking cessation in particular: Curry and colleagues (1998) found that a health care organization's providing full coverage of both a smoking cessation behavior change program and nicotine replacement therapy quadrupled members' demand for treatment, compared to providing only 50% coverage of both the behavior change program and NRT. (However, the quadrupling represented 2.4% of eligible members to 10%.)

The second barrier to treatment is a more subtle one: the "system's" failure to include smoking cessation among its covered services sends an implicit message to smokers (and others) that the organization's medical professionals do not deem cessation treatment worthwhile. Thus, MCO members may not want to use services for which they have to pay separately.

With most health care provided on a group basis, minority interests such as smoking cessation may not find a voice in the determination of plan benefits. (Only a minority of adults—fewer than a quarter—smoke, and not all of them want to quit.) This may lead to external pressure to force the provision of such services, possibly through lobbying by interested parties, such as the major voluntary health organizations, to get a state insurance commissioner to mandate coverage. Although this process can protect minority interests, it also risks creating a proliferation of cost-increasing services not widely used, or desired, by plan members.

Should a consensus develop that smoking cessation should be a component of ordinary health care coverage, however, policy measures definitely could be adopted to achieve the result. Legislators could act unilaterally to require such coverage. Although this might represent a good move for health care, it would create an unwieldy and unfortunate precedent, namely, legislating health care coverage piecemeal. A similar concern accompanied Congress's mandating health care providers not to discharge new mothers from the hospital the day after delivering a baby.

Similarly, if somewhat less objectionably (and assuming no conflict with ERISA), a state insurance commissioner could require coverage as a condition of a firm's authorization to sell policies in the state. Alternatively, an insurance commissioner could require the availability of smoking cessation treatment as optional coverage, included for a supplement to the membership premium. At either the state or federal level, government could get into the business of smoking cessation directly, covering it for Medicare or Medicaid, directly subsidizing consumers of products (e.g., NRT) or services (e.g., counseling). Recently, the French government decided to pay for NRT for indigent smokers.

Governments could employ other measures to expand the use of smoking cessation services and products, for example developing media campaigns to encourage cessation. Media campaigns are a staple of comprehensive state-based tobacco control programs, often addressing cessation directly or indirectly (National Cancer Policy Board 2000). Governments could subsidize the producers of cessation pharmaceuticals, either directly or indirectly, by easing the cost of developing such products (as is discussed in the second part of section 5). They could support increased reliance on HEDIS-like report cards that reward coverage of smoking cessation. The possibilities are numerous. The question is whether the resolve to do something about our modest collective investment in cessation exists in either government or the public that ostensibly directs its business.

Alternative Harm Reduction and Public Health Policy

Perhaps the most interesting policy question concerning smoking harm reduction, and ultimately possibly the most important, is how (or whether) regulators or policy makers will choose to deal with the profusion of new nicotine delivery technologies. Currently two types of innovations are altering the nicotine delivery landscape: pharmaceutical companies are bringing new generations of NRT to market, and tobacco companies are test-marketing innovative cigarettes and pseudo-cigarettes that yield reduced levels of certain toxins. As noted before and discussed elsewhere (Warner et al. 1997; Tobacco dependence 1998), these two approaches are subject to radically different governmental oversight, with the degree of oversight inversely related to the dangers posed by the products: NRT products—by far the least dangerous methods of delivering nicotine to humans—are heavily regulated as part of the FDA's responsibility for ensuring the safety and efficacy of drugs and drug delivery systems. The tobacco industry's innovations are labeled "cigarettes" by their purveyors and are introduced with no intent of subjecting them to the drug and device regulatory system.

The FDA is currently contemplating how to respond to this product class, an issue it has pondered since the FDA initiated a proposed regulation of tobacco products in the interests of child safety (FDA 1996). Although the Supreme Court rejected the agency's authority to regulate conventional tobacco products, the issue of the agency's role in regulating novel nicotine delivery devices produced by the tobacco industry remains open, especially products for which explicit or implicit health claims are being made. The agency commissioned the Institute of Medicine to study the scientific basis for regulation (Stratton et al. 2001). At present, no regulatory consideration is directed at cigarettes, the most dangerous form of nicotine delivery yet invented, one never subjected to any product regulation.

Two features of alternative nicotine-delivery systems (ANDS) determine their impact on public health. First and most obvious is their yield of chemicals. Most of the new-generation devices are likely less hazardous in this sense, simply because they reduce or eliminate tar and for the pharmaceutical products, carbon monoxide. Even conventional cigarettes may be made somewhat less hazardous through innovative treatments of tobacco. Consider, for example, Star Enterprise's low-nitrosamine cigarette, Advance (Fairclough 2000).

The second and far more complicated feature demonstrates why product yield reduction may not translate into public health benefit. For the cigarette smoker who would have continued smoking in their absence, lower-risk products almost certainly constitute risk reduction. For the smoker who would have quit smoking in the absence of ANDS, use of a "lower-risk" device may actually represent a net *increase* in risk (i.e., compared to smoking cessation). In the case of NRT products used long term, the addition to risk is probably small. In the case of products like Eclipse, with its high yield of carbon monoxide, the incremental risks could be substantial.

Comparison of use of an ANDS with complete cessation represents the easy case. Far more complicated is the situation in which a smoker uses both cigarettes and ANDS. Consider, for example, a smoker who uses nicotine gum for most of the day but who continues to smoke several cigarettes, although fewer than prior to the addition of gum. Is the gum merely a crutch, permitting continued smoking at a low level for a person who would have cut down or quit anyway? How about the smoker who has reduced daily cigarette consumption considerably without using any ANDS, the result perhaps of not being permitted to smoke at work? Use of ANDS during the workday presumably (although not necessarily) would represent an increase in this individual's disease risk.

Moreover, ANDS pose additional risk concerns. Might a novel nicotine-delivery device be sufficiently attractive to youths who currently eschew smoking to increase nicotine addiction in the next generation? How many of these newly addicted nicotine users would eventually graduate to cigarettes or other tobacco products? Alternatively, how many more youths would start smoking cigarettes in the belief that they could easily quit later using the ANDS?

These are the crucial public health questions confronting regulators and policy makers. Is the new device potentially risk-reducing in that it yields lower quantities of toxic substances? Does it emit new toxins? How would the device be used in practice by smokers (and possibly by nonsmokers as well)? Would it truly substitute for more hazardous smoking behaviors, or would it complement and possibly prolong smoking? Does a new product represent a technological improvement in nicotine delivery? Would its every-day use result in a net addition to or reduction in aggregate public health risk?

As difficult as these questions are, they represent only the first analytical stage of the policy makers' task. They must also determine how to regulate the development, introduction, and marketing of new nicotine-delivery devices. Should all new nicotine-delivery systems be subjected to the (or a novel) FDA drug or device regulatory process? Should newly approved ANDS be permitted on the market on a prescription-only basis or sold over the counter? Should some devices fall into this first category and others into the second? How should regulators control the marketing of new devices or processes, if at all? Should health claims, explicit or implicit, be regulated (Stratton et al. 2001)?

To illustrate the significance of marketing, consider the implications of Star Enterprise's advertising that its new cigarette, Advance, yields fewer nitrosamines than conventional cigarettes. Informed that most cigarette smoke contains nitrosamines and that nitrosamines are carcinogenic, would smokers preparing to quit flock to the new cigarette instead, believing that it would greatly reduce their risk of smoking-induced lung cancer? The net health consequences are unclear: for those smokers who would have continued smoking anyway, switching to Advance might well reduce risk. For smokers who would have quit, or former smokers induced to start smoking again by the availability of this purportedly "safer" product, the active marketing of a low-nitrosamine cigarette clearly would *increase* risk. The net impact would depend on the unpredictable balance between such effects.

In contemplating marketing restrictions, the FDA would need to consider the trade-off between the advantages and disadvantages of companies' advertising risk-reducing technologies. If, in the extreme case, Star was not permitted to advertise its removal of nitrosamines, and if other companies did not adopt the process, few smokers would benefit from this risk reduction because few would know to switch to the Star cigarette. On the other hand, smokers contemplating quitting would not lose their resolve, and former smokers would not be tempted to start up again. From a public health point of view, ideally the FDA might mandate the use of the nitrosamine-removal process in all cigarettes with no advertising permitted. But if the risk reduction could not be advertised, would the incentive to develop risk-reducing innovations decline substantially? The incentive to develop innovations that the FDA might require all cigarette manufacturers to adopt (such as a process removing nitrosamines) would remain strong. But would cigarette companies have adequate incentives to develop product-specific risk-reduction features that they could not advertise? Of course, this discussion about the desirability of permitting advertising ignores the legality, the constitutionality, of banning it.

In short, the situation confronting would-be regulators and policy makers is exceedingly complex. For several reasons, including a modest budget and the political fractiousness involved in dealing with tobacco products, the FDA undoubtedly views the challenge of addressing the situation with ambivalence at best. But as has been observed previously (Warner et al. 1997; Tobacco dependence 1998), failure to develop specific policies is tantamount to accepting today's de facto "policy": imposing a heavy regulatory burden on the safest nicotine-delivery devices, the pharmaceutical products, yet leaving the manufacturers of history's most deadly nicotine-delivery systems, cigarettes, free to introduce new cigarettes and pseudo-cigarettes at will.

The regulatory options available to the FDA are many. And at present, there are no institutional alternatives to the FDA. At a minimum, it seems reasonable to subject all new nicotine-delivery systems to regulatory review, regardless of industry of origin, including those designed by the tobacco industry. Working either within its existing authority or with new congressional authority to regulate tobacco products, the FDA must decide how heavy to make the regulatory burden. The strategic objective might be to make the review process thorough enough to ensure that only risk-reducing innovations successfully pass through it, but not so stringent that attempts to develop innovations are discouraged. Marketing policies must be developed as well. Regulators might permit unrestricted advertising of the most risk-reducing nicotine-delivery systems and heavily restricted marketing of those that reduce risk the least. Advertising of traditional cigarettes could fall within this guideline as well. Other marketing policies could also affect the use of new products. The FDA could impose restrictions on the time, place, and consumer age of purchase for some devices, with fewer or no restrictions on others. Of course, important constitutional issues must be addressed in developing such policies.

Henningfield and Fant (2000) have proposed a set of principles for dealing with novel nicotine-delivery techniques that might be characterized as the conservative ideal (see table 5.3). That is, they envision the use of ANDS with the unequivocal goals of reducing the damage wrought by tobacco and reducing, or at least not increasing, nicotine addiction—itself obviously desirable in light of remaining uncertainties about the health consequences of nicotine use per se (Benowitz 1998). Still, it is unclear precisely how these principles can be applied in practice, and thus how policy should guide the transition toward a reduced-risk environment. An enormous challenge confronting regulators in the real world is avoiding the paralysis that might accompany strict adherence to principles, or rules, that *require* that smoking cessation will not be impeded, or that nicotine addiction will not be increased in the aggregate. How can these outcomes be guaranteed? Is certainty essential to proceed with policy, or is a strong probability sufficient? (How strong?)

The complexity of the situation is demonstrated by a debate in which Henningfield is himself a central figure. As noted earlier, years ago Russell

Table 5.3. Henningfield and Fant's Principles for Regulation of Novel Nicotine-Delivery Technologies

1. The purpose of the indication or product must be to reduce the death and disease caused by tobacco.
2. The long-range goal for the indication or product should be to leave smokers both tobacco- and nicotine-free.
3. The product or approach should pose no added safety risk to the cigarette smoker, and safety data should be extensive.
4. The indication or product should not worsen the individual's level of nicotine dependence.
5. The product should not reduce the likelihood of eventual cessation of tobacco use.
6. The indication or product should not lead to increased population prevalence of nicotine dependence.
7. Its appeal to adolescents should be minimized so as to minimize the risk of adolescent misuse or abuse.
8. Marketing for the indication or product should provide consistent smoking cessation messages and offer help in quitting as well as help in terminating use.

From Henningfield and Fant 2000. Reprinted with permission of the authors.

(1976) advocated production of a medium-nicotine cigarette with low tar delivery.[6] More recently, Benowitz and Henningfield (1994) proposed a diametrically opposite approach: gradually phasing out nicotine from cigarettes and other tobacco products, a policy proposal designed to give addicted smokers the time to overcome their addictions, while ensuring that future generations of children would never become addicted to tobacco. The removal of nicotine is technologically simple. In the 1980s, Philip Morris introduced a "de-nicotined" cigarette named Next, using a process similar to that employed to take the caffeine out of coffee.

The Benowitz and Henningfield idea has had a mixed reception, with opponents concerned that it would lead to contemporary smokers' compensating for reduced nicotine yields by smoking additional cigarettes, among other techniques (Ferrence, Slades, Room, and Pope 2000). The advent of increasingly varied and sophisticated nicotine pharmaceuticals raises the prospect, however, that smokers could substitute "clean" nicotine for more intensive cigarette smoking, while trying to quit cigarettes (Warner et al. 1997; Henningfield, Benowitz, Slade, et al. 1998).

At the heart of any nicotine policy must lie the objective of minimizing damage to the public's health. As this brief review has demonstrated, the components of a nicotine regulation policy are numerous and interrelated in an exceedingly complicated manner. With so many of the essential questions confronting regulators unanswered and, what is worse, possibly not subject to definitive answers, the challenge facing regulators and policy makers is enormous. So, too, are the stakes.

Conclusion

Two factors have combined to force a re-evaluation of the traditional just-say-no approach to nicotine addiction: frustration with the limited ability (or willingness) of smokers to quit and the advent of an era of innovation in nicotine delivery. The objective of the smoking cessation community has always been harm reduction, but the combination of these two factors has dramatically expanded the options encompassed by the term. Because the new options fall short of eliminating subsequent risk from tobacco or other nicotine-yielding products, the term harm *reduction* has come into vogue.

This is a time of energy, creativity, and optimism, but a time too of caution and concern. Enchantment with the high-tech alternatives to just-say-no must always be tempered with recognition that cessation is and must remain the sine qua non of harm reduction. Smoking prevalence has declined gradually in the United States since the mid-1960s, and projections indicate that prevalence will continue to decline for at least the next quarter of a century, even assuming that nothing new appears in the domain of tobacco control. The range of possible declines depends heavily on rates of initiation of smoking by the next generations of children, as well as cessation rates among adults. If smoking cessation rates remain what they are today and initiation rates can be brought down to 20% (from 30% at present), prevalence will inevitably fall from its current rate of about 24% to 12%, driven by the sheer force of population demographics. However, if initiation climbs to 35%, prevalence will fall only to 21.5% (Mendez, Warner, and Courant 1998).

If alternatives to smoking cessation prove to be substitutes for cessation, harm reduction could backfire. If, on the other hand, the alternatives complement cessation, and perhaps eventually convert more smokers into quitters, harm reduction could usher in a bold new era of tobacco control that goes a long way toward taming the horrendous toll of tobacco. By omission or commission, policy will define the directions we take.

NOTES

1. There is one exception: state programs to reimburse smokers for cessation services. Although policies such as raising taxes and restricting smoking in public places will also encourage some adults to quit smoking, few public health professionals would publicly identify this outcome as an explicit objective, for fear of appearing paternalistic and violating adult autonomy. Rather, they call for higher taxes, for example, as a means of discouraging youth smoking (Warner et al. 1995), and clean indoor air laws as a way to protect nonsmokers (Brownson et al. 1997).

2. Technically, this should read "no *direct* discernible impact." Clearly, if all children renounced smoking hereafter, a significant number of adults likely would be induced to quit as a result. This would reduce adult mortality in the near term. The health effects on the children who do not smoke will not accrue until more than four decades hence.

3. No formal CEA of smoking cessation has included future health care cost savings from reduced disease as an offset to cessation treatment costs. Were such economic benefits included, there is reason to believe that many smoking cessation interventions would prove to be cost-saving, not merely cost-effective. (See Warner et al. 1996, whose cost-benefit analysis suggests this result.)

4. Strictly speaking, the media campaign may *not* be completely cost-ineffective for heavily addicted smokers requiring NRT to quit. If the campaign encourages such smokers to seek help in quitting from their physicians, or to try over-the-counter NRT on their own, subsequent cessations should be credited in part to the media campaign.

5. Evaluating the cost-effectiveness of the Agency for Health Care Policy & Research (AHCPR) guideline for smoking cessation, Cromwell et al. (1997) concluded that the *more* intensive interventions were more cost-effective than the less intensive. This is not necessarily inconsistent with what appears here to be the opposite conclusion. Cromwell et al. considered only clinical, physician-led interventions. The generalization in this chapter relates to broad categories of interventions, among which physician-directed interventions typically fall into the resource-intensive category (al-

though not always; brief physician counseling without NRT may constitute an exception).

6. The European Union has adopted a directive consistent with Russell's proposal, limiting machine-measured tar delivery to 12 mg. However, this limit may be lowered to 10 mg, with limits on nicotine (1 mg) and carbon monoxide (10 mg) added, if a 1998 European Commission proposal is adopted (Bates 2000).

REFERENCES

Ahlbom, A., U. A. Olsson, and G. Pershagen. 1997. Health hazards of moist snuff. Stockholm: (Swedish) National Board of Health and Welfare.

Altman, D. G., J. A. Flora, S. P. Fortmann, et al. 1987. The cost-effectiveness of three smoking cessation programs. *American Journal of Public Health* 77:162–165.

Associated Press. 2000. "Safer" cigarette may have toxins. October 4.

Bates, C. 2000. *Implications of European Commission tobacco product and branding regulation proposals.* London: Action on Smoking and Health, January 6.

Bayer, R., and G. M. Oppenheimer, eds. 1993. *Drug Policy: Illicit Drugs in a Free Society.* New York: Cambridge University Press.

Benowitz, N. L., ed. 1998. *Nicotine Safety and Toxicity.* New York: Oxford University Press.

Benowitz, N. L., and J. E. Henningfield. 1994. Establishing a nicotine threshold for addiction. *New England Journal of Medicine* 331:123–5.

Brownson, R. C., M. P. Eriksen, R. M. Davis, and K. E. Warner. 1997. Environmental tobacco smoke: Health effects and policies to reduce exposures. In *Annual Review of Public Health*, vol. 18. Edited by J. E. Fielding, L. B. Lave, and B. Starfield. Palo Alto, CA: Annual Reviews, Inc.

Chapman, S. 1985. Stop smoking clinics: A case for their abandonment. *Lancet* 1: 918–20.

Cromwell, J., W. J. Bartosch, M. C. Fiore, et al. 1997. Cost-effectiveness of the clinical practice recommendations in the AHCPR guideline for smoking cessation. Agency for Health Care Policy and Research. *JAMA* 278:1759–66.

Cummings, S. R., S. M. Rubin, and G. Oster. 1989. The cost-effectiveness of counseling smokers to quit. *JAMA* 261:75–9.

Curry, S. J., L. C. Grothaus, T. McAfee, et al. 1998. Use and cost effectiveness of smoking-cessation services under four insurance plans in a health maintenance organization. *New England Journal of Medicine* 339:673–9.

Eddy, D. M. 1992. David Eddy ranks the tests. *Harvard Health Letter*, July (suppl), 10–11.

Fagerstrom, K. O., R. Tejding, A. Westin, and E. Lunell. 1997. Aiding reduction of smoking with nicotine replacement medications: Hope for the recalcitrant smoker? *Tobacco Control* 6:311–6.

Fairclough, G. 2000. Smoking's next battleground. *Wall Street Journal*, October 2, B1, B4.

Ferrence, R., J. Slade, R. Room, and M. Pope, eds. 2000. *Nicotine and Public Health.* Washington, DC: American Public Health Association.

Fiscella, K., and P. Franks. 1996. Cost-effectiveness of the transdermal nicotine patch as an adjunct to physicians' smoking cessation counseling. *JAMA* 275:1247–51.

Flay, B. R. 1987. *Selling the Smokeless Society: Fifty-six Evaluated Mass Media Programs and Campaigns Worldwide*. Washington, DC: American Public Health Association.

Food and Drug Administration (FDA). 1996. Regulations restricting the sale and distribution of cigarettes and smokeless tobacco to protect children and adolescents; final rule. *Federal Register* 61(168) (28 August):44,396–45,318.

Giovino, G. A., S. L. Tomar, M. N. Reddy, et al. 1996. Attitudes, knowledge, and beliefs about low-yield cigarettes among adolescents and adults. In *The FTC Cigarette Test Method for Determining Tar, Nicotine, and Carbon Monoxide Yields of U.S. Cigarettes: Report of the NCI Expert Committee*, Washington, DC: U.S Department of Health and Human Services, Public Health Service, National Institutes of Health, National Cancer Institute, Smoking and Tobacco Program Monograph #7. NIH Publication No. 96–4028.

Glantz, S. A., J. Slade, L. A. Bero, et al. 1996. *The Cigarette Papers*. Berkeley: University of California Press.

Glasgow, R. E., R. C. Klesges, L. M. Lesges, et al. 1985. Long-term effects of a controlled smoking program: A 2-year follow-up. *Behavioral Therapy* 16:303–7.

Henningfield, J. E., N. L. Benowitz, J. Slade, et al. 1998. Reducing the addictiveness of cigarettes. *Tobacco Control* 7:281–93.

Henningfield, J. E., and R. V. Fant. 2000 Nicotine delivery systems: Implications for abuse potential, medications development, and public health. In *Nicotine and Public Health*. Edited by R. Ferrence, J. Slade, R. Room, and M. Pope. Washington, DC: American Public Health Association.

Holbrook, J. 1983. Tobacco smoking. In *Harrison's Principles of Internal Medicine*. 10th ed. Edited by R. G. Petersdorf. New York: McGraw-Hill.

Hughes, J. R., K. M. Cummings, and A. Hyland. 1999. Ability of smokers to reduce their smoking and its association with future smoking cessation. *Addiction* 94:109–14.

Hughes, J. R., M. G. Goldstein, R. D. Hurt, and S. Shiffman. 1999. Recent advances in the pharmacotherapy of smoking. *JAMA* 281:72–6.

Hwang, S. L. 1999. Latest move to make a safer smoke uses special tobacco. *Wall Street Journal*, 29 April, B1.

Koplan, JP. 1998. Managed care and approaches to tobacco control. *Tobacco Control* 1998; 7 (suppl. 1): S1–2.

Kozlowski, L. T., and J. L. Pillitteri. 1996. Compensation for nicotine by smokers of lower yield cigarettes. In *The FTC Cigarette Test Method for Determining Tar, Nicotine, and Carbon Monoxide Yields of U.S. Cigarettes: Report of the NCI Expert Committee*. Washington DC: U.S. Department of Health and Human Services, Public Health Service, National Institutes of Health, National Cancer Institute, Smoking and Tobacco Program Monograph #7. NIH Publication No. 96–4028.

Krumholz, H. M., B. J. Cohen, J. Tsevat, et al. 1993. Cost-effectiveness of a smoking cessation program after myocardial infarction. *Journal of the American College of Cardiology* 22:1697–1702.

Levi, F., S. Franceschi, C. La Vecchia, L. Randimbison, and V. C. Te. 1997. Lung carcinoma trends by histologic type in Vaud and Neuchatel, Switzerland, 1974–1994. *Cancer* 79:906–14.

McPhillips-Tangum, C. 1998. Results from the first annual survey on addressing tobacco in managed care. *Tobacco Control* 7 (suppl. 1): S11–3.

Mendez, D., K. E. Warner, and P. N. Courant. 1998. Has smoking cessation ceased? Expected trends in the prevalence of smoking in the United States. *American Journal of Epidemiology* 148:249–58.

Mintz, M. 1987. Tobacco lawyer said to concede risk. *Washington Post*, 2 December, F1.

Nadelmann, E. A. 1989. Drug prohibition in the United States: Costs, consequences, and alternatives. *Science* 245:939–47.

National Cancer Policy Board. 2000. *State Programs Can Reduce Tobacco Use*. Washington, DC: Institute of Medicine, National Research Council.

Oster, G., D. M. Huse, T. E. Delea, et al. 1986. Cost-effectiveness of nicotine gum as an adjunct to physician's advice against cigarette smoking. *JAMA* 256:1315–8.

Pauly, J. L., H. J. Lee, E. L. Hurley, K. M. Cummings, J. D. Lesses, and R. J. Streck. 1998. Glass fiber contamination of cigarette filters: an additional health risk to the smoker? *Cancer Epidemiology, Biomarkers, and Prevention* 7:967–79.

Prochaska, J. O., C. C. DiClemente, W. F. Velicer, and J. S. Rossi. 1993. Standardized, individualized, interactive and personalized self-help programs for smoking cessation. *Health Psychology* 12:399–405.

Reuter, P., G. Crawford, and J. Cave. 1988. *Sealing the Borders: The Effects of Increased Military Participation in Drug Interdiction*. R-3594-USDP. Santa Monica, CA: Rand.

R. J. Reynolds Tobacco Company. 1988. *New Cigarette Prototypes that Heat Instead of Burn Tobacco*. Winston-Salem, NC: R. J. Reynolds Tobacco Company.

Rodu, B. 1995. *For Smokers Only: How Smokeless Tobacco Can Save Your Life*. New York: Sulzberger & Graham.

Rodu, B., and P. Cole. 1999. Nicotine maintenance for inveterate smokers. *Technology* 6:17–21.

Russell, M.A.H. 1976. Low-tar, medium-nicotine cigarettes: A new approach to safer smoking. *British Medical Journal* 1:1430–3.

Samet, J. M. 1996. The changing cigarette and disease risk: Current status of the evidence. In *The FTC Cigarette Test Method for Determining Tar, Nicotine, and Carbon Monoxide Yields of U.S. Cigarettes: Report of the NCI Expert Committee*. Washington, DC: U.S. Department of Health and Human Services, Public Health Service, National Institutes of Health, National Cancer Institute, Smoking and Tobacco Program Monograph #7. NIH Publication No. 96–4028.

Schaler, J. A., and M. E. Schaler, eds. 1998. *Smoking: Who Has the Right?* Amherst, NY: Prometheus Books.

Scollo, M. 1998. The future regulation in Australia of products delivering nicotine: Deliberations, conclusions and recommendations following a one day symposium. Carlton South, Victoria, Australia: Victorian Smoking and Health Program.

Shiffman, S., K. M. Mason, and J. E. Henningfield. 1998. Tobacco dependence treatments: Review and prospectus. In *Annual Review of Public Health*, vol. 19. Edited by J. E. Fielding, L. B. Lave, and B. Starfield. Palo Alto, CA: Annual Reviews, Inc.

Slade, J. 1993. Nicotine delivery devices. In *Nicotine Addiction: Principles and Management*. Edited by C. T. Orleans and J. Slade. New York: Oxford University Press.

Stratton, K., P. Shetty, R. Wallace, and S. Bondurant, eds. 2001. *Clearing the Smoke: Assessing the Science Base for Tobacco Harm Reduction*. Washington: National Academy Press.

Strecher, V. J. 1999. Computer-tailored smoking cessation materials: A review and discussion. *Patient Education and Counseling* 36:107–17.

Sweanor, D. T. 1997. Regulation of tobacco and nicotine. In *The Tobacco Epidemic. Progress in Respiratory Research*, vol. 28. Edited by C. T. Bolliger, and K. O. Fagerstrom. Basel, Switzerland: Karger.

Tengs, T. O., M. E. Adams, J. S. Pliskin, et al. 1995. Five-hundred life-saving interventions and their cost-effectiveness. *Risk Analysis* 15:369–90.

Tilashalski, K., B. Rodu, and P. Cole. 1998. A pilot study of smokeless tobacco in smoking cessation. *American Journal of Medicine* 104:456–58.

Tillgren, P., B. J. Haglund, T. Ainetdin, et al. 1995. Effects of different intervention strategies in the implementation of a nationwide "quit and win" contest in Sweden. *Tobacco Control* 4:344–50.

Tillgren, P., M. Rosen, B. J. Haglund, et al. 1993. Cost-effectiveness of a tobacco "quit and win" contest in Sweden. *Health Policy* 26:43–53.

Tobacco dependence: Innovative regulatory approaches to reduce death and disease. 1998. *Food and Drug Law Journal* 53 (suppl. 1):1–137.

Tomar, S. L. 1996. Smokeless tobacco: A life saver? *Tobacco Control* 5:77–8.

U.S. Department of Health and Human Services (USDHHS). 1981. *The Health Consequences of Smoking: The Changing Cigarette. A Report of the Surgeon General*. Rockville, MD: U.S. Department of Health and Human Services, Public Health Service, Centers for Disease Control, Center for Health Promotion and Education, Office on Smoking and Health. DHHS Publication No. (PHS) 81–50156.

———. 1988. *The Health Consequences of Smoking: Nicotine Addiction. A Report of the Surgeon General*. Rockville, MD: U.S. Department of Health and Human Services, Public Health Service, Centers for Disease Control, Center for Health Promotion and Education, Office on Smoking and Health. DHHS Publication No. (CDC) 88–8406.

———. 1989. *Reducing the Health Consequences of Smoking: 25 Years of Progress. A Report of the Surgeon General*. Atlanta: U.S. Department of Health and Human Services, Public Health Service, Centers for Disease Control, National Center for Chronic Disease Prevention and Health Promotion, Office of Smoking and Health. DHHS Publication No. (CDC) 89–8411.

———. 1990. *The Health Benefits of Smoking Cessation. A Report of the Surgeon General*. Rockville, MD: U.S. Department of Health and Human Services, Public Health Service, Centers for Disease Control, Center for Chronic Disease Prevention and Health Promotion, Office of Smoking and Health. DHHS Publication No. (CDC) 90–8416.

———. 1996. *Smoking Cessation. Clinical Practice Guideline Number 18*. Rockville, MD: Public Health Service, Agency for Health Care Policy and Research, Centers for Disease Control and Prevention. AHCPR Publication No. 96–0692.

Warner, K. E. 1994. Nicotine replacement therapy in a public health context. *International Journal of Smoking Cessation* 3(1):1–2.

———. 1997. Cost-effectiveness of smoking cessation therapies: Interpretation of the evidence and implications for coverage. *PharmacoEconomics* 11:538–49.

———. 1998. Smoking out the incentives for tobacco control in managed care settings. *Tobacco Control* 7 (suppl 1):S50–4.

Warner, K. E., F. J. Chaloupka, P. J. Cook, et al. 1995. Criteria for determining an optimal cigarette tax. *Tobacco Control* 4:380–6.

Warner, K. E., J. Slade, and D. T. Sweanor. 1997. The emerging market for long-term nicotine maintenance. *JAMA* 278:1087–92.

Warner, K. E., R. J. Smith, D. G. Smith, and B. E. Fries. 1996. Health and economic implications of a worksite smoking-cessation program: A simulation analysis. *Journal of Occupational and Environmental Medicine* 38:981–92.

Warner, K. E., and P. A Warner. 1993. Is an ounce of prevention worth a pound of cure? Disease prevention in health care reform. *Journal of Ambulatory Care Management* 16(4):38–49.

Willner, J. S. 1983. Tobacco abuse and dependence. In *Family Medicine.* 2nd ed. Edited by R. B. Taylor. New York: Springer-Verlag.

Windsor, R. A., K. E. Warner, and G. R. Cutter. 1988. A cost-effectiveness analysis of self-help smoking cessation methods for pregnant women. *Public Health Reports* 103:83–8.

6

Reducing the Supply of
Tobacco to Youths

Nancy A. Rigotti

Preventing tobacco use by young people emerged as a major, if not *the* major, theme of tobacco control public policy in the 1990s for several reasons. From the public health perspective, prevention is more appealing than treatment as a remedy for harmful exposure. Conceptually, the simplest way to stop the harm of tobacco use is to prevent it from starting in the first place. This inevitably leads to a focus on youths because nearly 90% of smokers in the United States smoke their first cigarette before the age of 18 (USDHHS 1994). A youth-focused approach also has great political appeal. Protecting children from harm is a popular theme in American culture and electoral politics (Cismoski 1994). Because minors are supposedly too young to make rational decisions for themselves, American political tradition opens up additional policy options for tobacco control and permits government to regulate minors' behavior in ways that would not be acceptable if applied to adults. A youth-focused approach is also difficult for the tobacco industry to oppose because it is politically unacceptable for tobacco manufacturers to admit that they market to youths or that they want youths to use their products, even though previously secret tobacco industry documents provide ample evidence that they have done so.

The youth-focused strategy was not without controversy in the tobacco control community. Glantz (1996) and others pointed out its potential pitfalls, arguing that the message that young people shouldn't smoke inadvertently casts smoking as an "adult behavior," thereby transforming it into a "forbidden fruit" that would be even more appealing to young people seeking to rebel or appear more mature. The political downside was that a youth focus threatened to distract legislative and regulatory attention from clean indoor air policies, which were more broadly targeted and contributed to the steady decline in adult tobacco use during the 1980s (Americans for Non-smokers Rights 1998a). A youth-focused strategy will not reduce tobacco-related morbidity or mortality for decades, because of the time delay between the onset of tobacco use and the development of the diseases it causes. Most of the projected tobacco-related deaths for the first half of this century will occur among individuals who have already begun to smoke (World Health Organization [WHO] 1998). Even if youth tobacco initiation among the young stopped completely, it would take almost 40 years to reduce preva-lence of smoking by half (Levy, Cummings, and Hyland 2000). Tobacco use treatment can reduce tobacco-related mortality in the short term, and com-bining prevention and treatment is the optimal strategy. Yet treatment is not generally considered part of the youth-focused prevention approach.

Nonetheless, the youth focus was irresistible and became a dominant force in tobacco control public policy making in the 1990s. In this context, a new policy goal emerged: reducing the supply of tobacco to youths. Public health efforts to prevent tobacco use have traditionally aimed to reduce young peo-ple's *demand* for tobacco products by increasing the price of tobacco prod-ucts, restricting tobacco advertising and promotion, and providing school-based tobacco education. However, in order to start smoking, young people must not only want to smoke but also have a *supply* of tobacco products available to them. Reducing the supply of tobacco to youths, also phrased as reducing youths' access to tobacco products, became a new strategy for pre-venting tobacco use (Forster & Wolfson 1998; Rigotti 1999). Its underlying hypothesis was that fewer youths will use tobacco if they cannot obtain it from retailers or other sources (DiFranza 2000).

Policies with supply reduction as a goal remain widely advocated, enjoy strong public support, and are a cornerstone of youth-focused tobacco con-trol public policy efforts at the federal, state, and local levels (Forster & Wolfson 1998; Rigotti 1999). Because the supply-side approach to reducing youths' tobacco use is relatively new, evidence about its effectiveness is lim-ited. Questions about its effectiveness and appropriate role in the spectrum of tobacco control policy remain. The purpose of this chapter is review the record and consider the prospects for policies aimed at reducing youths' access to tobacco, which are a distinctive feature of the youth-focused strategy to tobacco control.

1. Sources of Tobacco for Youths

There is ample evidence that young people have ready access to tobacco. Adolescents consistently report in surveys that they have little difficulty obtaining tobacco products (USDHHS 1994; Forster & Wolfson 1998). The national school-based Monitoring the Future Surveys report that in each year from 1992 to 1997, 76%–78% of eighth graders and 89%–91% of tenth graders said that it would be "fairly easy" or "very easy" to get cigarettes if they wanted to obtain them (Monitoring the Future 2000). Small but statistically significant declines in the perceived availability of tobacco were observed for the first time in 1998 and persisted into 1999 for eighth, but not tenth graders. Even so, in 1999, 71.5% of eighth graders and 88.3% of tenth graders reported that cigarettes were easy to obtain.

Much is known about how and where teens obtain tobacco products (Cummings, Sciandra, Pechacek, Orlandi, and Lynn 1992; USDHHS 1996a; Forster, Wolfson, Murray, Wagenaar, and Claxton 1997; Forster & Wolfson 1998). Attention initially focused on commercial sources of tobacco products, which consist of sales to youths in stores and from vending machines, shoplifting of cigarettes from stores, and manufacturers' provision of free cigarette samples to youths. In surveys, youths consistently cite commercial sources, especially convenience stores, gas stations, and vending machines, as important sources of tobacco products (Forster & Wolfson 1998). Many studies that document the frequency at which retail stores sell cigarettes to minors who are making test purchase attempts (USDHHS 1994). One study that systematically assessed the sales of all types of tobacco products to underage teens found that cigars, chewing tobacco, and loose tobacco were sold to minors at the same rate as cigarettes (DiFranza, Coleman, and StCyr 1999).

Sales to minors are facilitated by self-service displays of tobacco products in stores, which minimize a young person's contact with a salesperson and encourage shoplifting (Forster et al. 1997; Tobacco Retailer Responsibility Initiative [TRRI] 1999). The sale of single cigarettes ("loosies") in low-income communities may also facilitate tobacco purchase by minors, who have less disposable income (Gemson et al. 1998; TRRI 1999). Vending machine sales account for only a small proportion of tobacco sales to youths, but they are relatively more important for younger teens, for whom over-the-counter tobacco purchase is more difficult. Youths could also purchase tobacco products through the mail or via the Internet (Williams, Montgomery, and Pasnik 1997). The extent to which this occurs is not known. Sales to youths via mail or Internet are facilitated by a low minimum order, as youths have less discretionary income, and by payment in forms other than credit cards, which youths are not likely to have (Malone and Bero 2000). Free samples of tobacco products are often distributed in the context of music concerts, car races, or other events sponsored by a tobacco company (TRRI 1999). These events attract a young audience and provide a venue in which it is easy for minors to obtain tobacco products.

The importance of noncommercial (or "social") sources of tobacco has been recognized more recently. Noncommercial sources include friends (usually older teens and young adults) and relatives (largely siblings but also parents and other relatives), who give tobacco to minors (Wolfson, Forster, Claxton, and Murray 1997a, Forster & Wolfson 1998). Underage youths also ask older teens and adults, especially young adults, to buy tobacco products for them. In one survey, 59% of 18- to 19-year-olds and 39% of 20- to 24-year-olds reported having been asked to provide tobacco to a minor in the past year (Ribisl, Norman, Howard-Pitney, and Howard 1999b). In Minnesota, 69% of smokers in eighth to tenth grades reported that they had provided tobacco to another teen in the past 30 days (Wolfson et al. 1997a). The students who gave to other teens were most likely to have obtained their own cigarettes from a commercial source. Thus, even the social sources of tobacco are at their root commercial. The cigarettes given to teens by friends and relatives initially had to be purchased (or stolen) from a commercial source by someone, although that person might not have been under age. Even so, the commercial versus social distinction is a useful way to describe the final step in the process that results in a tobacco product in the hands of a minor.

The relative importance of commercial and social sources varies according to a youth's age and smoking experience. Social sources are especially important for youths just starting to smoke, who do not yet need a consistent regular source of tobacco, and for younger teens, who have more difficulty buying tobacco for themselves. Emery and colleagues (1999) analyzed the source of cigarettes by youth's stage of adoption of smoking, using the 1996 California Tobacco Survey of adolescents. Experimenters (youths who had smoked <100 lifetime cigarettes) were most likely to be given cigarettes by others; established smokers (>100 lifetime cigarettes) usually purchased cigarettes themselves or through intermediaries. About 75% of experimenters, but only 17% of established smokers, reported that their usual source of cigarettes was others. Adolescents who reported daily cigarette smoking were more likely to purchase; those who did not smoke daily were usually given their cigarettes.

Basic economic theory postulates that if one supplier of a desired commodity stops, the incentive for another to enter the market will increase, as long as demand for the product remains strong (Jha and Chaloupka 1999). So social sources of cigarettes would become even more important as tobacco control efforts limit young people's access to tobacco from commercial sources (Rigotti 1999). Some data support this conclusion. In California, as the rates of tobacco sales to minors declined from 52% to 13% between 1994 and 1998, social sources increased and commercial sources decreased as the usual source of cigarettes for high school smokers (Ribisl et al. 1999a). There was no overall change in California youths' reports of their ease in obtaining tobacco products over the interval. In six Massachusetts communities, social sources of tobacco became more important as youths' perceived access to tobacco from commercial sources fell over 2 years (Rigotti et al. 1997).

The volume of tobacco products used by youths is huge. According to a recent estimate, youths under age 18 in the United States smoke 924 million packs of cigarettes per year. The sale of these cigarettes generates $1.86 billion in revenue, $222 million in federal tax revenues, $293 million in state tax revenues, and $480 million in tobacco company profits (DiFranza and Librett 1999). These figures illustrate the strong financial incentive that tobacco manufacturers and retailers have in continuing to sell tobacco eventually smoked by minors.

2. Policy Options for Reducing the Supply of Tobacco to Youths

Commercial Sources of Tobacco Products

Policies aimed at reducing the supply of tobacco to youths have focused on blocking their access to commercial sources of tobacco products. Policy options include (1) restricting or banning tobacco sales to minors, (2) mandating the conditions in which tobacco products can be sold, and (3) banning the distribution of free tobacco products to youths (or to anyone).

Because the major commercial source of tobacco to minors is over-the-counter tobacco sale, efforts to restrict or prohibit these sales have received the most attention. A policy whose goal is to block the commercial transfer of tobacco products from a retailer to a youth could be formulated in either of two ways. It could prohibit the *sale* of tobacco to individuals below a specified age or it could prohibit the *purchase* of tobacco by under-age individuals. These two approaches sound similar but have different enforcement implications. Banning tobacco sales to minors puts the responsibility for compliance on the retailer. Banning tobacco purchase puts the responsibility for compliance on the youth. Related to, but broader than, prohibiting the purchase of tobacco is a policy that prohibits the *possession* and/or *use* of tobacco products by minors. This approach keeps the onus for compliance on youths but extends beyond simple supply reduction.

The minimum age at which tobacco sale, purchase, possession, and use is permitted will affect tobacco's availability to youths. The current minimum age of tobacco sale is 18 years in nearly all states, but raising the minimum age to 19 or even 21 has been proposed. The potential value of a higher minimum age is suggested by analogy to the effects observed when the minimum drinking age was raised from 18 to 21 years in the United States in the 1980s. Rates of youth drinking and motor vehicle accidents fell, even though the minimum drinking age was poorly enforced and widely violated (Wagenaar and O'Malley 1991; Wagenaar and Wolfson 1994). Raising the minimum age for tobacco sale to 21 years would put tobacco on par with alcohol and permit better coordination of enforcement efforts. Even raising the minimum age of tobacco use to 19 years would, in theory, prevent high school seniors, who are usually no more than 18 years old, from legally buying tobacco and providing it to younger teens. This strategy should reduce the social availability and visibility of tobacco to high school students.

Limiting the conditions under which tobacco products can be sold could also limit the supply of tobacco to minors. One approach that has been used with alcohol is to limit the density of alcohol vendors (Mosher and Stewart 1999). Tobacco is more widely available than alcohol. Reducing the density of retail tobacco outlets, especially outlets where age-of-sale laws are not or cannot be enforced, might reduce the availability of tobacco to minors. An example is the prohibition of tobacco sales from vending machines, which cannot distinguish the age of the purchaser. Restricting tobacco vending machines to adults-only locales such as bars is a less comprehensive option. Tobacco sales could also be prohibited from categories of retail outlets that have poor compliance with age-of-sale laws, such as gas stations and convenience stores. It has even been suggested that tobacco sales be limited to government-run stores, as is the case for alcohol in some locales (Mosher and Stewart 1999; DiFranza 2000). Alternatively, retail tobacco outlets could be restricted from locations frequented by youths, such as schools, playgrounds, or residential facilities. Policies could establish a buffer zone around these facilities in which tobacco cannot be sold. Many state and local governments have adopted this approach to restrict alcohol sales (Mosher and Stewart 1999).

Alternatively, the conditions of tobacco product sale within stores could be limited. Two approaches are commonly suggested. One is to prohibit the sale of cigarettes in quantities less than a standard pack of 20 cigarettes. The sale of individual cigarettes, which are less expensive than a pack, is thought to make tobacco more affordable to youths, who have less disposable income. A second, widely advocated approach is to prohibit the free-standing displays of tobacco products in stores. Free-standing displays facilitate shoplifting of cigarettes by minors (Cummings, Hyland, Saunders-Martin, and Perla 1998–99). Retailers normally fight inventory loss due to shoplifting but have maintained self-service displays of cigarettes because tobacco companies pay them to do so (Feighery Ribisl, Achabal, and Tyebjee 1999). Presumably the fees paid to retailers more than compensate them for the lost inventory. Keeping tobacco products behind the counter rather than in free-standing displays also requires a longer period of contact between the store clerk and a minor, which might discourage minors from attempting to purchase tobacco and increase the likelihood that the clerk will refuse the sale.

Noncommercial Sources of Tobacco Products

Stopping the supply of tobacco to youths from noncommercial sources is more problematic. Policy options are likely to be more limited because of the private nature of the action: tobacco is obtained from an individual rather than a commercial source, the supplier is often a friend or relative, and tobacco is often (but not always) provided voluntarily. One option, analogous to alcohol policy, is to prohibit individuals from providing tobacco to minors. The act of providing tobacco to minors may already be banned by existing statutes that prohibit tobacco sales to minors or that prohibit adults from contributing to the delinquency of a minor (TRRI 1999). If not, a law that specifically banned the provision of tobacco to a minor by anyone could be adopted. But such a law is likely to be even more difficult to enforce effectively than existing bans on the commercial sale of tobacco to minors have been. Successful implementation would require a social consensus about the unacceptability of giving tobacco to youths or buying tobacco for youths. Whether this consensus exists is not clear.

A decrease in the social availability of tobacco to youths might also be a byproduct of more broadly targeted tobacco control policies, such as clean indoor air laws that prohibit smoking in public places, workplaces, and restaurants. By removing smoking from places that youths frequent, such as restaurants, community events, and school sporting events, clean indoor air laws could decrease the visibility of tobacco use and may reduce opportunities for youths to obtain tobacco from noncommercial sources. Raising the minimum age of legal tobacco sale to minors might also help to decrease the social availability of tobacco to youths by increasing the age difference between a teen requesting a tobacco purchase and the youngest adult who can legally buy as a proxy (DiFranza 2000; TRRI 1999). Given the difficulty in identifying policy approaches to reduce noncommercial sources of tobacco to youths, educational and persuasive efforts that aim to change social norms about the acceptability of providing tobacco to youths may be a starting point.

3. State and Local Government Actions to Reduce Tobacco Sales to Minors

To varying degrees, federal, state, and local governments have used legislative and regulatory means to block the supply of tobacco to minors from commercial sources. Legislative action has primarily been taken by state governments, followed by local communities. Every state currently has in place a law that prohibits the sale of tobacco to minors, and most already had a law in place before the dawn of the youth access movement in the 1980s (Forster & Wolfson 1998; DiFranza 1999). These statutes were left over from the now-defunct tobacco prohibition movement that banned tobacco use in many states in the late nineteenth and early twentieth centuries. Until the youth access movement, however, these laws were rarely enforced. DiFranza and colleagues (1987) first demonstrated retailers' poor compliance with the tobacco sales laws in 1987. Since then, the finding has been reproduced in multiple studies conducted in multiple states (Office of the Inspector General 1995). A 1994 summary of this work demonstrated that cigarettes and smokeless tobacco could be consistently bought by adolescents in test purchases at rates averaging 67% of attempts from stores and 88% of attempts from vending machines (USDHHS 1994). The purchase of tobacco products is easier for older adolescents and for girls/women (DiFranza, Savageau, and Aisquith 1996; Clark, Natanblut, Schumitt, Wolters, and Iachan 2000). A minor's race affected the success of purchase attempts in some but not all studies (Voorhees et al. 1997; Klonoff, Landrine, and Alcaraz 1997). Tobacco sales are more likely to occur after 5 PM than earlier in the day, on Saturdays more than other days, and when the clerk selling the tobacco is female (Clark et al. 2000). Tobacco sales to minors are less likely to occur if a store clerk asks a purchaser to display proof of age, although this is not a guarantee. Clerks sold tobacco to under-age youths 10.5% of the time when they were shown identification clearly indicating that a youth was under age (Clark et al. 2000).

The awareness of widespread noncompliance with existing laws banning tobacco sales to minors led to a series of public health responses taken primarily at the local community level (Rigotti 1999). Initially, the goal was to improve compliance with existing laws and regulations. Two strategies were tried. The first was to educate merchants about their responsibilities. The second was to enforce existing statutes more aggressively to create effective deterrents to retailers' sale of tobacco to minors. For a deterrent to work, there must be a credible threat that a sufficiently severe negative consequence will occur swiftly and certainly, and the threat must be perceived to persist over time (Ross 1992). To accomplish this end, enforcement programs tested merchant compliance proactively, using a "compliance check" or "test purchase" in which minors, supervised by adults, attempted to buy tobacco from a sample of stores or vending machines. Merchants who violated the law were fined and, for repeated offenses, could have their license to sell tobacco suspended. These enforcement programs were conducted primarily by public health officials and not by police, for whom enforcing tobacco sales laws had low priority.

New laws and regulations that went beyond existing laws were also proposed and passed. These generally strengthened existing statutes by incorporating provisions intended to facilitate enforcement. Expert groups and tobacco control advocates have generally agreed on a consistent set of provisions for a model tobacco access law: (Institute of Medicine 1994; Working Group 1994; Jacobson and Wasserman 1997; Forster & Wolfson 1998; Advocacy Institute 2000).

1. *Establish a minimum age* of at least 18 years for tobacco sales. A higher minimum age—19 or even 21 years—has been advocated by some, for the reasons already described.

2. *Require that retailers establish proof of age* by checking identification before selling tobacco to a young person. Illegal tobacco sales to minors are less likely to occur when a purchaser is asked for proof of age (Clark et al. 2000). This simple concept can be difficult to implement because of the time required for a clerk to look at a driver's license and calculate the customer's current age from the date of birth. Age verification slows commercial transactions, producing longer lines at the cash register and impatient customers. This problem is potentially amenable to a technological solution (TRRI 1999). Electronic price scanners used by large retail merchants can be programmed with tobacco "locks" that interrupt the transaction when a tobacco product bar code is scanned until birth date or age verification is entered. A state can design its drivers' licenses to allow retail store scanners to calculate age electronically.

3. *Create a tobacco sales licensing system* that allows tobacco retailers to be identified and informed of their legal responsibilities. Revenues generated from licensing can fund a government's enforcement program so that it is self-supporting and therefore does not depend on an annual allocation of state funds from the legislative or executive branches of state government. This approach increases the cost-effectiveness of enforcement as a tobacco control strategy.

4. *Require periodic proactive tests of retailers' compliance* with tobacco sales laws using the method of compliance checks or test buys. This method identifies retailers who are not complying with the law. Periodic monitoring of compliance is necessary to maintain retailer compliance, with advocates recommending testing each store several times per year (Advocacy Institute 2000). Setting a minimum acceptable standard of compliance is suggested as a way to ensure that en-

forcement efforts are sufficiently aggressive. Minimum compliance rates of 90% or more are most often suggested (Advocacy Institute 2000).

5. *Establish administrative or civil law penalties* for illegal tobacco sales that range from graduated fines to license revocation for repeat offenders. Administrative civil disposition of violations is considered appropriate to the nature of the offense and avoids costly, time-consuming, and unnecessary criminal prosecutions. Revocation of a license to sell tobacco is thought to provide a strong negative deterrent to tobacco sales, because tobacco sales are highly profitable and provide a substantial source of revenue for retailers, especially convenience stores. Penalties should be assessed against the store (e.g., the license holder) rather than the clerk.

6. *Prohibit self-service displays of tobacco products*, which facilitate shoplifting of cigarettes by minors (Cummings et al. 1998–99), as described earlier.

7. *Prohibit the sale of cigarettes in quantities less than a standard pack* (e.g., 20 cigarettes) because smaller quantities of cigarettes are more affordable to youths, who have less disposable income.

8. *Prohibit tobacco sales in vending machines*, which are a source of cigarettes especially for younger smokers, who have difficulty purchasing tobacco over the counter, or at least limit tobacco vending machines to adults-only venues such as bars.

9. *Prohibit distribution of free samples* of tobacco products, ideally to all individuals but at least to youths.

Laws with these provisions have been enacted at the state and local levels. According to the CDC's State Tobacco Activities Tracking & Evaluation (STATE) System database, at the end of 1999, all states banned tobacco sales to minors (CDC 2000). The minimum age of legal tobacco sale was 18 years in 47 states and the District of Columbia (DC), while 3 states (Alabama, Alaska, and Utah) set the higher limit of 19 years. In 33 states the legislation designated enforcement authority to a specified government department or agency. Laws in 47 states specify monetary fines for violations. Minimum penalties to businesses for first violations range from $0 to $500 with a median of $50. Maximum penalties for first violations range from $25 to $2,500, with a median of $250. In addition, 23 states and DC may suspend or revoke a business's license to sell retail tobacco products for violation of youth sales laws. State laws in 41 states and DC also put some restrictions on cigarette vending machines, with 19 states and DC banning vending machines in areas accessible to minors.

Local communities have also taken action to restrict tobacco sales to minors. As of 1995, over 400 towns had enacted local ordinances restricting youth access to tobacco (Siegel, Carol, Jordan, et al. 1997). By 2000, over 900 towns had enacted some form of youth access ordinance; this included 754 ordinances that restrict or ban tobacco sales in vending machines, 258 that prohibit distribution of free tobacco samples, 374 that require licensing of tobacco retailers, and 365 that prohibit self-service displays of tobacco products (Americans for Nonsmokers Rights Foundation, 2000). Local ordinances appear to be unequally distributed across the United States, with the bulk in four states—California, New Jersey, Massachusetts, and Minnesota. The most common types of ordinances require tobacco sellers to be licensed and those that ban self-service displays of tobacco products (Jacobsen et al. n.d.).

In general, local ordinances are more restrictive than the corresponding state law and frequently include provisions that facilitate enforcement. The spread of local ordinances has been hampered by the passage of state laws that preempt stronger local actions (Siegel et al. 1997). Many preemption laws are sponsored by the tobacco industry, which has adopted this state-level strategy to combat local ordinances of all types (DiFranza & Godshall 1996). In 1994, a working group of state attorneys general recommended that state legislatures not preempt local ordinances and cautioned them to be wary of solutions advanced by the tobacco industry (Working Group 1994). By 1997, however, 21 states had passed state laws preempting stronger local actions regarding youths' access to tobacco (Siegel et al. 1997).

Little is known about current levels of enforcement of either state and local laws. The most comprehensive data are from a 1997 survey of a stratified random sample of cities in 50 states. A low rate of enforcement of tobacco sales laws was found, with compliance checks conducted in a median of only 22% of cities in the preceding year. Even fewer cities had taken any action against any clerk or store that had sold tobacco illegally to a minor (Wolfson, Forster, Hannan, Sidebottom, Alesci, and Chen 1997b). Most current enforcement efforts operate at the community rather than state level.

In addition to these regulatory efforts, recommendations about "responsible retailing" practices for tobacco sales were made to retailers in 1994 by a working group of 12 state attorneys general (Working Group 1994). These recommendations encourage voluntary actions by retailers that would achieve many of the aims of model tobacco sales ordinances, such as requiring proof of age for tobacco sales, removing cigarette vending machines, keeping tobacco products behind the sales counter or in locked cases (e.g., avoiding self-service displays), not selling single cigarettes, posting signs to reinforce the tobacco sales law, developing effective training for employees on avoiding illegal tobacco sales to minors, and giving this training emphasis equal to alcohol sales training. In addition, they recommended that large or chain retailers use "secret shoppers" to monitor employee compliance with the law and reward employees who comply, a standard retailing practice for other products. Retailers are also urged to hold store managers accountable for their stores' compliance with tobacco sales laws, to program existing electronic price scanners with tobacco "locks" to help control tobacco sales and expedite the use of these scanners, and to remove in-store tobacco displays and promotional items. Retailers who preferred not to take these steps were urged to consider eliminating tobacco from their stores (TRRI 1999). The extent to which these recommendations had been adopted by 174 retailers in one New York state county in 1995 was assessed by a telephone survey (Cummings et al. 1998–99). Nearly all of the retailers had adopted practices such as educating employees about tobacco sales laws and posting signs stating that they do not sell tobacco to minors, but considerable room for improvement remained. Most retailers still sold tobacco in self-service displays, few rewarded employees who complied with tobacco sales laws, and even fewer had programmed electronic price scanners to prompt clerks to ask purchasers of tobacco products for age identification.

4. Federal Government Efforts to Reduce Tobacco Sales to Minors

Minors' access to tobacco was not addressed by federal government actions until the early 1990s. Since then, two actions—one legislative and one regulatory—have been taken, but only one survives.

Food and Drug Administration Regulations

In 1996 the FDA issued regulations designed to reduce minors smoking (USHDDS 1996b). These regulations included many of the provisions recommended in model tobacco sales ordinances. The FDA regulations established 18 as the national minimum age of tobacco sales, required vendors to verify the age of any purchaser under the age of 27, prohibited the sale of single cigarettes and distribution of free samples, and restricted cigarette vending machines and self-service displays of tobacco products to locations inaccessible to minors. Graded penalties were to be paid by the retailer, not the clerk. Fines ranged from $250 for a first offense to $10,000 for a fifth violation.

Only the age verification provisions of the FDA regulations ever took effect, starting on February 28, 1997. By the end of 1999, the FDA had mounted an extensive public education campaign and contracted with agencies in 43 states and U.S. territories to conduct the enforcement (Clark et al. 2000). Compliance checks were done by hiring youths ages 15 to 17 years who dressed age appropriately. Each carried a real identification card stating his or her true age that could be displayed if a clerk requested it. Stores that did not sell tobacco to a minor were sent a congratulatory letter; those who broke the law received a warning and, for repeated violations, a fine. Between 1997 and 1999, 151,301 compliance checks of 110,062 individual stores were conducted (93,071 in 1999 alone), with an overall violation rate of 27% (Clark et al. 2000). Compliance check results, reported by state, were posted on the FDA website, along with the names and addresses of stores that had been tested and the results of that test (FDA 2000). The violation rate by state ranged from a low of 9% in Maine to a high of 53% in Georgia (Adams 2000). The FDA did not conduct its compliance checks on a random sample of tobacco retailers in each state, and the agency urged caution in interpreting its violation rates. Still, it represented the largest and best-publicized nationally coordinated effort to stop the sale of tobacco to minors. It lasted less than 3 years. In March 2000, the entire FDA tobacco rule was voided by a Supreme Court ruling that the FDA had overstepped its regulatory authority in asserting jurisdiction over tobacco products. The impact, if any, of this temporary national program on youths' smoking behavior or perceived access to tobacco has not been assessed directly and will be difficult to distinguish from concurrent federal, state, and local efforts. Nonetheless, the end of the program clearly represents a lost opportunity to implement a nationally coordinated effort.

Synar Amendment

The second federal action was legislation, commonly known as the Synar amendment, that Congress passed in 1992 (Synar Law 1992). It requires states to take action to reduce the sale of tobacco to minors and mandates the Department of Health and Human Services (DHHS) to withhold federal Substance Abuse Prevention and Treatment Block grants from noncompliant states. According to the legislation, each state is required to have a law in effect that prohibits the sale or distribution of tobacco products to individuals under age 18 years and to enforce the laws "in a manner that can reasonably be expected to reduce the illegal sales of tobacco products to individuals under the age of 18 years." Enforcement must include annual random unannounced inspections to ensure compliance with the law, and these inspections are to be conducted in such a way as to provide a valid probability sample of the state's outlets accessible to youths. Congress required DHHS to reduce block grant funding to noncompliant states starting in 1994. No federal funds were allocated to states to pay for these mandated activities.

The implementation of the Synar amendment was rocky from the start. Although the law passed in 1992, the regulations implementing it did not go into effect until 1996, which effectively delayed the impact of the law by two years (USDHHS 1996c). Furthermore, as DiFranza (1999) has documented, the implementing regulations weakened the law as written. Rather than a uniform standard of compliance with state laws, each state is allowed to negotiate an individual goal and timeline with DHHS. Unlike the law, the regulations permit DHHS to use discretion in applying sanctions (e.g., withholding block grant funds to states) if it determines that unspecified "extraordinary circumstances" exist. The Synar regulations require each state to develop a plan to lower its rate of illegal sales to minors to 20% or less. This goal has been criticized by tobacco control advocates as insufficiently restrictive to meaningfully reduce the supply of tobacco to youths (DiFranza 1999). They advocate requiring states to achieve the more stringent goal of a 10% rate of illegal tobacco sales to minors. Finally, the Synar regulations require states to reach agreement with the Substance Abuse and Mental Health Services Administration (SAMHSA) on a time frame for achieving this goal and to submit an annual report to SAMHSA describing the state's activities to enforce its law (SAMHSA).

The CDC's STATE database reports on each state's negotiated target rate of illegal sales and its reported sales rate. In 1999, the median of the individual states' targets for illegal sales to minors was 25% (range, 20% to 45%). The median of sales rates reported to SAMHSA was 24.2% (range, 4.1% to 46.8%). In 1999, 20 states reported illegal tobacco sales rates of 20% or less, thereby reaching the target specified by the legislation. In contrast, only 11 states had reached the 20% sales rate goal in 1998. However, only three states reported illegal sales rates of 10% or less in 1999, which is the threshold preferred by tobacco control advocates. These data suggest slow progress in reducing illegal tobacco sales.

However, DiFranza questioned the validity of these data. He conducted a detailed audit of each state's 1997 SAMHSA application, which described events of 1995–96 (DiFranza 1999). His analysis concludes that the state compliance surveys are not sufficiently standardized to permit meaningful comparisons of illegal tobacco sales rates to minors among states or over time in individual states, a situation he describes as a "tremendous lost research opportunity" to compare the effectiveness of various enforcement methods. His analysis also compared the state reports against four prespecified criteria and documented substantial evidence of noncompliance with the statutory requirements of the Synar amendment. Fifteen states failed to document their enforcement inspections, and 18 failed to provide a single example of a violator being penalized. Although 19 states failed to meet statutory requirements, none was sanctioned by DHHS. He concluded that the flawed implementation of the Synar amendment had rendered it ineffective at that point.

Others have suggested that Synar law served as a catalyst to push states to enact tobacco sales laws. However, the efforts in some states were subverted because weak state laws were passed with clauses that preempted stronger local efforts (Forster & Wolfson 1998). Several factors hampered the implementation of the Synar amendment. A major one was its status as an unfunded federal mandate. However, DiFranza points out that a small portion of the funds that states now receive annually from the tobacco industry as part of the Master Settlement Agreement could be allocated to pay for standardized statewide compliance checks and enforcement of state laws in order to remove this barrier to optimal implementation of the Synar legislation (DiFranza 1999). Another barrier was the low priority law enforcement agencies assigned the enforcement efforts.

5. Impact of Youth Access Policies

The goal of the supply-side policies already described is to reduce young people's access to tobacco products. If youth access policies are effective, they should reduce the likelihood that retailers sell tobacco to minors (or that minors succeed in purchasing tobacco). This should decrease youths' perceived ease of access to tobacco products; demonstrating this end would indicate that the intermediate goal, reducing the commercial supply of tobacco to youths, has been achieved. The ultimate goal of supply reduction policy is to reduce the proportion of youths who use tobacco. Proving the validity of the supply-side hypothesis requires evidence that reducing the availability of tobacco products to young people decreases the proportion of them who use tobacco (DiFranza 2000). If youth access policies do affect smoking behavior, they could do so at several points in the progression from never smoking to daily smoking (Emery et al. 1999; Rigotti 1999). Reducing youths' access to tobacco products could reduce experimentation with cigarettes or it could act by blocking the transition from experimentation to regular tobacco use. Current youth access policies are more likely to stop the transition from occasional or experimental use to regular use because policies target the commercial sources of tobacco to youths rather than the social sources that are typically the source of a youth's first cigarettes. The assessment of the effectiveness of youth access policies has lagged behind the rapid pace of regulatory and legislative actions, but recently this information has begun to appear, as have reviews of the accumulated evidence (Forster & Wolfson 1998; Rigotti 1999; Stead & Lancaster 2000). This section describes what has been learned from these investigations.

Merchant Education

The initial public health strategy for improving compliance with tobacco sales laws was educational. It aimed to inform tobacco retailers about their legal responsibility not to sell tobacco to youths. The assumption was that merchants who were aware of these laws would comply with them, thereby blocking young people's access to tobacco from commercial sources. Both the public health community and tobacco industry have made these efforts, but there is no evidence that tobacco industry programs are effective (Americans for Nonsmokers Rights 1998b). The one published study, which assessed the Tobacco Institute's "It's the Law" campaign, found it to be ineffective (DiFranza et al. 1996). Merchant education efforts developed by the public health community have had better success in reducing the proportion of stores that sell tobacco to underage minors. However, they have not produced sustained improvement in merchant compliance, leading to the conclusion that merchant education alone does not work (Altman, Foster, Rasenick-Douss, and Tye 1989; Altman, Rasenick-Douss, Foster, and Tye 1991; Feighery, Altman, and Shaffer 1991; Keay, Woodruff, Wildey, and Kenney 1993).

More encouraging results have been seen in two studies that embedded merchant education in broader community programs focused on tobacco. A randomized controlled trial of four small rural California towns tested the effectiveness of merchant education as part of a community campaign to raise awareness about youths' access (Altman, Wheelis, McFarlane, Lee, and Fortmann 1999). An intensive 3-year community education program in two towns produced better improvement in merchant compliance (which rose from 25% to 100%) than occurred in two control towns, where compliance rose from 36% to only 61%. During the first two years of the study, tobacco use by seventh graders rose less in the towns receiving the intervention than in controls, but the effect was not sustained for the third year and there was no effect on tobacco use by older teens. Nonetheless, the study demonstrates the potential for merchant education to have a modest effect on teen smoking when included as part of a broader community intervention focused on youths' access issues. A second study randomized half of four pairs of eight Oregon towns to receive a community intervention whose objective was to mobilize positive reinforcement for not selling tobacco to youths (Biglan et al. 1995; Biglan et al. 1996). The intervention included merchant education as one component of a package that also included mobilization of community support, positive incentives for clerks who did not sell to minors in test buys, and feedback to merchants about the extent of their sales to minors. The community intervention reduced the rate of illegal tobacco sales to minors and increased the frequency at which clerks asked to see proof of age, but the effect of the community intervention on adolescent tobacco use was inconsistent and unimpressive (Biglan, Ary, Smolkowski, Duncan, and Black 2000).

Overall, the available data indicate that merchant education, by itself, is not a sufficient strategy for reducing youths' access to tobacco. A comprehensive community education and mobilization strategy appears more promising but is more resource-intensive, and its cost-effectiveness needs to assessed.

Active Enforcement of Tobacco Sales Laws

The disappointing results of merchant education led to a shift in public health strategy from education to active enforcement of tobacco sales laws using the compliance check or test buy method. Merchants who violated the law were fined and could have their license to sell tobacco suspended for repeated offenses. Both controlled and uncontrolled studies have demonstrated that active enforcement of tobacco sales laws changes retailer behavior by reducing the proportion of stores that sell tobacco to minors in a test buy (Feighery et al. 1991; Jason, Ji, Anes, and Birkhead 1991; DiFranza, Carlson, and Caisse 1992; Gemson et al. 1998). More frequent inspections produce better results (Cummings et al. 1998–99). Two randomized controlled trials have compared merchant education with enforcement. One, conducted in New York City, found enforcement to be more effective than merchant education (Gemson et al. 1998). Over a year, merchant compliance rose from 0% to 23% with education, compared with 0% to 53% with enforcement. However, a second controlled study in 12 upstate New York communities found no marginal benefit to adding enforcement to a merchant education effort (Cummings, Hyland, Saunders-Martin, Perla, Coppola, and Pechacek 1998). Retailer compliance increased from 36% to 74% over a year in towns with both education and enforcement, compared to 35% to 72% in towns with education only. The authors suggest that widespread publicity about the enforcement program gave merchants in the education-only towns the impression that the law was enforced in their towns.

Although enforcement programs reduce over-the-counter tobacco sales, they have little effect on vending machine sales (Feighery et al. 1991). The public health community advocates banning the sale of tobacco in vending machines, while the tobacco and vending machine industries prefer lesser measures such as restricting vending machines to adults-only locations or fitting them with locks that prevent cigarette purchase unless deactivated by an employee who presumably verifies a purchaser's age (Forster and Wolfson 1998). Locking devices have produced only modest reductions in vending machine sales to minors (Forster, Hourigan, and Kelder 1992; DiFranza et al. 1996). Vending machine bans appear to be essentially self-enforcing (Forster and Wolfson 1998) and represent a better strategy for achieving meaningful reduction in the availability of tobacco products.

Effect of Enforcement on Youths' Smoking

Active enforcement of tobacco sales laws can reduce tobacco sales to minors, but whether it achieves the ultimate goal of reducing young people's access to tobacco or tobacco use is less clear, in part because this is more difficult to study conclusively (Stead & Lancaster 2000). The results so far are mixed, with better results from uncontrolled studies than from controlled studies. Two uncontrolled studies conducted in single communities reported declines in adolescent smoking prevalence following enforcement programs that achieved high levels of merchant compliance (Jason et al. 1991; DiFranza et al. 1992). In Woodridge, Illinois, vigorous enforcement of a tobacco sales law, coupled with penalties for minors possessing tobacco, reduced illegal tobacco sales from 70% to 3% of purchase attempts. Over two years, seventh and eighth graders in the town reported a 50% decrease in experimentation with cigarettes and a 69% decline in the prevalence of regular smoking (Jason et al. 1991). Five years later, the prevalence of regular smoking by high school students was lower in Woodridge than in surrounding communities that did no enforcement (8% vs 16%) (Jason, Berk, Schnopp-Wyatt, and Talbot 1999). In Leominster, Massachusetts, a 44% decline in smoking prevalence among teenagers ages 12–13 was observed over two years following a law enforcement effort. A similar decrease was found for adolescents ages 16–17 years but not for 14- to 15-year-olds (DiFranza et al. 1992). A third uncontrolled study found only a nonsignificant reduction in teen tobacco use (25% to 20%) following adoption of a local ordinance in Everett, Washington (Hinds 1992).

Two published controlled studies have not replicated the dramatic results of the uncontrolled studies. One controlled study compared three Massachusetts communities that enforced a tobacco sales law with three matched control communities that did no enforcement (Rigotti et al. 1997). Over two years, merchant compliance with the law improved significantly more in the towns that enforced the law (increasing from 35% to 82%) than in towns that did not (28% to 45%), but enforcement was not associated with a fall in high school students' self-reported access to tobacco products or tobacco use. This study was the first to demonstrate that compliance checks overstate the true level of merchant compliance with tobacco sales laws and do not directly assess the ease with which young people can obtain tobacco products. It suggested that blocking the supply of tobacco to minors would require a more intensive or longer-lasting enforcement program than the two-year effort that was tested.

In contrast, a small effect on youths' smoking was reported in a randomized controlled trial conducted in 14 small rural Minnesota towns (Forster et al. 1998). Seven towns were randomly assigned a community organizer to mobilize citizens to adopt and enforce tobacco sales laws. Seven control towns did not receive this assistance. After 32 months, all seven towns receiving the intervention passed comprehensive local ordinances to limit youths' access to tobacco. Tobacco use by students in grades 8–10 increased in all 14 towns over 3 years, but the increase was smaller in the seven intervention towns than in the seven controls. The difference in daily smoking prevalence between groups was statistically significant, although corresponding differences in weekly or monthly smoking prevalence were not. Students in the intervention towns made fewer attempts to purchase tobacco illegally and perceived that that they had less access to commercial (but not social) sources of tobacco. However, changes in merchant compliance measured in test buys did not differ between groups, rising from 61% to 95% in towns receiving the intervention and from 58% to 88% in controls. The authors suggest that the effect on youths' smoking was attributable not to the enforcement per se, but to a more general effect of community organizing that changed young people's perceptions about the availability of tobacco and led them to make fewer attempts to purchase tobacco. The intervention in the Minnesota study was more comprehensive than the law enforcement approach used in the Massachusetts study, and whether the results of the Minnesota trial could have been achieved with a less comprehensive intervention is unclear. The Minnesota study also achieved a higher level of merchant compliance than the Massachusetts study, which may also have contributed to its stronger effect on youths' smoking.

Both studies raised questions about the accuracy of compliance checks as measures of young people's ease of access to tobacco products. Several reasons have been advanced to explain why compliance tests may overestimate the true level of merchant compliance with tobacco sales laws. Youths in compliance checks are not allowed to behave as real under-age smokers might; for example, they do not carry tobacco, lie about their age, show false proof-of-age identification, dress to appear older, shoplift tobacco, or try to buy tobacco from a store where they are known or where their friends work as clerks (Rigotti 1999; DiFranza & Rigotti 1999). One small study has tested the importance of having a minor tell the truth about his or her age during a test purchase attempt (Hyland, Cummings, and Seiwell 2000). The same under-age youth visited the same store on different days and either told the truth about her age or was allowed to lie. The rate of merchant compliance fell only slightly, from 63% to 55%, when lying about age was permitted. The effect was not greater because most of the time the store clerk failed to ask a minor's age at all. The authors conclude that getting a clerk to ask about age or ask for identification would have greater effect than permitting youths to lie about their age.

Another reason why compliance checks may underestimate youths' perceived access to tobacco products is inherent in the measurement method, which assesses the proportion of retailers who sell tobacco to a minor who visits many stores. In real life, under-age smokers probably learn which retailers sell tobacco to minors and try to buy only from these stores (DiFranza & Rigotti 1999). Theoretically, a single retailer could be sufficient to supply tobacco to a community's youths even if the great majority of retailers do not break the law (Rigotti 1999). A further limitation of compliance tests as commonly done is that usually only one test per store is done. A few studies have tested individual stores more than once (DiFranza, Savageu, and Aisquith 1996). They have found that the reliability of the test is low; for example, many stores that do not sell tobacco to a minor on a single test will do so if tested more than once. A single test of each merchant will overestimate a community's compliance rate with age-of-sale laws. Therefore, reducing the supply of tobacco to young people may require a higher merchant compliance rate than the 82% achieved by the Massachusetts study. Merchant compliance rates exceeded 90% in Woodridge, Illinois, the most successful example of youth access policy that has been reported. Consequently, it has been hypothesized that merchant compliance rates need to reach and remain at that level for a sufficient period of time to reduce the availability of tobacco to youth (DiFranza 2000).

Secondary Analyses of Population Surveys

At a macroscopic level, secondary analyses of data from large population surveys provide additional evidence concerning the effect of youths' access laws. These studies compare youth tobacco use rates between communities with and without youth access laws, controlling for the potentially confounding effect of other tobacco control policies. Three studies have analyzed cross-sectional data. Using national survey data from over 100,000 adolescents, Chaloupka and Grossman (1996) found no relationship between the presence of a youth access law and youths' smoking prevalence, although they did find that communities with clean indoor air ordinances or higher cigarette prices had lower teen cigarette consumption. In contrast, Lewit and colleagues (1997) found a relationship between policies limiting minors' access to tobacco and youths' smoking in an analysis of over 15,000 ninth graders surveyed as part of a large community intervention trial. Wasserman and colleagues (1991) found no relationship between living in a state with a youth access law and adolescent cigarette consumption.

One study has used a prospective cohort study design, which permits an inference about cause and effect. Siegel and colleagues (1999) followed a population-based sample of 592 Massachusetts youths who did not smoke and were 12–15 years old in 1993. Four years later, youths who lived in communities with a local tobacco sales ordinance at baseline were 40% less likely to progress toward established smoking (>100 lifetime cigarettes) than those who lived in communities without laws. This longitudinal study is consistent with an interpretation that local tobacco sales laws led to less teen smoking initiation. This conclusion is limited by the fact that the statistical significance of the effect became borderline after adjustment for multiple factors known to affect youths' smoking, although the odds ratio did not change. Curiously, youths who lived in towns with local sales laws reported having no more difficulty obtaining tobacco than those living in towns without the laws, suggesting that the effect of the law was not mediated through reduced access to tobacco products. The authors suggest that the effect might be mediated indirectly by factors such as the community mobilization and public attention that generally accompanies the passage of a youth access law. Although the results are not definitive, the study does provide evidence that tobacco sales laws may influence youths' smoking behavior, although the process may not be as straightforward as originally envisioned.

The studies have an important limitation: they have no data about whether the laws were actually enforced. Given what is known about the low level of compliance with the laws in the absence of enforcement and the low level of enforcement of the laws in general, it is likely that these studies largely assess the effect of unenforced youth access laws and underestimate the potential impact of these ordinances if adequately enforced. The studies cannot be interpreted as providing a true test of the supply reduction hypothesis, for it is unclear that the supply of tobacco to minors was substantially reduced.

Summary of the Evidence

The first wave of studies to examine the impact of tobacco sales laws assessed intermediate endpoints (merchant compliance with laws) and clearly demonstrated that enforcing the laws changed retailer behavior. Enforcement must continue to be done regularly to remain effective. The relative effectiveness of different penalties as deterrents to selling tobacco to minors has not been systematically studied (Stead and Lancaster 2000).

The second wave of studies uses youth access to tobacco and tobacco use as outcomes. These studies have yet to provide conclusive evidence that interventions using retailer education or law enforcement alone can change the ease with which young people obtain tobacco products. Because interventions have not been able to interrupt the supply of tobacco to minors, it is not surprising that they have not been clearly shown to reduce youth's tobacco use (Rigotti 1999; DiFranza 2000; Stead and Lancaster 2000). Existing studies have not been able to provide a rigorous test of the supply reduction hypothesis (e.g., that reducing the supply of tobacco to youths from all, or at least commercial, sources will reduce adolescent tobacco use) because it has proved difficult to mount interventions that substantially reduce the supply of tobacco to minors. These studies have also demonstrated the limitations of the compliance test methodology for assessing the availability of tobacco to youths—and even for assessing retailers' compliance with age-of-sale laws. Stronger or longer-lasting interventions that achieve high levels of merchant compliance may be able to achieve sufficient supply reduction to provide a true test of the hypothesis. Yet composition of such interventions remains to be defined. At best, blocking commercial sources may only slow the flow of tobacco to youths so long as substantial compensation by noncommercial tobacco sources occurs.

These data should not be interpreted to indicate that supply reduction policies have no value, only that supply reduction is more difficult to achieve than originally envisioned. In retrospect, this is not surprising, given what we know about the success of policies to reduce the supply of alcohol and other addictive drugs. Economic theory predicts that, even if one supplier is stopped, a new supplier will enter the market as long as demand for a commodity persists. For this reason, a World Bank review of global tobacco strategies concluded that measures to reduce tobacco supply were much less promising than those that reduce demand (Jha and Chaloupka 1999).

Despite the inherent limits of supply reduction strategies, the studies of youth access policies do contain some promising findings. Modest effects on youth tobacco use have been demonstrated in two randomized controlled studies employing multicomponent community-focused interventions that included, but were broader in scope than, simple retailer education or law enforcement (Forster et al. 1998; Altman et al. 1999). In both cases, the interventions blunted a rise in minors' tobacco use rather than producing a decline. Nonetheless, they provide evidence that restricting access to tobacco can discourage youths' tobacco use as part of a broader strategy. They also suggest that comprehensive interventions targeting both commercial and noncommercial tobacco sources may be necessary to achieve the goal of reducing young people's access to tobacco and tobacco use. The exact nature, intensity, duration, and cost-effectiveness of these interventions are undefined.

The impact of the two federal actions of the late 1990s, the FDA regulations and the Synar law, is more difficult to assess. The independent effect of each is difficult to disentangle because both were implemented at roughly the same time. The FDA regulations were enforced from 1997 to 2000, while the Synar regulations were finally implemented in 1996. Although no clear causal relationship can be determined, shortly thereafter, in 1998 and 1999, the ease with which a national sample of teenagers reported being able to obtain tobacco products fell slightly but significantly after years of stability (Monitoring the Future 2000). It was a small change, and only time will tell if it represents the start of a new trend. Perhaps that the change was the result of the FDA regulation implementation, with its attendant publicity, as well as the effect of Synar implementation and increasing state and local actions. The combined youth access effort may have reached a critical mass and begun to have an effect on reducing the supply of tobacco to youths. Definitive proof is needed, but the trend is a hopeful sign.

Finally, as in all policy efforts, there is the possibility of negative consequences. Tightening the supply of tobacco would likely lead some to seek alternative sources. One outcome could be a black market that would supply cigarettes to under-age youths. For example, young adults legally able to buy tobacco could be paid by under-age youths to buy tobacco for them. If a black market did emerge, these "tobacco dealers" would presumably charge prices higher than retail prices, thereby effectively raising the cost of smoking to young people. The increase in "cost" of tobacco would reduce demand, which is not necessarily a negative effect, although a black market itself is an undesirable development. This consequence of supply reduction efforts has not been reported, but it is critical to remain alert for the possibility of inadvertent negative consequences of youth access policies.

6. Emerging Issues/Strategies

Two new issues have recently emerged and need further attention from policy makers interested in reducing the supply of tobacco to youths.

Reducing Social Sources of Tobacco for Youths

The importance of noncommercial tobacco sources for youths was recognized only recently, and interventions to block the supply of tobacco through these channels have just begun to be developed. Public policy options are essentially undefined. At present, the interventions being tested are educational and persuasive rather than regulatory. One pilot effort consisted of a mass media campaign whose goal was to persuade adults not to provide cigarettes to under-age youths. (Ribisl, Tencati, Feighery, and Flora 1999c) Public service announcements and slides shown at movie theaters targeted young adults in one California town. A survey of 18- to 30-year-olds conducted after the campaign showed that it reached 27% of respondents in the target audience but failed to alter their intentions to provide tobacco to youths or their confidence in their ability to refuse such a request. The researchers conclude that mass media messages need to be supplemented with more intensive interpersonal interventions to be effective. An ongoing project in Minnesota is testing a broad community mobilization strategy whose goal is to create tobacco-free environments for youths and adults. The intervention has generated smoke-free ordinances in restaurants, public parks and playgrounds, and sports venues. Investigators hypothesize that these environments will provide fewer opportunities for youths to exchange tobacco with each other and with adult smokers, as well producing fewer adult and youth models for tobacco use. A randomized controlled trial is testing the impact of the intervention on, among other outcomes, youths' reports of the availability of tobacco from social sources (Forster 2000).

Prohibiting Tobacco Purchase, Possession, or Use

Until recently, state and local laws attempting to stop the supply of tobacco to minors focused exclusively on the seller, not the buyer, of tobacco products. These laws prohibited the sale of tobacco to under-age youths but not the purchase of tobacco by those youths. In contrast, alcohol laws have generally prohibited both the sale and the purchase/possession/use of alcohol. This has changed, as laws passed under the label of "youth access" increasingly prohibit the minors' purchase, possession, or use of tobacco. Unlike the older laws that focused on the seller, these laws were not initiated by tobacco control advocates, and their value as tools of tobacco control policy is controversial. At present, there are essentially no data on which to judge the benefit or harm of these laws.

Nonetheless, laws that prohibit minors' tobacco use, purchase, or possession have spread rapidly at the state and local level. At the end of 1999, according to the CDC's STATE database, 36 states prohibited the purchase of tobacco products by minors, 31 prohibited tobacco possession by minors, and 18 prohibited use of tobacco products by minors. All but seven states had at least one of these provisions. Thirty-five states specify penalties for minors for violations: misdemeanors, petty offenses, civil offenses, or fines. Among the 28 states that specify monetary amounts for first violations, the minimum fine ranges from \$0 to \$200, with a median of \$2.50. Maximum fines range from \$50 to \$1,000, with a median of \$50. At the local level, 266 town ordinances restrict the use, possession, or purchase of tobacco products by minors (Americans for Nonsmokers Rights Foundation 2000). Much less is known about the extent to which these laws are enforced. One systematic study of enforcement in 1,000 cities across 50 states revealed that minors were more likely to be cited for violating purchase or possession laws than retailers were to be cited for selling tobacco to minors (Wolfson et al. 1997b).

Though data are lacking, numerous rationales have been advanced in support of laws that ban tobacco purchase, possession, and use (Cismoski 1994; Institute of Medicine 1994). The first is fairness, an issue often raised by tobacco retailers and manufacturers. They argue that if retailers can be punished for selling tobacco to under-age youths, it is only fair for youths to be punished for buying. A second rationale is that penalizing youths for purchasing or using tobacco products will communicate the clear message to young people that society is serious about them not smoking (e.g., "If tobacco is so bad, it would be illegal for me to use it"). In this context, analogy is often made to alcohol, another addictive drug whose supply to youths is restricted widely by laws that ban purchase, possession, and use. Third, some school officials and law enforcement officers support youths possession or use laws as a way to keep students from gathering to smoke just off school grounds and modeling tobacco use for other teens. They hope that the risk of a penalty for being seen smoking will drive under-age smokers underground, making tobacco use less visible and perhaps also reducing by individual smokers' tobacco consumption. A fourth rationale is that penalizing minors for possession or using tobacco could deter young people from using tobacco. To be successful as a deterrent, these laws need to be enforced and have penalties relevant to teens. Suggested penalties include suspension or postponement of driving privileges (a consequence that should be immediately relevant to youths), community service, or fines. Potentially, an offense provides the opportunity to intervene to reduce a young person's smoking (e.g., required participation in education/cessation program). It has also been suggested that awareness of penalties for tobacco use may also give a young nonsmoker more ammunition for resisting peer pressure to smoke.

In contrast, tobacco control advocates' opinions about tobacco purchase, possession, and use laws vary from uncertainty to outright opposition. The fact that tobacco manufacturers and retailers support the laws makes them suspect as ineffective or, worse, as "Trojan horses" that will prove counterproductive to tobacco control efforts. The primary argument against the laws is that they shift responsibility from the merchants who sell tobacco to youths who have "succumbed to the sophisticated and well-funded efforts of the tobacco industry to attract and addict them" (Cismoski 1994; TRRI 1999,

47). They are seen as part of a broader tobacco industry strategy to shift blame from manufacturers and sellers to users and lead enforcement to concentrate on youths rather than on retailers (Mosher 1995). Similar arguments have been made about alcohol laws (Mosher 1995). There is some evidence to support this. A survey of enforcement practices of youth access laws in a national sample of cities found that a median of 38% had cited a minor for purchase or possession of tobacco in the past year, yet only 22% had conducted a compliance check of retailers and even fewer had cited any violators (Wolfson et al. 1997b).

At a theoretical level, some argue that penalizing youths for tobacco use is inconsistent with the rationale for restricting minors' access to tobacco in the first place. Tobacco, a legal product for adults, is restricted among youths because young people are viewed as too immature to make a responsible decision about using it, particularly because they may not fully appreciate the risk of lifelong tobacco addiction. If a person is too immature to make this decision, then the state should not hold that person responsible for attempting to make the decision anyway. Given these assumptions, it is more appropriate to focus on the adults (e.g., sellers) than on the under-age users (Cismoski 1994; TRRI 1999). Of course, these arguments would also apply to alcohol, and alcohol possession laws are widely accepted, although some alcohol policy makers make the same argument that the appropriate focus of supply reduction is the seller, not the user (Mosher 1995). Some have also argued that enforcement programs targeting under-age purchasers cannot be effective deterrents on theoretical grounds. For a deterrent to be effective, that there must be a credible ongoing threat that a violator will be caught. The chance that a youth will be penalized for tobacco use, possession, or purchase is low (Mosher 1995).

Laws prohibiting underage tobacco purchase, use, or possession also raise civil liberty concerns because of their potential to be applied discriminately. Universal enforcement is unlikely because of the frequency of minors' tobacco use. The risk is that law enforcement agents will use these laws as a reason to stop, question, or cite a youth for a reason unrelated to the potential tobacco use. This will subvert the aim of the law, engender disrespect for the law, and do nothing to reduce teen tobacco use.(Cismoski 1994) At a practical level, laws that criminalize under-age purchasers have the drawback of making enforcement programs more difficult to implement. Merchant compliance programs cannot be done legally when the under-age purchaser is criminalized by a youth possession law, unless special arrangements are made.

Some have argued that possession ordinances have symbolic value and that the lack of sanctions against tobacco possession implies that society tolerates the behavior. An Institute of Medicine report counters this by arguing that the many other laws restricting sales of tobacco, such as those requiring warning labels on tobacco products, and prohibiting tobacco use in certain venues, clearly communicate society's disapproval of tobacco use (Institute of Medicine 1994). Some have made the case that tobacco and alcohol should be treated similarly and that youths' possession of tobacco should be banned if we also prohibit their possession of alcohol. Others counter that alcohol, unlike tobacco, is intoxicating and leads to immediate harms such as motor vehicle accidents, which tobacco does not cause, even though in the long run tobacco-related mortality is greater (Cismoski 1994). Cismoski argues further that laws not meant to be enforced (or unable to be enforced) only engender disrespect for laws in general. Finally, others argue that these laws make tobacco a "forbidden fruit," adding to the attractiveness of tobacco products for rebellious teens.

The rapid spread of this controversial new approach, coupled with the lack of actual evidence about its effect, makes careful empirical study a critical need. Some work has begun. One study, for example, randomly assigned 10 Illinois towns to fine or not fine minors for tobacco possession. The study will compare the smoking rates of middle school students in these towns (Jason 2000). So far, however, there are no published reports evaluating the new laws that penalize minors for tobacco possession, purchase, or use.

Conclusion

Efforts to reduce youths' access to tobacco abounded in the 1990s, culminating in landmark federal regulatory and legislative actions (the FDA regulations and Synar amendment, respectively) and a host of state and local actions. At present, there is no conclusive evidence that supply reduction efforts achieve the goal of reducing youths' smoking, largely because of the difficulty in actually reducing the supply of tobacco products to youths. Reducing the supply from commercial sources has proved more difficult than originally envisioned. When it succeeds, young people are partially able to compensate by shifting to social sources of tobacco that are less amenable to policy solutions. Viewed in the context of drug and alcohol supply reduction policies, the results are not surprising. It is difficult to shut off the supply of a desired or addicting drug, even for drugs that are illegal and whose use carries greater legal consequences than tobacco use. Clearly, supply reduction has limits. That doesn't mean that the approach should be abandoned, rather that it cannot stand alone, without coexisting demand reduction strategies. In a sense, even the distinction between supply and demand side approaches is artificial because supply-side controls ultimately work by reducing demand. If a youth cannot easily buy tobacco in a store, the cost of obtaining a tobacco product is effectively increased for that youth, whether cost is measured in dollars or time and effort spent. The higher "cost" of tobacco should reduce the youth's demand for tobacco and ultimately his or her consumption.

Assuming that policies that aim to reduce youths' access to tobacco are neither completely effective nor completely ineffective—that there is some benefit—there is no reason not to include them as a component of a comprehensive tobacco control policy strategy. Tobacco sales laws and enforcement programs should not be viewed as a magic bullet, but as one aspect of a comprehensive tobacco prevention strategy. For policy makers, the issue then is determining the relative emphasis on different policies. This should depend on the relative cost-effectiveness of alternative tobacco control policies. How much needs to be spent to get a positive effect and how positive is that effect in comparison to the cost? DiFranza has outlined a self-financing enforcement system funded by tobacco licensing fees that can offset the costs (DiFranza, Celebucki, and Seo 1998). Even so, the benefits of enforcement on youths' tobacco use need clearer definition. These benefits extend beyond supply reduction. Youth access policies may help to change social norms about the acceptability of tobacco use in general and thereby contribute indirectly to reducing tobacco use at all ages.

At the federal level, the demise of the FDA's tobacco regulations represents a tremendous lost opportunity to mount and evaluate a nationally coordinated effort. The Synar law and regulations remain. Despite their limitations, they do provide an opportunity to mount a national effort, especially if the implementation and enforcement can be optimized.

Finally, continued scrutiny of these policies is a critical need. Newer supply-side approaches that penalize youths especially deserve careful study, for reasonable arguments have been made that they may have inadvertent negative consequences. Until we know that they are not counterproductive, it would be preferable for policy makers to avoid adopting them and keep the focus of enforcement on tobacco retailers. Additionally, efforts to reduce young people's supply of tobacco from noncommercial or social sources are just starting and deserve far more attention. In the end, much remains to be learned about the full effects of youth access policies, but enough is known to endorse their inclusion as part of comprehensive programs that attempt to reduce both the supply of and demand for tobacco products by youths.

REFERENCES

Adams, C. 2000. FDA checks find children can buy tobacco products a quarter of the time. *Wall Street Journal Interactive Edition*, 24 January.

Advocacy Institute. 2000. Policies to reduce youth access to tobacco. In *Making the Case: State Tobacco Control Policy Briefing Papers*. Washington, DC: Advocacy Institute.

Altman, D. G., V. Foster, L. Rasenick-Douss, and J. B. Tye. 1989. Reducing the illegal sales of cigarettes to minors. *JAMA* 261:80–3.

Altman, D. G., L. Rasenick-Douss, V. Foster, and J. B. Tye. 1991. Sustained effects of an educational program to reduce sales of cigarettes to minors. *American Journal of Public Health* 81:891–3.

Altman, D. G., A. Y. Wheelis, M. McFarlane, H. Lee, and S. P. Fortmann. 1999. The relationship between tobacco access and use among adolescents: A four community study. *Social Science Medicine* 48:759–75.

Americans for Nonsmokers Rights Foundation. 2000. Local Tobacco Control Ordinance Database. Berkeley: Americans for Nonsmokers Rights. June 5.

Americans for Nonsmokers Rights. 1998a. Clean indoor air as a youth protection strategy. *ANR Update* 17(1):1–3.

———. 1998b. Tobacco industry "prevention" programs. Online. Available: http://www.no-smoke.org/youth.html.

Biglan, A., D. V. Ary, V. Koehn, et al. 1996. Mobilizing positive reinforcement in communities to reduce youth access to tobacco. *American Journal of Public Health* 24:625–63.

Biglan, A., D. V. Ary, K. Smolkowski, T. E. Duncan, and C. Black. 2000. A randomized controlled trial of a community intervention to prevent adolescent tobacco use. *Tobacco Control* 9:24.

Biglan, A., J. Henderson, D. Humphrey, et al. 1995. Mobilising positive reinforcement to reduce youth access to tobacco. *Tobacco Control* 4:42–8.

Centers for Disease Control and Prevention (CDC). 2000. State Tobacco Activities Tracking & Evaluation System.

Chaloupka, F., and M. Grossman. 1996. Price, tobacco control policies, and youth smoking. Cambridge, MA: National Bureau of Economic Research. NBER Working Paper 5740 (NBER Working Paper Series).

Cismoski, J. 1994. Blinded by the light: The folly of tobacco possession laws against minors. *Wisconsin Medical Journal* 4:591–8.

Clark, P. I., S. L. Natanblut, C. L. Schmitt, C. Wolters, and R. Iachan. 2000. Factors associated with tobacco sales to minors: Lessons learned from the FDA compliance checks. *JAMA* 284:729–34.

Cummings, K. M., A. Hyland, T. Saunders-Martin, and J. Perla. 1998–99. What retailers are doing to prevent tobacco sales to minors. *International Quarterly of Community Health Education* 18:1999–2008.

Cummings, K. M., A. Hyland, T. Saunders-Martin, J. Perla, P. R. Coppola, and T. F. Pechacek. 1998 Evaluation of an enforcement program to reduce tobacco sales to minors. *American Journal of Public Health* 88:932–936.

Cummings, K. M., E. Sciandra, T. F. Pechacek, M. Orlandi, and W. R. Lynn. 1992. Where teenagers get their cigarettes: A survey of the purchasing habits of 13–16 year olds in 12 U.S. communities. *Tobacco Control* 1:264–7.

DiFranza, J. R. 1999. Are the federal and state governments complying with the Synar Amendment? *Archives of Pediatric Adolescent Medicine* 153:1089–97.

———. 2000. Youth access: The baby and the bath water. *Tobacco Control* 9:120–1.

DiFranza, J. R., R. R. Carlson, and R. E. Caisse. 1992. Reducing youth access to tobacco. *Tobacco Control* 1:58.

DiFranza, J. R., C. Celebucki, and H. G. Seo. 1998. A model for the efficient and effective enforcement of tobacco sales laws. *American Journal of Public Health* 88: 1100–1.

DiFranza, J. R., M. Coleman, D. StCyr. 1999. A comparison of the advertising and accessibility of cigars, cigarettes, chewing tobacco and loose tobacco. *Preventive Medicine* 29:321–6.

DiFranza, J. R., and W. T. Godshall. 1996. Tobacco industry efforts hindering enforcement of the ban on tobacco sales to minors: Actions speak louder than words. *Tobacco Control* 5:127–31.

DiFranza, J. R., and J. J. Librett. 1999. State and federal revenues from tobacco consumed by minors. *American Journal of Public Health* 89:1106–8.

DiFranza, J. R., B. D. Norwood, D. W. Garner, and J. B. Tye. 1987. Legislative efforts to protect children from tobacco. *JAMA* 257:3387–9.

DiFranza, J. R., and N. A. Rigotti. 1999. Impediments to the enforcement of youth access laws at the community level. *Tobacco Control* 8:152–5.

DiFranza, J. R., J. A. Savageau, and B. F. Aisquith. 1996. Youth access to tobacco: The effects of age, gender, vending machine locks, and "It's the Law" programs. *American Journal of Public Health* 86:221–4.

Emery, S., E. A. Gilpin, M. M. White, and J. P. Pierce. 1999. How adolescents get their cigarettes: Implications for policies on access and price. *Journal of National Cancer Institute* 91:184–6.

Feighery, E., D. G. Altman, and G. Shaffer. 1991. The effects of combining education and enforcement to reduce tobacco sales to minors. A study of four northern California communities. *JAMA* 266:3168–71.

Feighery, E. C., K. M. Ribisl, D. D. Achabal, and T. Tyebjee. 1999. Retail trade incentives: How tobacco industry practices compare with those of other industries. *American Journal of Public Health* 89:1564–66.

Food and Drug Administration (FDA). 2000. Children & Tobacco Compliance-Checker. Online. Available: http://www.fda.gov/opacom/campaigns/tobacco/compliancechecker.html Visited February 15, 2000.

Forster, J. L. 2000. Project for a Tobacco Free Future fact sheet. Presented at Tobacco and Youth Research Meeting, National Cancer Institute, Denver, CO, June 2000.

Forster, J. L., M. E. Hourigan, and S. Kelder. 1992. Locking devices on cigarette vending machines: Evaluation of a city ordinance. *American Journal Public Health* 82:1217–9.

Forster, J. L., D. M. Murray, M. Wolfson, T. M. Blaine, A. C. Wagenaar, and D. J. Hennrikus. 1998. The effects of community policies to reduce youth access to tobacco. *American Journal Public Health* 88:1193–8.

Forster, J. L., and M. Wolfson. 1998. Youth access to tobacco: Policies and politics. *Annual Review of Public Health* 19:203–35.

Forster, J. L., M. Wolfson, D. M. Murray, A. C. Wagenaar, and A. J. Claxton. 1997. Perceived and measured availability of tobacco to youths in 14 Minnesota communities: The TPOP study. *American Journal of Preventive Medicine* 13:167–74.

Gemson, D. H., H. L. Moats, B. X. Watkins, M. L. Ganz, S. Robinson, and E. Healton. 1998. Laying down the law: Reducing illegal tobacco sales to minors in central Harlem. *American Journal of Public Health* 88:936–9.

Glantz, S. A. 1996. Preventing tobacco use—The youth access trap. *American Journal of Public Health* 86:156–7.

Hinds, M. W. 1992. Impact of local ordinance banning tobacco sales to minors. *Public Health Representative* 82:1217–21.

Hyland, A., K. M. Cummings, and M. Seiwell. 2000. The impact of untruthful age reporting during tobacco compliance checks. *Journal of Public Health Management and Practice* 6:115–8.

Institute of Medicine. 1994. *Growing Up Tobacco Free: Preventing Nicotine Addiction in Children and Youths*. Edited by B. Lynch and R. Bonnie. Washington, DC: National Academy Press.

Jacobsen, P. D., P. M. Lantz, K. E. Warner, J. Wasserman, H. A. Pollack, and A. Ahlstrom. n.d. *Reducing Teen Tobacco Use: Meeting the Challenge*. Unpublished manuscript.

Jacobson, P. D., and J. Wasserman. 1997. *Tobacco Control Laws: Implementation and Enforcement*. Santa Monica, CA: RAND.

Jason, L. A. 2000. *The Effects of Enforcement and Possession Laws on Youth Prevalence*. Project summary, Robert Wood Johnson Foundation Substance Abuse Policy Research Program. Online. Available: http://www.phs.wfubmc.edu/sshp/rwj

Jason, L. A., M. Berk, D. L. Schnopp-Wyatt, and B. Talbot. 1999. Effects of enforcement of youth access laws on smoking prevalence. *American Journal of Community Psychology* 27:143–60.

Jason, L. A., P. Y. Ji, M. D. Anes, and S. H. Birkhead. 1991. Active enforcement of cigarette control laws in the prevention of cigarette sales to minors. *JAMA* 266: 3159–61.

Jha, P., and F. J. Chaloupka. 1999. *Curbing the Epidemic: Governments and the Economics of Tobacco Control*. Washington, DC: World Bank.

Keay, K. D., S. I. Woodruff, M. B. Wildey, and E. M. Kenney. 1993. Effect of a retailer intervention on cigarette sales to minors in San Diego County, California. *Tobacco Control* 2:145–51.

Klonoff, E. A., H. Landrine, and R. Alcaraz. 1997. Experimental analysis of sociocultural variables in sales of cigarettes to minors. *American Journal of Public Health* 87: 823–6.

Levy, D. T., K. M. Cummings, and A. Hyland. 2000. A simulation of the effects of youth initiation policies on overall cigarette use. *American Journal of Public Health* 90:1311–4.

Lewit, E. M., A. Hyland, N. Kerrebrock, and K. M. Cummings. 1997. Price, public policy, and smoking in young people. *Tobacco Control* 6 (suppl. 2):S17–24.

Malone, R. E., and L. A. Bero. 2000. Cigars, youth, and the internet link. *American Journal of Public Health* 90:790–2.

Monitoring the Future Study. 2000. Online. Available: http://monitoring the future. org/data. June 5.

Mosher, J. F. 1995. The merchants, not the customers: Resisting the alcohol and tobacco industries' strategy to blame young people for illegal alcohol and tobacco sales. *Journal of Public Health Policy* 16:412–31.

Mosher, J. F., and K. Stewart. 1999. *Regulatory Strategies for Preventing Youth Access to Alcohol: Best Practices*. Rockville, MD: Pacific Institute for Research and Evaluation.

Office of the Inspector General. 1995. State oversight of tobacco sales to minors. Washington, DC: Department of Health and Human Services. OEI-02–94-00270. April.

Ribisl, K. M., B. Howard-Pitney, K. A. Howard, G. J. Norman, L. Rohrback, and J. Unger. 1999a. *Social sources I: More California youth now get their cigarettes from social sources than retail sources*. Presented at American Public Health Association meeting, November.

Ribisl, K. M., G. J. Norman, B. Howard-Pitney, and K. A. Howard. 1999b. Which adults do underaged youth ask for cigarettes? *American Journal of Public Health* 89: 1561–64.

Ribisl, K. M., E. Tencati, E. Feighery, and J. Flora. 1999c. *Evaluation of a media campaign to prevent adults from providing tobacco to minors*. Presented at American Public Health Association meeting, November.

Rigotti, N. A. 1999. Youth access to tobacco. *Nicotine & Tobacco Research* 1:S93–7.

Rigotti, N. A., J. R. DiFranza, Y. C. Chang, T. Tisdale, B. Kemp, and D. E. Singer. 1997. The effect of enforcing tobacco sales laws on adolescents' access to tobacco and smoking behavior. *New English Journal of Medicine* 337:1044–51.

Ross, H. 1992. *Confronting Drunk Driving: Social Policy for Saving Lives*. New Haven, CT: Yale University Press.

Siegel, M., L. Biener, and N. A. Rigotti. 1999. The effect of local tobacco sales laws on adolescent smoking initiation. *Preventive Medicine* 29:334–42.

Siegel, M., J. Carol, J. Jordan, et al. 1997. Preemption in tobacco control. Review of an emerging public health problem. *JAMA* 278:858–63.

Stead L. F., and T. Lancaster. 2000. A systematic review of interventions for preventing tobacco sales to minors. *Tobacco Control* 9:169–76.

Substance Abuse and Mental Health Services Administration (SAMHSA). Implementing the SAMHSA tobacco regulation for the substance abuse prevention and treatment block grant. Online. Available: http://www.samhsa.gov/centers/csap/csap.html.

Synar Law. 1992. State Law Regarding Sale of Tobacco Products to Individuals Under Age of 18. *U.S. Code*. Vol. 42, sec. 1926.

Tobacco Retailer Responsibility Initiative. 1999. *Preventing Teenage Access to Tobacco. A Report to the National Association of Attorneys General*. Waltham, MA: Institute for Health Policy, Heller Graduate School, Brandeis University.

U.S. Department of Health and Human Services (USDHHS). 1994. *Preventing Tobacco Use Among Young People: A Report of the Surgeon General*. Atlanta, GA: U.S. Department of Health and Human Services.

———. 1996a. Accessibility of tobacco products to youths aged 12–17 years—United States, 1989 and 1993. *Morbidity and Mortality Weekly Report* 45:125–30.

———. 1996b. Food and Drug Administration: Regulations restricting the sale and distribution of cigarettes and smokeless tobacco to protect children and adolescents; final rule. *Code of Federal Regulation*. Vol. 21, part 801, et al. *Federal Register* 61:44,396–45,318.

————. 1996c. Substance Abuse and Mental Health Services Administration: Tobacco regulation for substance abuse prevention and treatment block grants; final rule. *Federal Register* 13:1491–1509.

Voorhees, C. C., R. T. Swank, F. A. Stillman, D. X. Harris, H. W. Watson, and D. M. Becker. 1997. Cigarette sales to African-American and white minors in low-income areas of Baltimore. *American Journal of Public Health* 87:652–54.

Wagenaar, A., and D. O'Malley. 1991. Effects of minimum drinking age laws on alcohol use, related behaviors, and traffic crash involvement among American youth, 1976–1987. *Journal of Studies on Alcohol* 52:478–91.

Wagenaar, A., and M. Wolfson. 1994. Enforcement of the legal minimum drinking age in the United States. *Journal of Public Health Policy* 15:37–53.

Wasserman, J., W. G. Manning, J. P. Newhouse, and J. D. Winkler. 1991. The effects of excise taxes and regulations on cigarette smoking. *Journal of Health Economics* 10:43–64.

Williams, W. S., K. Montgomery, and S. Pasnik. 1997. *Alcohol and Tobacco on the Web: New Threats to Youth.* Washington, DC: Center for Media Education.

Wolfson, M., J. L. Forster, A. J. Claxton, and D. M. Murray. 1997a. Adolescent smokers' provision of tobacco to other adolescents. *American Journal of Public Health* 87: 649–51.

Wolfson, M., J. L. Forster, P. J. Hannan, A. Sidebottom, N. Alesci, and V. Chen. 1997b. *Enforcement of laws regulating youth access to tobacco: Preliminary results.* Paper presented at the Annual Meeting of the Robert Wood Johnson Foundation Substance Abuse Policy Research Program, December, San Antonio, Texas.

Working Group of State Attorneys General. 1994. *No Sale: Youth, Tobacco and Responsible Retailing. Developing Responsible Retail Sales Practices and Legislation to Reduce Illegal Tobacco Sales to Minors.* Washington, DC: National Association of Attorneys General.

World Health Organization. 1998. *Guidelines for Controlling and Monitoring the Tobacco Epidemic.* Geneva, Switzerland: World Health Organization.

7

The Third Wave of
Tobacco Tort Litigation

Robert L. Rabin

In a quiet way, tobacco tort litigation emerged as a challenge to the tobacco industry in the mid-1950s at the height of the popularity of smoking—long before a more pervasive regulatory attack on the industry was envisioned by even the most ardent of antitobacco activists. At the time, roughly half the adult population in the United States smoked. There were no limitations on advertising; indeed, tobacco was among the leading industry advertisers on television and radio and in the print media. Similarly, there were no limitations on where smoking might take place, no enforcement of bans on sales to minors, minimal excise taxes, and no public health reports on the risks of smoking. Against this backdrop the initial cancer scare based on scientific data triggered the first wave of lawsuits against tobacco manufacturers (Rabin 1993).

By now, the consequent total lack of success in the courthouse over the course of almost forty years, involving two waves of litigation, is a familiar story.[1] At the end of that period, tobacco observers on all sides awaited with great anticipation the U.S. Supreme Court's decision in the 1992 case of *Cipollone v. Liggett Group, Inc.,*[2] addressing the question of whether the 1965 cigarette labeling act preempted state tort claims based on negligent failure to warn. The preemption defense, along with assumption of risk, had been the hallmarks of industry success in fending off the second wave of tort claimants. *Cipollone* was the case, many thought, that would indicate whether a breakthrough would finally occur against Fortress Tobacco. And immediately after the Court concurred with the industry's preemption claim, it appeared that yet another wave of tort litigation might be a long time in coming.

As it happened, less than two years later, the industry was under assault from two formidable directions: private class action tort litigation and state health care reimbursement suits (Pringle 1998). Within the relatively short span of another five years, the industry had entered into multibillion dollar settlements in the state litigation, remained precariously positioned in the class action litigation, and faced an uncertain future in the newly rejuvenated individual tort suits. A clearly discernible third wave of tobacco-related claims showed no signs of abating and raised the specter of unpredictable liability—the industry's nightmare of potential catastrophic loss—far more vividly than ever before.

In this chapter, I will discuss the developments that so dramatically challenged the industry's long success on the litigation front. As I will indicate, the industry had to contend with two convergent and unexpected circumstances: the revelation of highly damaging internal documents tracing a pattern of industry concealment and misrepresentation of tobacco-related health information, and the adoption by adversaries of a new litigation strategy, based on aggregating claims rather than proceeding on a case-by-case basis. Nonetheless, the resulting turnabout in industry fortunes on the litigation front is far more ambiguous than it first appears. This ambiguity—a mixed "scorecard" of successes and defeats—offers insights that I will also discuss into the institutional strengths and weaknesses of the tort system generally as a medium for achieving broader public health goals. That discussion, in turn, will lead me to some general observations about the future course of tobacco tort litigation.

1. Prelude

When the U.S. Supreme Court decided *Cipollone* in 1992, reading the federal cigarette labeling act to preempt state tort suits based on a post-1965 negligent failure to warn, its pronouncement had all the trappings of a monumental setback for tobacco tort litigation. From the time the case was filed on August 1, 1983, *Cipollone* had the aura of the best effort that could be launched against the industry. Rose Cipollone's lawyer, Marc Edell, was an energetic young litigator who had accumulated highly relevant experience in successfully handling asbestos cases. He was associated with a law firm that appeared willing to bankroll the case at a level that at least began to match the virtually unlimited resources the industry had typically made available to defend prior litigation. The case was initially tried before Judge H. Lee Sarokin, an activist federal jurist who made no bones about his antipathy toward the tobacco industry. The applicable products liability precedents in the forum state of New Jersey were as plaintiff-favorable as any corpus of common law principles in the country. And, despite a subsequent court of appeals decision overturning Sarokin's rejection of the preemption defense, when the case finally reached the Supreme Court, after still another round of lower court decisions, it was against the background of an unprecedented $400,000 jury award in favor of the plaintiff. In this context, the Supreme Court's authoritative decision to preempt the applicability of post-1965 negligent failure to warn claims seemed particularly devastating.

Even the glimmer of light left open by the Court, in remanding the case for still further consideration, appeared to be illusory. The Court had clearly indicated that the preemption defense would reach only claims of *negligent* failure to warn, not fraud or conscious misrepresentation on the part of the industry. On this score, Edell had managed to gain access to internal industry documents and testimony of former industry employees to an extent then unprecedented in the forty-year history of litigation against the industry—documents and testimony indicating that the industry had discouraged internal efforts to take cognizance of the health risks of smoking and to develop a safer cigarette (Daynard and Morin 1988; Kelder and Daynard 1997). Even so, to be actionable, any claim of fraud or misrepresentation by the industry would still require reliance on the part of the plaintiff—and the major thrust of the classic defense case against tobacco litigants, including Rose Cipollone, was that they were well aware of the health risks of tobacco yet continued to smoke popular brand cigarettes. In other words, no reliance on industry conduct. Indeed, after hearing all the evidence, the jury in *Cipollone* had found Rose more at fault than the defendant and had awarded damages only to her husband on his collateral claim—a legally suspect move by the jury in itself. Viewed in this context, the *Cipollone* decision appeared to leave little room for successful maneuver by plaintiffs in future cases.

Moreover, entirely apart from the blizzard of legal arguments, a clear-eyed view of the financial side of the litigation suggested the daunting prospects that prospective tort claimants faced. Over the course of eight years of bitter litigation, the *Cipollone* case had required an investment of some $3 million on the plaintiff's side. Indeed, after the Supreme Court's remand, when Edell indicated his intention to proceed on a fraud theory, his law firm simply refused to sink further resources into the case and instructed him to close shop. Even if future litigants might realize some economies by piggybacking on Edell's efforts, there was no reason to believe that the litigation would come cheap. On this score, the defense's willingness to spend the then-staggering sum of some $75 million on the case was perhaps an even more alarming warning signal of resolve than the plaintiff's expenditures (Mather 1998).

As a consequence, forty years of tort litigation against the industry appeared to have reached a dead end. Ironically, in an important sense, it was the *Cipollone* jury verdict rather than the Supreme Court opinion that struck the most foreboding note. Through two waves of tobacco litigation, the industry had successfully argued initially that smokers would have continued to smoke even if they had knowledge of the health risks involved and, later, that smokers continued to smoke in full possession of that knowledge. Despite the award to Rose Cipollone's husband—an aberration in any event, since technically he could only prevail if she were entitled to damages—the jury had once again, in this best-presented of cases, failed to side with the smoker. Moreover, implicit in the jury's finding that Rose Cipollone chose to continue smoking, despite knowledge of the risks to her health, was a rejection of Edell's further argument that addiction negated her freedom of choice. If, in fact, a jury would refuse to find that a tobacco plaintiff was a deserving victim when the addiction argument was a centerpiece of the case, and if a jury was unmoved by testimony that the industry had curtailed efforts to market a safer cigarette and cut off health-related research—if the smoker's conduct, in the final analysis, was still perceived by jurors as a stubborn refusal to quit, negating any claim for damages—then even apart from the preemption hurdle, it did not auger well for the future of tobacco tort litigation. The industry appeared to maintain its aura of invincibility.

2. A Third Wave Emerges

Out of this unpromising setting, within the short span of two years, sprang a newly energized two-pronged litigation initiative that would press the industry as it had never been challenged before. On the tort side, a nationwide class action against the industry, the much-publicized *Castano v. American Tobacco Co.*,[3] in effect could be regarded as a consolidated version of two earlier generations of smoking litigation, that is, the aggregation of individual claims for harm into one massive tort challenge to the industry. The second assault similarly built on the allegedly tortious conduct of the industry, but with a novel structural twist to the claims—a strategy that focused sharply on the public health dimension of tobacco use. These latter claims, brought by states beginning with Mississippi, sought reimbursement from the industry for the Medicaid and related health care costs that smoking imposed on government welfare programs.

What accounted for this sudden revitalization of litigation? What triggered this renewed sense of resolve and surge of initiative? Two principal factors converged: (1) heightened optimism about the prospects of consolidating tobacco claims, and (2) continuing new revelations of industry efforts to conceal and misrepresent tobacco-related health concerns.

Case Aggregation

Prior to midcentury, aggregation of large numbers of tort claims was unknown. After a moment's reflection, this comes as no surprise. Motor vehicle accidents, slip-and-fall cases, malpractice suits, defectively manufactured product claims—the grist of the torts mill—did not come in large bunches from one aberrant act. In fact, the vast preponderance of accidental-harm victims suffer individual injuries to this day.

The first serious qualification to this state of affairs came with the rise of commercial aviation. An airline crash in the modern era could well claim hundreds of lives. Even so, an ensuing mass tort settlement in an air disaster was characterized by certain singular features. All of the victims typically suffered precisely the same fate (death) under the same circumstances (no need to examine possible plaintiff-contributing behavior on an individual basis) from a single wrongful act. As a consequence, the *theoretical* concern about consolidating claims of tort victims—the inconsistency between consolidating claims and the traditionally particularistic inquiry into whether the plaintiff was "deserving" and the defendant was a "wrongdoer"—was put to rest.

By extension, the exceptional status of airline cases came to incorporate, in the 1980s, an occasional disastrous hotel fire (the DuPont Plaza in San Juan, the MGM Grand in Las Vegas) or skywalk collapse (the Hyatt skywalk in Kansas City). But the predominant categories of tort liability remained firmly grounded in case-by-case inquiry—inquiry into the respective fault of a defendant and a plaintiff, a determination of individual causation, and an assessment of personal harm. No wonder, then, that the ritualized morality play of tobacco litigation proceeded through two generations without a hint of the possibility of clustering cases.

The first successful foray into case aggregation of mass toxic harms came in the widely noted *In re "Agent Orange" Prod. Liab. Litig.*[4] Filed in 1978, the case eventually was transferred to Federal District Court Judge Jack Weinstein, who had developed a substantial reputation for being open to innovative claims. Agent Orange was a herbicide containing dioxin that had been widely used as a defoliant in Vietnam. By the late 1970s, veterans of the jungle fighting claimed to be suffering from a variety of disorders allegedly resulting from exposure to the spraying and sued the chemical manufacturers of Agent Orange in a case consolidated for class treatment after transfer of ongoing cases by the federal Multidistrict Litigation Panel. After much pretrial maneuvering, the case—involving a class of some 250,000 veterans—eventually settled in 1984, with the eight manufacturers of Agent Orange agreeing to pay $180 million to the claimants under an allocation plan devised by a special master. Appeals of Judge Weinstein's settlement order, and his equally controversial decision to dismiss all opt-out claims, eventually came to naught. Despite the wide array of injuries to those in the claimant class and the highly disparate circumstances under which the individual injuries occurred, *Agent Orange* stood as testimony to the possibilities of aggregating mass toxic cases (Schuck 1987).

Ten years later, as the cadre of mass tort lawyers contemplated a third wave of tobacco litigation, *Agent Orange* did not stand alone. Either through resort to class action or less formal methods of case consolidation, toxic harm and related product defect claims had been aggregated in a growing number of publicized incidents: asbestos, DES, Dalkon Shield, Shiley heart valve, Bendectin, breast implants, to name only the most familiar (Hensler, Pace, Dombey-Moore, Giddens, Gross, and Moller 2000; Advisory Group on Civil Rules 1999).

These efforts at consolidating cases did not always succeed. Judge Robert Parker, for example, had by 1990 devised multiple plans for consolidating asbestos claims—the most staggeringly burdensome of all ongoing mass tort controversies—only to experience reversal by a Fifth Circuit Court of Appeals staunchly committed to a traditional model of individual due process.[5] But the consolidation strategy had become increasingly familiar. If not all mass tort claimants had suffered the same injuries under like circumstances, still the possibility existed of creating subclasses of injury victims—categorized by type of harm and perhaps mode of exposure—and relying on representative named parties. An innovative judge, like Jack Weinstein or Robert Parker, might be persuaded to adopt such an approach, and if the certification withstood appeal, litigants—particularly those armed with evidence of industry deceit or disregard of health concerns—anticipated a favorable reception in the forum of public opinion, the jury room.

But the great appeal of the consolidation strategy to tobacco lawyers turned not just on the estimation of a favorable legal climate. First and foremost, consolidation created the opportunity to level the playing field in tobacco tort cases. Tobacco lawyers were well aware of the industry wisdom leaked to the press during the second wave of litigation and frequently cited thereafter; boastfully, an anonymous industry lawyer remarked that the no-holds-barred defense strategy made the litigation "extremely burdensome and expensive for plaintiffs' lawyers. . . . To paraphrase General George Patton, the way we won these cases was not by spending all of Reynolds' money, but by making (the enemy) spend all his."

The filing of *Castano* was in fact announced with a flourish: 60 leading plaintiffs' attorneys were contributing $100,000 each on the front end to establish a $6 million "war chest" to launch the litigation. Clearly, a cooperatively financed tobacco tort venture drawing on the resources of so many well-established plaintiffs' lawyers marked a sharp departure from the past.

Just as clearly, such an undertaking made financial sense only if the prospective reward for success was a huge mega-verdict (or settlement). A class action estimated by some to include 45 million addicted smokers filled the bill. Even recovery limited to the most modest of claims, medical monitoring—a claim linked nicely to the addiction theory, it should be noted—would reach awesome proportions with the multiplier effect of such an enormous class.

In addition, a class action had the great virtue of economy of scale in trial preparation. Rather than repetitive individual efforts to document the defendants' course of conduct, a single concentrated narrative of industry wrongdoing might be constructed. Correspondingly, a single effort at characterizing the conduct (as "fraudulent," "willful misconduct," or whatever) for purposes of claiming punitive damages might suffice. In the same vein, instead of repeated reinvention of the causal relation wheel, the massive epidemiological evidence on tobacco-related harms and the physiological findings on nicotine addiction could be presented once as a single coherent story, serving as a foundation for the millions of individual claims.

Clearly, somewhere down the line a greater degree of particularity would be necessary. Every toxic tort lawyer recognizes the distinction between generic causation and individual causation, and the concomitant necessity to show that the individual client has the type of lung cancer that in fact shows a significant relationship to tobacco use in the epidemiological studies. Similarly, the concept of reliance arguably breaks down into what a particular plaintiff knew at a given time. Nonetheless, economies of scale loomed large. It might not be necessary to proceed beyond a generic showing of malevolent conduct and causal relation. At that point, the industry, facing the prospect of catastrophic loss, might be amenable to settlement. Or, even if the industry remained combative, a sympathetic judge might create subclasses in a fashion that captured many of the economies of scale promised by consolidation. The main point was to avoid the staggering costs and delay intrinsic to staging the morality play of industry versus individual smoker over and over again.

The state health care reimbursement cases constitute an interesting variation on this theme. Once again, aggregation is the leit motif—the states sought reimbursement for total expenditures related to health care for smokers under state welfare programs such as Medicaid. As plaintiffs, the state attorneys general obviously operated on a far more level playing field than the personal injury lawyers who traditionally had represented smokers in individual cases. In reality, the states retained private attorneys on a contingent fee basis to take the lead in document searches, retention of expert witnesses, and pretrial motion work, and, in virtually all cases, these private attorneys also assumed responsibility for the pretrial litigation costs. Once again, the anticipated economies of scale from developing a single narrative of industry misconduct and relying on causal inferences drawn from a comparison of statistical aggregations developed through epidemiological studies, rather than delving into the causal nexus in individual cases—assuming a court would rely on such aggregations—were critical to the novel conception of third-party recovery. In addition, the states leaned heavily on the expertise and financial resources of a small number of enterprising personal injury lawyers (Pringle 1998).

Aggregation, in fact, also had a substantive thrust. If the state filed case-by-case claims for reimbursement, they would be characterized as tantamount to subrogation suits, and the industry's formidable assumed risk defense could be used as a counter to the liability claims. By contrast, consolidation underscored the state's contention that it was suing in its own right for the aggregate economic harm it suffered as a consequence of the industry's wrongful conduct. The downside risk was that a claim for economic cost recovery by the state lacked the grounding in precedent that a tort/subrogation approach would offer. But in early 1994, riding a wave of anti-industry feeling and mass tort optimism, let alone the prospect of mega-recovery through consolidating claims, the climate seemed right for undertaking a new challenge to Big Tobacco—in particular, as the evidence mounted that the industry had long maintained a stonewall of silence about its own understanding of the public health concerns associated with tobacco use (Pringle 1998).

Revelations

In a sense, the newly emerging third wave picked up on the unfinished business of *Cipollone*. As I have suggested, Rose Cipollone's lawyer had engaged in a valiant effort through pretrial discovery, not without some success, to penetrate the inner recesses of industry strategizing about tobacco marketing and promotion. But circumstances conspired against Edell. Because he was exploring uncharted territory, he proceeded without a sharply defined notion of what pathway would prove most promising. Nor did he have the good fortune to be blessed with corporate renegades and dissidents who might have undermined the industry's determined commitment to secrecy about its practices. In part due to these circumstances, Edell's effort remained a circumscribed attack that never really engaged an audience beyond professional tobacco tort observers.

That was soon to change, however. Two whistleblowers in particular shredded the industry's carefully constructed veil of silence. Merrell Williams, a paralegal who had worked for a Kentucky law firm representing Brown & Williamson, began copying internal documents prior to his dismissal by the firm in early 1992. Jeffrey Wigand, the head of research and development at

Brown & Williamson, was fired in March 1993 after a tempestuous four years of bitter disagreement with the company over its failure to take a forthright stance on the health risks of smoking.

In both instances, the revelations that came to light focused particularly on the openly disingenuous stance of industry executives about the addictive properties of nicotine (Pringle 1998). Two examples came to be frequently quoted. In a 1963 internal memo, a top industry lawyer remarked, "We are, then, in the business of selling nicotine, an addictive product." And a high-ranking research scientist (at Philip Morris) said, "Think of the cigarette as a storage container for one day's supply of nicotine" (Levin 1989).

In early 1994, both the Williams cache of documents and Wigand's testimony became public, finding their way into the *New York Times*, the *Wall Street Journal*, congressional hearings on tobacco before the Waxman committee, and the hands of anti-tobacco activists (and subsequently onto Web sites). To make matters worse for the industry, these revelations came almost simultaneously with a widely viewed television documentary *Day One*, in February 1994, accusing the industry of spiking the nicotine content of tobacco, and another media "event," televised congressional hearings in April 1994 in which seven chief executives of the leading tobacco companies disavowed any knowledge of the addictive properties of nicotine.

These developments triggered a wave of revulsion against the industry in the public and political spheres that did not go unnoticed by the cadres of personal injury lawyers in the process of preparing the Mississippi Medicaid and *Castano* class action suits. By spring 1994, when both these litigation ventures had been filed, these new entrants into the ranks of antitobacco litigants were convinced that the industry was vulnerable as never before.

This point requires elaboration: the first two waves of tobacco litigation, apart from the vastly greater litigation resources available to the industry, were in essence a morality play staged before American juries. On this stage, defense lawyers were consistently able to counter claimants' efforts to characterize the industry as coldly indifferent to public health concerns—and motivated by a relentless pursuit of profits—by chastising plaintiffs for suing when they smoked with knowledge of the risks involved in doing so (Rabin 1993).

The success of this defense strategy clearly turned on juries concluding *on balance* that plaintiffs were more responsible than defendants for their health problems. In mid-1994, as the tale of industry deceit unfolded, it appeared to be time for a reassessment: jurors, reflecting a growing public indignation against "Big Tobacco" might finally come around to regarding industry machinations as trumping smokers' weakness of will (Cupp 1998).

Still another related factor came into play. Through two waves of tobacco litigation, plaintiffs based their claims on the industry's failure to warn of the *health risks* of smoking; correspondingly, the defense argued that smokers were aware of those risks. The emerging revelations paved the way for a singular shift of focus initially foreshadowed in *Cipollone*. Although the internal memoranda offered a harvest of documentation on industry efforts to suppress or color health-related findings, tobacco executives seemed preoccupied with the addictive properties of nicotine—perhaps not surprisingly, in view of addiction being the gateway to habitual smoking.

For the plaintiffs' lawyers, nicotine addiction, as a focal point, opened possibilities that had been tentatively explored by Edell (and a handful of other plaintiffs' lawyers) in the waning days of the second wave, but that had never been developed into the centerpiece of the litigation. But now, perhaps the centrality of nicotine addiction in the internal documents of the industry would lend force, in the minds of jurors, to the argument that smokers were virtually powerless to quit smoking (negating freedom of choice). And it could surely be argued that plaintiffs were not aware of the addictive properties of nicotine to anywhere near the same extent that the smoking public knew about the health risks of smoking—and hence did not assume the risk of continuing to smoke.

If the addictive properties of nicotine were a focal point of the documents, they by no means exhausted the possibilities apparent to plaintiffs' attorneys. Powerlessness took another form, as well. Even if adult smokers were cognizant of the risks associated with smoking, it has long been established that the vast majority of smokers develop the habit as youths; in other words, at a particularly impressionable stage of life. Here, the documents again suggested an opening for plaintiffs, because an identifiable theme was industry efforts to encourage youth smoking through advertising and promotion strategies.

Finally, the revelations of industry deceit and misrepresentation not only revitalized the assessment of the prospects of prevailing but also bolstered the financial incentive to litigate. As the documents multiplied, and the aura of cynical manipulation and misrepresentation grew, the likelihood of characterizing the industry conduct as fraudulent and consciously indifferent to public health gave rise to the possibility of the greatest prize of all—punitive damages.

3. Four Pathways

A new era had begun. Buoyed by the optimism over the industry's newly perceived vulnerability, tobacco litigators proceeded along four distinct pathways. In one venture, a number of state class action tort suits were filed after the Fifth Circuit Court of Appeals decertified the nationwide class action in

Castano but left open the prospect of better success in refiling at the state level (Kearns 1999). Along a second route, the Mississippi state health care reimbursement case created a blueprint that eventually came to be employed in virtually every state, with a significant variation in a few states, particularly Florida, which enacted legislative versions of the cost recovery strategy (Pringle 1998). Within this same category, another interesting variant was a series of filings by private health insurers and union health plans based on similar allegations of economic loss resulting from expenditures for treatment of smoking-related harm (Geyelin 1999a). A third initiative arose out of the developing evidence of secondhand smoke harm to nonsmokers, generating an especially prominent case, *Broin v. Philip Morris Companies, Inc.*,[6] involving a class action by flight attendants who sued the tobacco industry for alleged work-related harm from exposure to tobacco smoke. And finally, after a brief hiatus, tobacco tort litigation came full circle with a surge in filings of individual tort claims—a surge reflecting, in part, the uncertainty surrounding the *Castano* class action strategy and, in part, a broader sense that the new climate of anti-industry sentiment called for reassessment even along the pathway that had previously proven to be an impenetrable thicket for tobacco litigants (Rabin 1999).

Castano and Its Progeny

Although the *Castano* class potentially represented about 40 million claimants, the case was in a sense narrowly conceived. Rather than resorting to the conventional claim for health-related damages from smoking, the *Castano* lawyers made nicotine addiction the centerpiece of their case. The class was framed to include smokers medically diagnosed as addicted and those who had been medically advised to quit but had not yet done so. This narrower characterization of the harm resulting from industry conduct linked nicely with the developing evidence that tobacco executives engaged in a disingenuous pattern of conduct, in which they strove to conceal and misrepresent information about the addictive properties of nicotine—indeed, in which they appeared to manipulate the content of nicotine in tobacco products.

As I mentioned earlier, focusing on addiction also constituted a direct challenge to the principal industry defenses. To begin, the addictive character of nicotine was less familiar to smokers than the health effects of tobacco. In addition, the addiction argument served as a direct rebuttal to the freedom of choice defense. And any apparent modesty in requesting only addiction-related recovery would not go unrewarded; the consequent compensatory damage claims for medical monitoring, emotional distress, and disgorgement of profits, however much they might have been overshadowed in size by a health effects claim, would reach staggering proportions when multiplied by some 40 million injury claimants, even if recoverable only in part. Moreover, this sum would be without regard to the corresponding claim that the industry efforts at concealment and misrepresentation warranted punitive damages.

In denying the industry's effort to get the case dismissed, the trial judge found the technical requirements of Rule 23(b)(3) of the Federal Rules of Civil Procedures dealing with class actions satisfied—in essence, finding that questions common to the class predominated over individual questions and that the class action was a superior vehicle for litigating the questions. He reached these conclusions (and certified the class) as to two critical issues: (1) whether the industry had engaged in a fraudulent course of conduct, and (2) if so, whether punitive damages were warranted. With regard to more particular issues of individual reliance and case-by-case need for medical monitoring, he decided to resolve these claims at a later stage—perhaps through carving out subclasses. By resorting to this bifurcated approach, the judge held that foundational issues of industry responsibility could be tried in consolidated fashion.[7]

With hindsight, the Fifth Circuit's refusal to uphold the class certification may have been inevitable. But a critical contemporaneous decision by the Seventh Circuit Court of Appeals on the propriety of class action treatment of mass tort cases almost certainly sealed the fate of *Castano* on appeal. In *The Matter of Rhone-Poulenc Rorer, Inc.,*[8] Judge Richard Posner, writing for a panel of the appellate court, decertified a class action brought by hemophiliacs suffering from AIDS against blood solids manufacturers. The plaintiff class based their argument for liability on an alleged failure to take reasonable care in guarding against the known risks of hepatitis (care that would have also protected hemophiliacs from contracting AIDS) and in failing to take adequate care with respect to donors. Judge Posner reasoned that the claims were based on state law that varied from state to state, creating potentially significant difficulties in trying the cases in consolidated fashion ("choice of law" problems). And, he added, certification would unfairly require the industry, which had in fact won 12 of the 13 individual trials that had taken place, possibly to stake its very existence on one roll of the dice—prematurely, in his view, for further individual trials might indicate that mass certification was unnecessary.

These arguments clearly resonated with the appellate court in the *Castano* case, which cited and quoted *Rhone-Poulenc* repeatedly in its opinion. Publicly, at least, the *Castano* plaintiffs group took the choice of law concern to be the gist of the Fifth Circuit's decertification decision, and accordingly went on to file "son of *Castano*" cases in a number of state courts, each of which would have to apply only the law of its own jurisdiction. A careful reading of the *Castano* opinion, though, seems to belie this narrow interpretation (Kearns 1999).

In my view, the *Castano* court saw a considerable number of knotty problems raised by consolidation—among others, the arguably individual determinations of reliance, comparative fault, consumer expectations, and actual damages—that would need to be confronted at some stage, even if they could be disregarded in an initial phase of the trial. And most significantly of all, these issues potentially would have to be faced for some 40 million claims generated by *Castano* itself, against the backdrop of perhaps 100 or so ongoing individual claims at the time *Castano* was decided—claims that might go away or remain at about the same quantitative level if tobacco cases continued to be brought individually.

The aftermath of *Castano* largely bears out this reading. Virtually all of the second-round *Castano* cases were either dismissed or have languished in state courts, in contradiction of the notion that choice of law is the essence of the tobacco consolidation concern. As of early 2001, class certification of post-*Castano* cases had been granted and upheld in only one state (Louisiana) but denied or remained in doubt in 25 others (Geyelin and Fairclough 2000; Van Voris 2001).

One notable outlier has been *R. J. Reynolds Tobacco Co. v. Engle,*[9] an initially little-noticed Florida state court class action, filed independently of *Castano* (but roughly contemporaneously) by an attorney team with no links to the *Castano* group, who ignored the addiction theory and instead relied on the traditional disease-related basis for claiming injury. In 1996, a Florida intermediate court of appeals upheld the certification of a class of some 300,000–700,000 Florida smokers suffering from tobacco-related disease. When the state supreme court refused to hear an appeal by the tobacco industry defendants, the stage was set for a phase one trial of the issues deemed suitable by the trial court judge for class disposition: whether the industry had engaged in deceptive conduct, whether the epidemiological evidence established a causal link between smoking and a variety of diseases from which members of the class suffered, and whether punitive damages were warranted. After the jury answered each of these questions in the affirmative, the same jury engaged in subsequent phase two determinations, in mid-1999, that three class representative plaintiffs were entitled to $12.7 million in compensatory damages and, in mid-2000, that punitive damages for the entire class were warranted in the astronomical sum of $144.8 billion.[10] In spring 2001, the case remained on appeal.

Whether the plaintiffs' victory in the *Engle* case will survive is highly uncertain. Massive punitive damage awards are routinely cut back on appeal, and this award also bears the strikingly unorthodox feature of appearing to put the cart before the horse: ordinarily both the size of a punitive damage award and its allocation would be based on initial determination of individual compensatory damage award claims—a set of determinations, in this case, that (barring settlement) will not be resolved until claims by all members of the class have taken place. More fundamentally, the sheer prospect of hundreds of thousands of trials, or more realistically, the monumental task of subclassing batches of cases for efficient disposition in a fashion consistent with due process, could lead the appellate courts to overturn the *Engle* case altogether, although any such appellate intervention would seem to have been likely before the mammoth, and protracted, case proceeded this far. In sum, whether *Engle* will have staying power remains to be seen.

With the significant exception of *Engle*, the *Castano* returns—from the traditional tort perspective of success at trial or favorable settlement—can be regarded as modest at best for the present. If *Castano* itself seemed doomed from the outset by inevitable appeal to a conservative Fifth Circuit Court of Appeals, one may ask why a consortium of high-powered plaintiffs' attorneys invested so much time and money in the case. It is speculation, of course, but a real possibility is that the team was in essence engaged in high stakes poker—that is, gambling that certification at the trial court level (which did in fact occur) would create sufficient unpredictability about a potentially catastrophic loss to persuade the industry finally to consider the prospect of settlement. Interestingly, this was precisely the course that unfolded in the contemporaneous state health care litigation, spearheaded by the rival group of plaintiffs' attorneys retained by the states.

The State Health Care Reimbursement Cases

The pioneering venture in the state health care reimbursement litigation, the Mississippi case, was filed less than two months after *Castano*, in May 1994. In some ways, the two efforts to recover for aggregated claims shared an affinity beyond nearly simultaneous filing. Both were undertaken by attorneys experienced in asbestos litigation and convinced that the unfolding revelations of industry indifference to public health concerns could be translated— in tobacco, as in asbestos—into mass industry liability (Pringle 1998). But the health care reimbursement claim, which would soon be replicated in one state after another across the nation, rested on a very different premise from *Castano*. Although the reimbursement claim rested on precisely the same tort-type conduct, the state's theory of recovery was in fact not based on products liability law, for the state was not a "direct" victim suffering from tobacco-related disease. Instead, Mississippi, and the states that were to follow its lead, argued for relief on equitable grounds such as unjust enrichment (Pringle 1998).

In essence, the states' legal theories—which later came to include statutorily based claims, such as violation of consumer protection laws—asserted that the industry's deceptive and misleading conduct constituted a wrong against the public as well as against individual smokers. In arguing unjust enrichment, the claim was for restitution of public tax funds allocated for treating impecunious smokers whose health problems were allegedly the industry's responsibility. A similar theory—wrongfully profiting at the expense of the public—undergirded claims of conspiracy and consumer fraud, particularly those industry tactics aimed at making smoking attractive to underage youths (Ciresi 1999).

In reality, these theories were largely untested, and the claim that the state's interest was independent of and distinct from the individual smoker's generally rested on a shaky foundation. Consider, for example, the claim of unjust enrichment. The industry was only "unjustly enriched," presumably, if it profited from harm for which it should have been held legally responsible. But this sounds suspiciously circular: industry responsibility presupposes smoker nonresponsibility, which is precisely the issue at the core of the individual cases. Similarly, a conspiracy claim rests on the wrongful imposition of harm on the public, where "wrongful" once again arguably raises individual issues of reliance and comparative responsibility, even if the tobacco companies misrepresented health information. Moreover, in purely economic terms, the claim for recovery of health care costs would seem to be interlocked with the excise tax payments levied on the industry, if not—as some economists argued—the net health cost savings to social welfare programs from premature deaths of smokers as well (Viscusi 1999; Schwartz 1999).

Untested or not, the theories of recovery multiplied, finally including deceptive advertising, antitrust violations, federal RICO (racketeering) claims, unfair competition, a variety of fraud allegations, and in at least two states (Florida and Massachusetts) statutory claims based on the enactment of specific health care cost recovery legislation. By summer 1997, the number of states bringing suit had grown to 40, with virtually every still-uncommitted state considering action; Blue Cross and labor union insurers were devising parallel lawsuits; and, in California, cities and counties had joined in the fray (Geyelin 1998; Weinstein 1998).

Then, after months of rumors, in June 1997 the states and the major tobacco companies reached a "global settlement," in reality, a detailed legislative proposal that was presented to Congress as an effort to virtually extinguish the tobacco wars. The tobacco industry, which for more than forty years had proudly proclaimed its invincibility from product liability, was now prepared to underwrite the largest civil settlement ever, paying $368.5 billion over 25 years to bring an end to the third wave of aggregate claims. In addition, the proposed legislative package would have bound the industry to an array of public health proposals, including acknowledgment of FDA jurisdiction to engage in constrained regulation of nicotine; agreement to a "look back" provision under which the industry would be subject to fines linked to failure to reduce underage smoking according to targeted goal and timelines; and bans on billboard advertising, use of human and cartoon figures in ads, and brand-name sponsorship of sporting events and promotional merchandise (Geyelin 1997b).

Beyond doubt, the June 1997 agreement is a testament to the awesome threat posed by the litigation strategy. What the industry was willing to buy, at a considerable price, was relief from litigation uncertainty. This latter point is underscored by the concessions offered by the antitobacco forces in the proposal; in other words, the industry's quid pro quo. Under the plan, the state health care reimbursement suits would have been settled and the industry would have been granted immunity from all other forms of class action. Thus, in one fell swoop, the industry would have eliminated its greatest nightmare—the prospect of catastrophic loss from a cluster of state recoupments, certified classes of tort claimants, or third-party sources such as Blue Cross or union health plans, successfully convincing juries that the industry's past course of conduct warranted potential multibillion dollar recoveries in compensatory and punitive damages for the legions of injury victims represented in the particular cases. Moreover, under still another provision in the settlement plan, there would have been no punitive damages allowed in individual cases for industry conduct prior to the enactment by Congress of the legislation. Once again, this provision directly targeted a massive source of uncertainty—the prospect of a breakthrough in individual cases with one jury after another reacting with vehemence against the narrative of industry deceit. A third provision would have capped the total annual liability for awards on future individual claims at $5 billion, a considerable sum, but nonetheless a fixed cap that would contribute from yet another perspective to the predictability that the industry sought (*New York Times* 1997).

There were other restrictions on litigation as well, but the point is clear. The state health care cases may have rested on dubious theoretical premises. But a realistic assessment of the threat presented by potential catastrophic loss litigation requires more than just finely honed theoretical analysis. By mid-1997, the industry faced the prospect of being sued by virtually every state in the country, represented on a retainer basis by a cadre of the most experienced and skilled tobacco lawyers, pressing a variety of common law and statutory claims. Other third-party claims lurked in the background. The documents told a tale of industry deceit and indifference to public health considerations. Could trial court judges in every, or virtually all, state health care recovery cases be counted on to enter summary judgment, or would the industry be at the mercy of juries exposed to the tale of industry wrongdoing?

At that point, a variety of scenarios seemed possible in the attorneys general suits, some of which foretold financial disaster. The son of *Castano* cases might be going against the plaintiffs, but the battle was far from over and proceeding in many forums; here, too, the scenario of a plaintiff-sympathetic trial judge and an inflamed jury was not beyond the realm of possibility. And even on the individual litigation front, as I will discuss later, the document cache appeared to have triggered a revitalized effort to test jury sympathies, with punitive damages as the prize for success. A considerable measure of predictability and future certainty on all these fronts seemed worth buying at a substantial price, particularly if the financial burden could be spread over a number of years and passed on to future smokers through graduated price increases.

What the negotiating parties failed to recognize was that once their "settlement" reached the halls of Congress, it would take on a life of its own. Almost immediately, as the wave of anti-industry public sentiment crested, a far more draconian legislative proposal emerged. The McCain bill would have obligated the industry to pay $516 billion over 25 years, and, even more strikingly, the bill incorporated virtually all of the earlier negotiated public health provisions while eliminating the industry's hard-fought quid pro quo—the litigation immunity provisions. Perhaps inevitably, a reversal of the legislative tide occurred, bolstered by an urgent industry advertising blitz and the backing of industry congressional supporters. And, in the end, no federal legislation was enacted (Rosenbaum 1998).

As the congressional battle waxed and waned, the industry—perhaps as a strategy to promote a new image in timely fashion—settled individually with the four states that were closest to trial and that, with one exception (Texas), probably presented the greatest threat of a litigation setback: Mississippi, Florida, Texas, and Minnesota. In the absence of these settlements, one might well have concluded, as the congressional deliberations collapsed in June 1998, that the third-wave aggregation strategy had yielded precious little beyond massive additional documentation of industry wrongdoing.

But the four individual state settlements did amount to some $40 billion, to be paid out over 25 years. And within a year, in November 1998, the industry and the 46 remaining states had negotiated a $206 billion settlement of all outstanding state health care reimbursement claims, considerably less in industry payout than the failed June 1997 agreement, but, on the other hand, the agreement contained none of the immunity provisions from class action litigation and punitive damages included in that earlier package (Meier 1998).

In the end, it is hard to assess the significance, if any, of the health care reimbursement litigation. The so-called Master Settlement, which extinguished any further liability of the industry to the states, contained a scaled-back version of the public health provisions in the earlier 1997 agreement, with some remaining restrictions on advertising and promotion aimed at the youth market: billboard advertising was banned and brand name sponsorship of recreational activities was limited, among other things. But no longer were there any provisions for industry "look back" penalties if scheduled reductions in teenage smoking were not met. No longer was there any mention of acknowledging FDA jurisdiction—a separate battleground then before the Supreme Court, which subsequently ruled against the FDA, on the agency's independent assertion of regulatory authority.[11] No longer was there certainty that the costs of smoking would rise appreciably; estimates were that, as a result of the settlement, the price of a pack of cigarettes would rise a relatively modest 35 cents over five years, and the agreement contained set-off provisions for federal tax increases and product sales downturns that served as potential further qualifiers. Indeed, no longer was there any assurance that the states would spend a significant proportion of the industry payments on smoking reduction programs. To the contrary, by early 2000 it was clear that the states were earmarking the funds for a variety of projects unrelated to tobacco control and, in many instances, bearing no relationship to public health concerns (Winter 2001). Many argued, with some justification, that the major beneficiaries of the Master Settlement were the plaintiffs' lawyers, who stood to realize billions in attorneys' fees (Weinstein 2001).

Secondhand Smoke Claims

Surprisingly, the earliest tobacco class action effort, commenced at the tail end of the second wave in 1991, was an action filed on behalf of nonsmoking flight attendants alleging secondhand smoke injuries. The flight attendants claimed to be suffering from tobacco-related disease from harm in the workplace—the airline cabins where they were regularly exposed to tobacco-using passengers prior to the 1990 ban on in-flight smoking.

Broin v. Philip Morris Companies, Inc.[12] was a bold effort, launched in Florida state court by the same husband and wife team, the Rosenblatts, who would later file the Florida state court class action on behalf of direct victims of smoking-related disease, the Engle case (discussed previously). Broin was given very little chance of succeeding when it was filed (Geyelin 1997). This was before Castano, let alone any indication that the aggregation technique might generally supplant case-by-case litigation. Moreover, secondhand smoke harm had not yet attracted the general attention that it would after the publication of the 1992 Environmental Protection Agency report designating it as a known human lung carcinogen with no established safe level of exposure (U.S. Environmental Protection Agency 1992).

Bold as it might seem, *Broin* had major points in its favor: first and foremost, a sympathetic plaintiff class (flight attendants) that could not be tarred with the assumed risk defense. Imagery also seemed likely to work against the industry. Virtually everyone was familiar with the smoke-filled ambience of the smoking section of an airplane and could identify with the sustained, confined exposure of the flight attendants. On the other hand, even after the publication of the EPA report, the epidemiological data on workplace exposure remained thin; the strongest association between secondhand smoke and pulmonary disease was household exposure, especially of young children, which obviously had no direct bearing on the plaintiffs' case.

But before any of these issues on the merits of the case became salient, there was the threshold question of nationwide class certification. To the surprise of most observers, the trial court's refusal to certify was reversed by the Florida appellate court, and the *Broin* class was certified for trial.[13] The court of appeals, in a brief opinion, made the matter seem clear-cut: generic causation and industry course of conduct were questions common to the class, as was an assessment of the egregiousness of defendants' conduct. Any choice of law problems and individual issues of damages could be decided at a later stage, the court remarked, perhaps by recourse to subclassing, notwithstanding some 60,000 potential claims nationwide.

Whether *Broin* would have survived trial is open to serious question. As the court of appeals' opinion approving the parties' subsequent settlement makes clear, the defense had arguments of real substance on the merits: no generic causation, no fraud as to secondhand smoke claimants, preclusion of suit by the statute of limitations, among others.[14] But in the midst of trial, before these issues could be addressed, a $349 million settlement was announced. The tobacco industry had once again demonstrated its vulnerability, just as it did in the roughly contemporaneous settlements of the four state Medicaid cases in Mississippi, Florida, Texas, and Minnesota.

On closer inspection, the significance to be attached to the *Broin* settlement is far less clear. Like the individual state agreements, it came in the midst of the industry's effort to build a positive image in support of the congressional debate over a global tobacco settlement. It involved not a penny of compensation to the flight attendants themselves; rather, it set up a scientific research foundation (and made concessions on the statute of limitations and the burden of proof in any individual flight attendant cases that might be brought in the future). Perhaps most important, it is highly problematic whether it has any wider applicability. In the individual workplace secondhand smoke cases that followed *Broin*—lung cancer claims brought by a barber for long-term exposure in his shop and by a nurse who worked for many years in a veterans' hospital—the industry made no concessions and prevailed before the juries (*Wall Street Journal* 1999). And other occupational groups that might be consolidated are not likely to replicate the widely shared exposure characteristics of the flight attendants, who themselves were still highly vulnerable to a no-causation defense. Thus, in the aftermath of *Broin*, it seems dubious whether secondhand smoke litigation plows new ground that will prove to be fertile.

Coming Full Circle—A Reprise on the Individual Claims

The first chink in the industry's armor on the familiar battleground of individual litigation came in a 1996 case, *Carter v. Brown & Williamson* in which a Florida trial lawyer, Woody Wilner, convinced a state court jury that the industry's responsibility exceeded that of his client, although he did not argue that his client was without fault. In a similarly modest vein, Wilner made no claim for punitive damages, despite introducing evidence of the tobacco company's efforts to conceal health-related information. The jury responded affirmatively, entering a verdict of $750,000 in compensatory damages for the plaintiff's lung cancer.

Wilner's success, and his stated resolve to bring an endless succession of similar cases against the industry, caught the attention of tobacco tort observers, many of whom had written the individual cases off as historical anachronisms in light of the new wave of aggregation claims. Now, however, as the first rush of enthusiasm for consolidation gave way to the grimmer prospect of a long and uncertain struggle in the courts, the simplicity of multiple presentations of *Carter*, virtually without end—reflecting the recast version of the long-standing morality play of individual litigation—offered new hope to tobacco activists.

Soon, however, reality was to set in. Within the span of two years, Wilner won another case, *Widdick v. Brown & Williamson*, but he also failed to convince juries that the industry should be held responsible for the health effects of his clients' smoking in another pair of Florida cases. His scorecard was mixed, and so too were the signals sent by the handful of jury verdicts in other individual cases in the years immediately following *Carter*. In fact, within the short span of three months, between March and May 1999, juries awarded blockbuster verdicts of $50 million in punitive damages in a California case, *Henley v. Philip Morris, Inc.*, and $85 million in an Oregon case, *Williams-Branch v. Philip Morris, Inc.* (reduced by the trial judges, to $25 million and $32.8 million, respectively, but upheld otherwise). But a Tennessee jury rejected the claims of three tobacco litigants (represented by Wilner) and a Kansas jury did likewise. By mid-2000, another multimillion dollar California jury award had been registered, but so too had defense verdicts before juries in Mississippi and New York; and all of the pro-plaintiff outcomes remained on appeal (Geyelin and Fairclough 2000) except for *Carter*, in which the plaintiff's award was finally upheld.[15] The industry was clearly still contesting these lawsuits on all fronts with vigor (Rabin 1999).

If we put aside the outcomes in individual cases, what were the critical differences, if any, in the single-plaintiff tobacco tort suits being brought in the third wave from those brought earlier? In a word, the distinction is in the documents. By the late 1990s, a tobacco litigator could build a case against the industry on the voluminous document discovery in the state health care cost recovery suits and the class action litigation, as well as the earlier caches of whistleblower revelations. A narrative could be woven beginning with tobacco officials discussing, in clandestine fashion, the targeting of teenagers before they had developed to maturity and the retention of the adult market through the addictive powers of nicotine. In *Henley*, for example, the plaintiff's attorney put together a package of 790 damning industry documents, and, although the trial judge allowed only 10 to be introduced, this was sufficient to trigger a punitive damage award from the jury of $50 million, more than twice the punitives that the plaintiff had, in fact, sought.

Moreover, the reinvention of the wheel, in terms of strategy, was now a thing of the past. Plaintiffs' attorneys drew not just on the same now-public documents, but consulted among each other on micromanagement issues: which documents to rely on, what lines of argument to pursue, what expert witnesses to call. By 1999, in fact, the Tobacco Trial Lawyers Association had been formed, an organization dedicated to networking and coordination among those involved in tobacco trial litigation. Earlier efforts of Marc Edell, in *Cipollone*, to penetrate the inner recesses of industry marketing strategies, and of Richard Daynard, chair of the Tobacco Products Liability Project, to coordinate information exchanges among tobacco lawyers, had but scratched the surface. Without the industry documents and the initial indications of success in the courthouse, it was almost impossible to stand up to the industry on its own terms, case by case, litigant by litigant. Now all of that was in the process of change.

In retrospect, *Cipollone* had proven to be only a minor setback. The documents served as the foundation for fraud and deceit claims that, as mentioned, had been left open by the Supreme Court opinion. Moreover, the court had addressed only preemption of negligent failure to warn. Liability for product design defect, based on failure to develop a reasonably safe alternative (in those courts that would not rule as a matter of law that the industry had done everything that could be expected to develop a safe cigarette), complemented misrepresentation claims, as well as failure to warn before 1965, as avenues for reaching the jury, where now, anything might happen.

But as the early returns indicate, if massive liability judgments now seemed a possibility as never in the past, the industry still remained armed with effective weapons. Relying on the strongly individualistic strand in American culture, it could still muster freedom of choice as a powerful defense, especially as the industry shifts ground and confesses to its past machinations, arguing, instead, that it has now reformed its ways under new "enlightened leadership" (Bragg 2000). If the documents come to be viewed as a matter of only historical interest, and if the industry concedes that addiction means it is very hard but nonetheless possible to quit—and this plaintiff, unlike so many other ex-smokers knowledgeable of the health risks, did not demonstrate the requisite will power—a freedom of choice defense may be newly energized.

Another shift in grounds, away from a defense that eventually became an embarrassment, has now taken place. From the outset of the litigation, the industry argued that the causal link between smoking and allegedly tobacco-related diseases had never been conclusively established: correlation is not causation. This argument, too, finally became an albatross, not just because of the voluminous epidemiological findings but also because of the hypocrisy revealed in the documents. But the relevance of the documentary evidence can be contested once general causation is conceded. And the concession of generic causation does not close the door on arguing that the particular plaintiff before the court has a type of lung cancer not associated strongly with smoking, or died from an independent disease, or died from lung cancer but was massively exposed to asbestos, and so forth. Because of the long latency of tobacco-related disease, the plaintiff's life history often creates the possibility of multiple causes of life-threatening illness.

These latter considerations bring us back full circle to the matter of cost. As in the first two waves of litigation, expert witnesses are central to trying a tobacco tort case. The documents do not change this critical feature of the cases. The etiology of tobacco-related disease frequently requires the testimony of a pathologist, a pharmacologist, an oncologist, and, in its broader dimensions, an epidemiologist, an addiction specialist, and public health experts. Aside from the health perspective, a case may call for experts in marketing and promotion and product design aspects of the claim. And, as long as the plaintiff's risk-taking proclivities remain an element of the defense strategy, a laundry list of character witnesses from the plaintiff's past—with corresponding pretrial deposition and interrogatory costs—is likely to be a staple of the cases. The documents, as a somewhat standardized package, go part of the way toward reducing the costs of tobacco tort litigation, but only part of the way. The cases are likely to remain expensive and time-consuming propositions as long as they are vigorously contested by the industry.

4. A Public Health Perspective on the
Tobacco Tort Litigation

Studies indicate that more than 400,000 premature deaths occur annually in the United States as a result of tobacco use. This enormous figure accounts for the major attention paid to the problem in the public health community. But what is the "appropriate" level of mortality and serious disease from smoking? None at all? The numbers that would nonetheless occur if smokers were fully informed of the health risks of smoking? And in assessing the case for regulatory intervention, how does addiction fit into the picture? Or the fact that most smokers take up the habit at an immature age?

These bedrock philosophical questions about how much smoking a society should tolerate take us far beyond the scope of this chapter (Goodin 1991; Sullum 1998). Nonetheless, it is possible to discuss the contribution of tort liability to the control of smoking along a number of dimensions. In traditional tort terms, the litigation can be evaluated from a deterrence perspective. From a broader public health vantage point, the litigation can be viewed as one among many strategies currently employed to reduce smoking—and the question can be asked whether tort has a positive interactive effect with these other approaches (LeBel and Ausness 1999). Finally, tort can be evaluated in terms of its secondary consequences as a medium for educating the public (Schuck 1995). In the following discussion, I will consider each of these perspectives.

Tort as a Regulatory Regime: Deterrence

For a generation now, a principal theme in tort theory has been the articulation of the deterrent role of tort (Calabresi 1970; Landes and Posner 1987). This theme has been particularly evident in the modern development of strict liability in tort for product injuries, the domain that includes smoking-related harm. For example, consider the design of a power tool that results in a number of serious head injuries every year because the mechanism for securing the wood is inadequately fastened to hold it in place when subjected to extreme pressure. The deterrence goal is said to be served by imposing the costs of resulting injuries on the manufacturer on the grounds that a liability rule will create incentives to adopt a safer design or to provide adequate warnings that inform the user of the risks associated with the product as designed. The prospect of tort damages compensating the injury victim is meant to lead the manufacturer to "optimize" the cost of injuries by taking all reasonable additional design or warning precautions, that is, those that yield benefits in injury reduction exceeding the costs of greater safety.

Transposed to the tobacco arena, deterrence theory has provided the underlying foundation for claims of inadequate warning and defectively dangerous design. In the former instance, the argument from a tort perspective has been that imposing liability on tobacco manufacturers would create incentives to warn the public more adequately of the health and addiction risks of smoking. In the latter case, the claim would be that liability would create incentives to take all reasonable steps to manufacture a safer cigarette (Hanson and Logue 1998). Tobacco manufacturers, in turn, argue in essence that smokers are the better cost avoiders because they are fully aware of the risks of smoking and can decide for themselves whether those risks are outweighed by the satisfaction derived from smoking. A market system such as ours, the argument goes, does not seek to eliminate accidental harm—we do, after all, build high-speed roads and allow risky activities such as skiing—but rather to reach the socially optimal level of risk related activity by allocating injury costs to the party best able to take cost-efficient measures for reducing injury.

This is the theory. In the real world of tobacco litigation, however, deterrence considerations operate so haphazardly as to lose virtually all meaning. The major costs imposed on the tobacco industry through nearly a half century of litigation have been the $206 billion settlement with the states (and the associated billions in earlier settlements with four individual states) and the untold millions in paying the industry lawyers' bills to contest liability on all fronts—estimated in mid-2000 at about $900 million annually (Geyelin and Fairclough 2000). The former cost (the state settlements) bears no rational relationship to any intelligible notion of appropriate deterrence. It represents nothing more than the political outcome of what the traffic would bear after four years of jousting with the states over reimbursement of public health care costs (supplemented later in the litigation by a variety of unfair business practice claims). Similarly, the massive litigation costs of a half-century of tort warfare conform to no fine-tuned theoretical objective of internalizing accident costs.

This is not to say that the massive financial expenditures imposed on the industry to buy a measure of peace have had no regulatory effect on smoking. To the extent that these costs are internalized in the price of tobacco products sold in the future, they are reflected in price increases and affect demand for tobacco. Reportedly, sharp price increases beginning in late 1998 after the multistate settlement resulted in a drop in domestic cigarette consumption of about 7% in 1999 (Geyelin and Fairclough 2000). Rather, the point is that the costs bear no particular relationship to the goal of imposing on the industry a burden that reflects its proper responsibility for the disease-related harm associated with smoking.

Nothing about the recent mixed record of litigation success against the industry in the third wave changes this conclusion. If these victories stand on appeal, they will sharply underscore the massive uncertainty and potential for catastrophic loss arising from punitive damage awards. But these punitive damage awards, in turn, reflect no more than isolated resolutions of the morality play of victim versus industry in which a particular jury decides to "send a message" to the industry. Again, a string of these awards will affect price and consequent demand. Indeed, a groundswell of individual awards or even a single multibillion dollar aggregate award might threaten the financial viability of the industry. However, this affords no clear signal whether, from a public health or economic efficiency perspective, tobacco litigation is having the desired impact on smoking. In fact, insolvency itself would arguably have only a minimal impact on the availability of tobacco, albeit perhaps under a rather different regime of promotion and distribution after corporate reorganization.

In any event, it seems apparent that tort liability is an exceedingly blunt weapon for doing battle with tobacco on the consumer demand front. Clearly, the industry can no longer stand behind its long-running boast that not a penny has been paid out in tort liability, not after the state settlements and the still-uncertain bill of continuing individual litigation. But the boast was always illusory in a sense. From the outset of the first wave, the industry spared no litigation expense in battling tort liability. Then, as now, the costs of litigation had some impact on the price of tobacco; now, it is far larger, and in the future it could be exorbitant. At no time, however, have litigation-associated costs operated as a rational scheme, from a regulatory perspective, in affecting the demand for the product. Put another way, tort is a haphazard public health strategy because it is powerfully influenced, in the tobacco arena, by ever-changing normative judgments about the scruples of the contestants and extraordinary investments of lawyering activity in attempting to stage an effective appeal to moral sensibilities. It is not a forward-looking strategic device that is likely to fine-tune behavior through the medium of liability awards.

Tort and Complementary Control Strategies

In the years immediately preceding the third wave, state and local governments enacted a wide range of regulatory controls over tobacco. By the mid-1990s, many localities across the nation had adopted restrictions on smoking in public places; states and localities had enacted a wide variety of new controls on retail sales and possession of cigarettes by minors; some states had adopted significant excise tax increases on tobacco; many communities were restricting advertising of tobacco products; some states were engaged in counteradvertising campaigns; and, at the federal level, modest measures in some of these areas were on the books.

For my purposes, the question is how tobacco tort litigation intersects with this broad array of regulatory strategies. In one sense, the public health aims and accomplishments of these initiatives highlight the limitations of tort as a regulatory strategy. Because recent data indicate that smoking among teenagers is on the rise—and it is well established that smoking initiation is largely a youth phenomenon—a powerful case can be made that reducing underage smoking is the most salient of tobacco control goals. There is little reason to think that tort litigation contributes much in a direct sense to achieving this objective. Tort awards translate into money judgments to smoking victims rather than compelling retailers to check the age of cigarette purchasers, dictating the character of tobacco advertising, or punishing the possession of cigarettes.

At the same time, however, one may argue that tort has had an indirect sanctioning effect. As already discussed, when the industry expends large sums on defense and in resolving liability controversies, these costs of doing business lead to increases in the price of cigarettes—most apparent, perhaps, in the recent state health cost reimbursement settlements with the states—which would have a positive impact on reducing minors' smoking. Similarly, as mentioned, the settlements with the states did provide for limited controls on advertising and promotion, as well as generate revenues that will be used in some instances to fund counteradvertising. In the larger scheme of things, however, it is difficult to make the case for any major inroad in teenage smoking as a result of tort liability. Barring a series of catastrophic judgments against the industry that would create a dramatic upward spiral in the price of tobacco, youths' smoking will likely diminish only when a fine-tuned approach is developed for integrating some combination of stricter retail enforcement, tax increases, and educational initiatives that make smoking appear less "cool."

For adult smokers, arguably the most effective long-term public health measures are the increasingly stringent controls on smoking in the workplace and in places of public accommodation. These controls are likely to lessen the potential impact of secondhand smoke harm, particularly on heavily exposed co-workers and service providers. At the same time, these restrictions may change habitual behavior of smokers themselves over time: as smoking becomes increasingly time-and place-proscribed, the tobacco habit may become more attenuated for any but the most hardcore smokers. In this sphere of conduct control, tobacco tort litigation, in contrast to legislative activity, has no immediately apparent complementary role to play—again, putting aside the indirect and somewhat haphazard effect of catastrophic tort awards that might dramatically increase the cost of tobacco or force the industry into bankruptcy.

Educational Effects

In recent years, public opinion polls have consistently indicated that the public—including the smoking public—is well aware of the health risks of smoking. Indeed, the industry has used this information to its own end in the tort litigation, as a buttress to its argument that smokers assume the risk of smoking-related disease. In my view, however, tobacco tort proponents cannot lay claim to a significant role in creating a risk-informed public. As far back as 1954, when the *Reader's Digest* triggered the first smoking-related cancer scare through graphic summation of the initial scientific studies of the relationship between lung cancer and smoking, the media has played a key role in publishing health findings on tobacco. In addition, beginning with the U.S Surgeon General's Report of 1964, the federal government has played an important complementary role. In fact, prior to the filing of *Castano* and the health care reimbursement suits, tobacco tort litigation was a distinctly low-visibility enterprise, and by the time those third-wave ventures were filed, the health risks of tobacco were already common knowledge.

By contrast, the addictive properties of nicotine had received less attention through the early 1990s; as discussed earlier, third-wave litigation has capitalized on this perceived information gap. But here, too, the educational role of tort is hard to assess. The whistleblower-leaked documents that provided support for *Castano* and the state heath care reimbursement suits were simultaneously distributed to leading news media, congressional representatives, the FDA, and public health activists. In particular, as mentioned, the joint appearance of tobacco executives before the Waxman committee, in which they avowed ignorance of the effects of nicotine, focused nationwide attention on nicotine addiction, as did the TV documentary, *Day One*. Thus, it seems fair to say that by the mid-1990s the channels of public communication of health information about the risks of tobacco were filled to overflowing, making it impossible to identify a singularly influential source.

Nonetheless, a meaningful distinction can be drawn between the key sources of public information about the health risks of tobacco and, beginning in 1993, the most salient source of information on the unfolding narrative concerning the industry's pattern of concealing and misrepresenting its own understanding of those health risks over a period of some thirty years. On this latter score, the determined efforts at pretrial discovery in litigation— such as that pursued by the state of Minnesota in its health care reimbursement suit—did in fact stand out as a source of public information. As in the earlier case of asbestos, the full story of conscious industry disregard for the health effects of its profit-making activity might never have become a part of the public record in the absence of the tort litigation.

If this is correct, tort law (in the tobacco context) is most assuredly public law, not so much because of its social welfare character as a compensatory mechanism or for its regulatory character as a medium for establishing proper incentives for safety, but for its contribution to the unfolding documentation of public affairs.

5. Concluding Thoughts

For the past twenty years the specter of asbestos has haunted the tobacco industry. Not without reason. The similar pathology of lung disease associated with the two products, and the synergistic health effects from joint exposure, led attorneys from both the plaintiffs' and defendants' asbestos bar, among others, to migrate into tobacco plaintiff representation—and to pose a far more sophisticated challenge to the industry than did the less experienced personal injury lawyers who predominated in the earlier cases. And just as in asbestos, the tobacco litigation took an alarming turn for the industry when enterprising pretrial discovery contributed substantially to uncovering a pattern of deceit and misrepresentation about the health risks inherent in its product.

If the battleground of asbestos produced more formidable adversaries for the tobacco industry, it also, more dauntingly, yielded alarming lessons. Once the asbestos producers began to settle cases, a stream became a raging river; a seemingly endless number of claims were filed that soon reduced even the most profitable firms, such as Johns Manville, to insolvency (Brodeur 1985). From the outset of the first wave of tobacco suits, the stark numbers—the legions of potential lung cancer claimants—energized the industry to avoid settling at virtually any cost. But the asbestos debacle stiffened this sense of resolve. It also shaped the industry strategy. Asbestos had sealed its fate by settling cases that were indistinguishable from literally hundreds of thousands of other cases. No industry could withstand such an onslaught. And so, in the third wave the tobacco industry continued to pursue its no-holds-barred strategy in the individual cases, while attempting to "seal off" its aggregate liability (to public entities) through once-and-forever settlement.

In the future, if the tobacco industry can put its past misdeeds behind it, and persuade most—not necessarily all—juries that it is repentant, the prospects for once again prevailing on a freedom of choice line of defense are not necessarily bad. Here the tobacco story sharply diverges from asbestos: smokers, unlike asbestos claimants, do not bear the mantle of innocent victims—unless the addiction argument, coupled with youthful initiation prevails. Correspondingly, tobacco continues to sell its product, on the premise that risk is often intermixed with pleasure in life, unlike asbestos, which was removed from the market once its hazards were revealed.

From a public health perspective the lesson seems clear. Litigation is a highly unpredictable ally in the movement to reduce tobacco use. The premise of tort is that injury victims should recover only if they are "deserving." To be sure, one or more multibillion dollar liability awards always remain a possibility in the continuing saga of mass tort litigation against the industry. But it is a possibility that could just as well never come to pass. Public health proponents, confronting over 400,000 premature deaths a year from smoking, have little reason to rest their hopes for dramatic inroads in their war against tobacco-related disease on tort conceptions of victimization. Strategies aimed at reducing access to tobacco and its attractiveness to the teenage population through controls on sales and promotion, tax increases, and counteradvertising offer no magic solution either, but they may serve as more reliable allies than tort litigation in directly addressing the tobacco control problem.

NOTES

1. The first wave of tobacco tort litigation lasted from 1954 to 1965. Encouraged by developments in the products liability area and the replacement of contributory negligence as a total bar to liability by comparative negligence regimes in virtually every state, a second wave transpired between 1983 and 1992 (Rabin 1993).

2. *Cipollone v. Liggett Group, Inc.*, 505 U.S. 504 (1992).

3. *Castano v. American Tobacco Co.*, 160 F.R.D. 544 (E.D. La. 1995), *rev'd*, 84 F.3d 734 (5th Cir. 1996).

4. *In re Agent Orange Prod. Liab. Litig.*, 597 F.Supp. 740 (E.D.N.Y. 1984), *aff'd*, 818 F.2d 145 (2nd Cir. 1987), *cert. denied sub nom. Pickney v. Dow Chemical Co.*, 484 U.S. 1004 (1988).

5. *Cimino v. Raymark Industries, Inc.*, 151 F.3d 297 (5th Cir. 1998).

6. *Broin v. Philip Morris Companies, Inc.*, 641 So.2d 888 (Fla.App. 1994), *review denied*, 654 So.2d 919 (Fla. 1995).

7. *Castano*, 160 F.R.D. at 544.

8. *The Matter of Rhone-Poulenc Rorer Inc.*, 51 F.3d 1293 (7th Cir. 1995).

9. *R. J. Reynolds Tobacco Co. v. Engle*, 672 So.2d 39 (Fla. Dist. Ct. App. 1996), *review denied*, 682 So.2d 1100 (Fla. 1996).

10. No. 94-08273 (Fla, 11th Cir. Ct. 2000).

11. *Brown & Williamson Tobacco Corp. v. Food & Drug Admin.*, 153 F.3d 155 (4th Cir. 1998), *aff'd* 529 U.S. 120 (2000).

12. *Broin*, 641 So.2d at 888.

13. *Broin*, 641 So.2d at 888.

14. *Ramos v. Philip Morris Companies, Inc.*, 743 So.2d 24 (Fla.App. 1999).

15. 25 Fla. L. Weekly 51072 (Fla. Nov. 22, 2000), rehearing denied (Jan. 19, 2001).

REFERENCES

Advisory Group on Civil Rules, and Working Group on Mass Torts. 1999. *Report on Mass Tort Litigation.* Washington, D.C.: Government Printing Office.

Bragg, R. 2000. Tobacco industry has changed its ways, executive says. *New York Times,* 13 June, A24.

Brodeur, P. 1985. *Outrageous Misconduct: The Asbestos Industry On Trial.* New York: Pantheon Books.

Calabresi, G. 1970. *The Costs of Accidents: A Legal and Economic Analysis.* New Haven, Conn.: Yale University Press.

Ciresi, M. V. 1999. An account of the legal strategies that ended an era of tobacco industry immunity. *William Mitchell Law Review* 25:439–446.

Cupp, R. L., Jr. 1998. A morality play's third act: Revisiting addiction, fraud, and consumer choice in "Third Wave" tobacco litigation. *University of Kansas Law Review* 46:465–94.

Daynard, R. A., and L. Morin. 1988. The *Cipollone* Documents. *Trial,* November.

Geyelin, M. 1997a. Flight-attendants tobacco trial nears. *Wall Street Journal,* 2 June, B7.

———. 1997b. The settlement: Terms of the tobacco pact. *Wall Street Journal,* 23 June, B10.

———. 1998. Second wind: Is Big Tobacco reeling? Maybe not; it wins new rounds in court. *Wall Street Journal,* 5 June, A1.

———. 1999a. Tobacco firms win in union-fund trial. *Wall Street Journal,* 19 March, A3.

Geyelin, M., and G. Fairclough. 2000. Taking a hit: Yes, $145 billion deals a huge blow, but not a killing one. *Wall Street Journal,* 17 July, A1.

Goodin, R. E. 1989. *No Smoking: The Ethical Issues.* Chicago: University of Chicago Press.

Hanson, J. D., and K. D. Logue. 1998. The costs of cigarettes: The economic case for ex post incentive-based regulation. *Yale Law Jounal* 108:1162.

Hensler, D. R., N. M. Pace, B. Dombey-Moore, B. Giddens, J. Gross, and E. Moller. 2000. *Class Action Dilemmas: Pursuing Public Goals for Private Gain.* Santa Monica, Cal.: RAND.

Kearns, S. E. 1999. Decertification of statewide tobacco class actions. *New York University Law Review* 74:1336–75.

Kelder, G. E., Jr., and R. A. Daynard. 1997. The role of litigation in the effective control of the sale and use of tobacco. *Stanford Law and Policy Review* 8:63–87.

Landes, W. M., and R. A. Posner. 1987. *The Economic Structure of Tort Law.* Cambridge, Mass.: Harvard University Press.

Lebel, P. A., and R. C. Ausness. 1999. Toward justice in tobacco policymaking: A critique of Hanson and Logue and an alternative approach to the costs of cigarettes. *Georgia Law Review* 33:693–719.

Levin, M. 1989. Tobacco industry unharmed by landmark defeat in smoker death case. *Los Angeles Times*, 31 December, A41.

Mather, L. 1998. Theorizing about trial courts: Lawyers, policymaking, and tobacco litigation. *Law and Social Inquiry* 23:897–940.

Meier, B. 1998. Cigarette makers and states draft a $206 billion deal. *New York Times*, 14 November, A1.

New York Times. 1997. Excerpts from agreement between states and tobacco industry. 23 June, B8.

Pringle, P. 1998. *Cornered: Big Tobacco at the Bar of Justice.* New York: Henry Holt.

Rabin, R. L. 1993. Institutional and historical perspectives on tobacco tort liability. In *Smoking Policy: Law, Politics, and Culture.* Edited by R. L. Rabin and S. D. Sugarman. New York: Oxford University Press.

———. 1999. The uncertain future of tobacco tort litigation in the United States. *Tort Law Review* 7:91–95.

Rosenbaum, D. E. 1998. Senate approves limiting fees lawyers get in tobacco cases. *New York Times*, 17 June, A1.

Schuck, P. H. 1987. *Agent Orange on Trial: Mass Toxic Disasters in the Courts.* Cambridge, Mass.: Belknap Press of Harvard University Press.

———. 1995. Mass torts: An institutional evolutionist perspective. *Cornell Law Review* 80:941–65.

Schwartz, G. T. 1999. Tobacco, liability, and Viscusi. *Cumberland Law Review* 29:555–68.

Sullum, J. 1998. *For Your Own Good:The Anti-Smoking Crusade and The Tyranny of Public Health.* New York:Free Press.

U.S. Environmental Protection Agency (EPA). 1992. *Respiratory Health Effects of Passive Smoking: Lung Cancer and Other Disorders.* Washington D.C.: Government Printing Office.

Van Voris, B. 2001. What's tobacco future in the Bush era? *National Law Journal*, 5 February, A1.

Viscusi, W. K. 1999. A post mortem on the cigarette settlement. *Cumberland Law Review* 29:523–54.

Wall Street Journal. 1999. Tobacco industry ruled not liable in Mississippi case. 23 June, A12.

Weinstein, H. 2001. Fees of anti-tobacco attorneys criticized. *Los Angeles Times.* 15 March, C1.

Weinstein, H. 1998. California and West 5 tobacco lawsuits to consolidate common allegations for State Trial Court: Plaintiffs and cigarette companies agree on the action. *Los Angeles Times*, 21 July, A3.

Winter, G. 2001. State officials are faulted on anti-tobacco programs. *New York Times.* 11 January, A20.

8

Clean Indoor Air Restrictions: Progress and Promise

Peter D. Jacobson & Lisa M. Zapawa

For the past 25 years, the enactment of strong clean indoor air laws has been a primary goal of the tobacco control movement. From a legislative perspective, the issue has been how to translate increasingly broad public support for clean indoor air restrictions into laws that protect the public from the harms of environmental tobacco smoke (ETS, also known as passive or secondhand smoke) without unduly burdening individual rights to consume a legal product.[1]

Even today, when smoking in public places is highly regulated in many states, the debate over the scope of that regulation is far from settled. That the state has the right to regulate smoking to secure the public's health is beyond question. The policy debate is about when, how, and under what circumstances the state should exercise that power (Jacobson, Wasserman, and Raube 1993).

In this chapter, we review the extent to which the goal of enacting strong clean indoor air laws has been achieved and how effective the laws have been. We begin with a discussion of the justifications for clean indoor air laws, followed by arguments against them. In the second section, we describe recent trends in the enactment of federal, state, and local clean indoor air laws. We also discuss how those laws have diffused across jurisdictions and the rise of voluntary smoking restrictions. Then, we discuss what is known about the effectiveness of clean indoor air laws in reducing the tobacco-related health costs to employers and employees, in helping smokers quit altogether, and in encouraging the voluntary adoption of no-smoking policies. The final section discusses the prospects for future policy development and the rationale for collective public health intervention—in contrast to reliance on market-based approaches—at a time of far-reaching changes in civil norms regarding smoking in public places. The chapter concludes by considering strategies policy makers and tobacco control advocates might pursue to take advantage of changes in civil norms regarding smoking in public places.

With the increasing opposition to tobacco control measures from libertarians and conservatives, it is timely to reassess the public health justification for more stringent regulation of clean indoor air. This reassessment will consider whether, at least in some instances, market forces are driving adoption of clean indoor air policies and compliance with them—suggesting a limited need for additional government intervention.

1. The Debate Over Regulating Smoking in Public Places

Antismoking legislation of the late nineteenth century was based largely on moral opposition to smoking. By the mid-1920s, the economic benefits associated with tobacco production and consumption overwhelmed these objections. All state antismoking laws were repealed by 1927, leaving the antismoking movement politically moribund until scientific evidence of tobacco's health hazards emerged in the 1950s and 1960s.

In recent years, the primary argument justifying regulation of tobacco products has been the health costs and risks associated with tobacco use. Antismoking advocates have successfully invoked evidence that ETS presents sufficient health hazards to third parties to justify governmental intervention. When the tobacco industry was the primary opponent to governmental intervention, these arguments were compelling. But support for regulation has recently been submitted to more rigorous questioning by the counterarguments from conservative and libertarian think tanks. Thus, it is especially important to consider in detail the contours of the debate over the rationale for regulating smoking in public places.

Justifications for Clean Indoor Air Laws

The justification favoring clean indoor air laws rests on a combination of scientific, moral, and public policy grounds.[2] Advocates claim that the clear social and health gains from clean indoor air restrictions far outweigh the intrusion upon individual liberties.

Scientific Arguments   The most recent scientific debate on smoking concerns the effects of ETS. In 1990, the Environmental Protection Agency (EPA) released a draft report that reviewed 24 epidemiological studies. The EPA concluded that passive smoking causes 3,000 lung cancer deaths each year (EPA 1992), corroborating an earlier report on passive smoking from the surgeon general (USDHHS 1986).

The adverse health outcomes related to secondhand smoke exposure have been the primary justification behind restrictions on smoking in public venues (Jacobson et al. 1993; Sullum 1998). In the early 1990s, the nation's leading scientific research organizations released definitive statements emphasizing the need to reduce the public's exposure to ETS. In 1991, the CDC's National Institute for Occupational Safety and Health (NIOSH) issued a bulletin recommending that secondhand smoke be reduced to the lowest feasible concentration in the workplace (EPA 1992). Reviews of the scientific data relating to the dangers of secondhand smoke by the National Academy of Sciences, the U.S. Public Health Service, the EPA, NIOSH, and the American Heart Association all separately concluded that exposure to ETS at the levels that often occur in U.S. homes and worksites is associated with lung cancer, cardiovascular disease, stroke, and other illnesses in nonsmokers (Burns et al. 1992; California EPA 1997; Bonita et al. 1999).

Employees are at especially high risk of harm from ETS, given their constant exposure in places that allow smoking. For example, ETS exacerbates problems of chronic cardiovascular disease (Mannino, Siegel, Rose, Nkuchia, and Etzel 1997), can lead to ischemic stroke (Bonita et al. 1999), and peripheral vascular disease (Andrews 1983). And ETS exposure in enclosed spaces, such as bars, restaurants, and airplanes, where there appears to be an elevated lung cancer risk for workers, is of particular concern (Siegel 1993). Airline attendants recently won a $300 million settlement from the tobacco industry as a result of ETS exposure.[3] Data also show that there are higher levels of workplace ETS exposure in younger people, men, African Americans, individuals with lower educational levels, and rural workers (Brownson, Eriksen, Davis, and Warner 1997).

Risk studies by the EPA consistently rank indoor air pollution as one of the most important environmental risks to the public's health (EPA 1993). Human exposure to indoor air pollutants is often substantially greater than outdoor exposure to the same substances. The aerosol particles from ETS are concentrated indoors and remain long after each cigarette has been extinguished. These risks are of particular concern as people are estimated to spend up to 90% of their time indoors (EPA 1993).

Conceptual Arguments   In addition to the scientific arguments, advocates also offer conceptual justifications for clean indoor air laws. For instance, Arno, Brandt, Gostin, and Morgan (1996) offer three justifications for regulating tobacco: risk to public health or safety, risk assumed by children and adolescents, and risk assumed by consenting adults.

For the first justification, common sense dictates that the protection of third parties, especially nonsmokers, from the harmful effects of ETS must outweigh the individual's right to smoke anywhere he or she pleases. Limiting the public spaces where an individual can smoke is not a significant intrusion upon individual liberties, especially when balanced against the public's right to breathe clean air. To the extent that exposure to ETS is a public health hazard, it becomes the government's responsibility to protect the public from such exposure. Nonsmokers have the right to be protected from ETS in public places, including privately owned businesses (such as stores and malls) that are open to the public. This justification is even stronger when applied to employees, who cannot avoid exposure to ETS if smoking is permitted.

The second justification is generally noncontroversial as the public supports attempts to reduce adolescent smoking and exposure to ETS. Though determining which public places are frequented by children might well be contested, there is little question that clean indoor air laws should apply to schools, day care centers, and transportation facilities.

The third justification—the risk to consenting adults—is the most controversial of the conceptual arguments for regulation because of its paternalistic tone. It is certainly accurate to say that governmental paternalism is least justified to protect a consenting adult from engaging in risky behavior. Clean indoor air acts are thus difficult to defend if the primary rationale is to prevent adults from harming themselves (Sullum 1998; Scanlon 1999). For several reasons, however, clean indoor air laws do not present unjustified paternalism.

First, the laws' primary rationale is to protect third persons, not to prohibit an adult from smoking. Smokers may be inconvenienced, but they can still smoke outside or in nonpublic places. Second, laws are not dictating personal choices; they are merely limiting the effects of those choices on the public. In this way, the case for regulating tobacco is stronger than the case for laws requiring seatbelts or motorcycle helmets, which have also been challenged as paternalistic. The courts have traditionally upheld such laws as not unduly intruding into personal freedoms when balanced against the benefits to the community. With seatbelt and helmet laws, individuals are compelled to take an action they might otherwise not take. Clean indoor air laws merely prohibit smoking in certain public venues. Third, as Arno et al. (1996) argue, the addictive nature of nicotine and the industry's concerted efforts to hide evidence of tobacco's harms from the public undermine the claim of paternalism. It is generally agreed that government has a right to intervene to prevent drug addiction or harms from personal choices not freely made.

Clean indoor air laws can also be justified as a mechanism for assisting smokers who would like to quit. Surveys consistently show that most smokers regret their decision to smoke cigarettes and would like to quit (Saad 2000). Far from being purely paternalistic, clean indoor air laws may therefore be instrumental in facilitating the decision to quit (see, e.g., Feinberg 1989; Sorensen, Rigotti, Rosen, Pinney, and Prible 1991; Scanlon 1999).

Certainly, clean indoor air laws may be hard on smokers, especially if they are addicted. But this hardship does not justify subjecting nonsmokers to ETS. Smokers can easily avoid the conflict by smoking outside. By contrast, if indoor smoking is allowed, those who object to ETS exposure would be forced to avoid the public space altogether. Some might argue that this conflict could be resolved through common courtesy, with smokers simply putting out their cigarettes (or not lighting up in the first place) when asked. There are several objections to this solution. First, not all nonsmokers are aware of the dangers of ETS. Second, some might be too shy or intimidated to ask. Finally, experience suggests that not all smokers are in fact responsive to such courteous requests. Common courtesy does not substitute for stringent laws (Davis, Boyd, and Schoenborn 1990).

The Case against Clean Indoor Air Laws

The arguments favoring regulation have largely propelled recent regulatory restrictions, but they are not universally accepted as an adequate justification for intervening in the market. Recently, a backlash against clean indoor air laws has emerged from critics outside the tobacco industry. The central claims of opponents to ETS regulation are that smoking is a matter of individual choice and that market arrangements should determine where people smoke, not the government.

In the past few years, conservative and libertarian scholars have built on and expanded traditional tobacco industry arguments against governmental intervention.[4] Even if the recent commentators are raising arguments that are no different in substance from those the tobacco industry has been making since the late 1980s (Jacobson et al. 1993), the source of the arguments can no longer be dismissed as disingenuous tobacco interests. More important, these commentators have the means and ability to disseminate their ideas to influence policy. To date, there is no indication of any radical public opinion shifts resulting from opponents' arguments,[5] but the battle for regulations is now facing stronger opposition than it ever has before.

Reliance on the Market   In general, opponents believe that the market should determine the proper role of smoking in society. In particular, there is the problem of whose rights are allowed to dictate what is legislated. This is the traditional public health dilemma of whether the individual's right to smoke and take responsibility for his or her own health is outweighed by the public's right to clean air. Similarly, there is the underlying philosophical question of how far the government, at any level, should be allowed to limit individual freedoms for the sake of public health. Framed somewhat differently, the issue is how much weight the majority's opinion should be given relative to protecting the rights of the minority.

The market-driven argument is that if a majority of the American public does not smoke and is annoyed by the presence of secondhand smoke, they will make their preferences known through their patronage and spending habits. This would allow some private businesses to cater to those who oppose exposure to ETS, while permitting other private businesses to cater to those who are indifferent to the risks posed by ETS. Instead of an all or nothing solution, the market power exercised by those who avoid places that permit smoking will dictate the number and types of voluntary smoking restrictions that are implemented.

Advocates of market-driven sanctions often point to the hotel industry as an example. Relatively few laws mandate nonsmoking rooms, yet most of the hotels in the United States offer nonsmoking floors or rooms, though many continue to permit smoking in other public sections of the hotel. In this particular example, critics argue that the market is successfully gauging the preferences of the consumers. As we describe later, there is also recent evidence of expanding voluntary smoking restrictions among business establishments.

Personal Choice   Most forcefully, opponents of clean indoor air restrictions have argued that smoking is a matter of personal choice for adults that should not be subject to governmental interference (see, e.g., Tollison and Wagner 1991; Sullum 1998). These commentators actively oppose smoking regulations on conceptual grounds as unjustified governmental paternalism. Supporters of the tobacco industry also argue that smokers retain certain rights in pursuing personal social behavior and cannot be discriminated against for their tobacco use.

In recent years, the opponents of tobacco regulation have accused the tobacco control movement of being intolerant and tyrannical. To these critics, smokers are unfairly treated as social outcasts (Sullum 1998). They see antismoking advocates not only as paternalistic but also as ultimately favoring a naively prohibitionist approach to smoking, a policy no more likely to be successful than the previous attempt to ban alcohol in the 1920s and 1930s.

Sullum (1998) addresses an important aspect of the public's desire to regulate tobacco products—the irritation factor. Regardless of the specific harms from ETS, most nonsmokers find ETS irritating and unwelcome and support regulation for that reason. To Sullum, the problem with irritation as a justification for regulation is the absence of choice:

> By stepping in and imposing the same smoking policy on everyone, the government destroys diversity—the potential to satisfy a wide variety of tastes and preferences, not just the majority's. If someone tried to open a large restaurant in New York City that catered exclusively to smokers, he would be breaking the law. . . . Although I have no desire to eat in such a restaurant . . . , I think it's a shame that no one can. In a free society it's especially troubling that tobacco's opponents seek to foreclose these options as a way of pressuring smokers into quitting. (p. 179)[6,7]

Essentially, Sullum is arguing that a policy environment allowing for a diversity of market standards regarding acceptable smoking behavior is preferable to a uniform antismoking policy. In this, he combines the philosophical and the market arguments into a plea for a more pluralistic and flexible policy environment.

Scientific Arguments   Much of the opposition to tobacco control laws is for philosophical reasons, but a few commentators nonetheless challenge certain aspects of the scientific evidence and regulations based on that evidence. For instance, Levy and Marimont (1998) and Gori and Luik (1999) challenge the EPA data on ETS. The standard critique of the EPA's ETS findings is that EPA selectively included studies that favored its position and ignored those that did not, and used a *p* value (a standard measure of statistical significance) of .10 instead of the generally accepted .05. Beyond that, the odds ratios were small by epidemiological standards (less than a relative risk of 2) and the use of meta-analysis for such disparate studies was inappropriate.[8] Levy and Marimont (1998) offer a concerted attack on the broader estimates of direct and indirect harm from tobacco use, arguing that current estimates over-classify diseases as being smoking-related. In their view, a more accurate estimate would be closer to 255,000 people killed per year rather that the 400,000 routinely reported. More importantly, they note that 60% of these premature deaths occur at age 70 or older.[9] Thus, Levy and Marimont (1998) conclude that the government has vastly overstated the harms from tobacco, particularly the age at which tobacco is likely to cause death.

Summary

For most of the 1990s, the "interventionists" had the upper hand, forcing opponents of tobacco control to show that the justifications for intervention were either incorrect or insufficient. Despite the absence of any radical public opinion shifts, new interest groups have now embraced the battle against regulation, and the interventionists have found their arguments under increasing attack.

Clean indoor air laws present the traditional public health dilemma of whether the individual's rights to smoke and take responsibility for his or her own health are outweighed by the public's right to clean air. Similarly, there is the underlying philosophical question regarding how far the government, at any level, should be allowed to legislate in the name of public health while limiting individual freedoms. Framed somewhat differently, the issue is how much weight the opinion and welfare of the majority should be given relative to the need to protect the rights of the minority.

In contrast to opponents' pure libertarian arguments, we believe that government should act to discourage smoking in public places to protect nonsmokers from being exposed to cancer-causing chemicals. It follows that government should not condone smoking and should use its powers to make smoking in public as difficult as possible. One need not ascribe to a prohibitionist approach (which we reject) to suggest that some products are so harmful that governmental neutrality is neither obligatory nor desirable. Just as public policy seeks to marginalize illicit substance use, it is appropriate for government to design policy mechanisms to marginalize tobacco use. The enactment of such restrictions represents an expression of the majority's desire to occupy the same public space without the presence of tobacco smoke.[10]

In our view, the case against clean indoor air laws fails on numerous grounds. For one thing, the market rationale may be responsive to consumer preferences but does nothing to protect employees from ETS. For another, the scientific basis for regulating smoking in public places is far stronger than critics contend. Recent studies continue to demonstrate the health problems associated with ETS (Bonita et al. 1999). Finally, because smokers are not being asked or required to give up smoking, the minor intrusion on where they can smoke is far outweighed by the harm to third persons from allowing smoking in public places.

Applying a market rationale to public places, such as restaurants, workplaces, and the myriad of other facilities open to the public, remains problematic. First, not many public facilities are arranged like hotels where it is feasible to accommodate both smokers' and nonsmokers' wishes. In a restaurant, on public transportation, or in a mall, for example, it would be difficult to isolate exposure to ETS from nonsmokers. In many cases, there is no economically feasible way to accomplish separate air supplies through separate ventilation systems.

Second, reliance solely on the market's desire to please the consumer is probably not going to address the matter completely, or perhaps even adequately, especially given evidence that common courtesy is not an effective strategy (Davis et al. 1990). As we have already seen, less than complete bans on smoking in public places do not provide complete protection from the hazards of ETS exposure.

Third, it is often difficult for nonsmokers to convey the proper market signal to merchants to encourage voluntary restrictions. Even if effectively conveyed, the tobacco industry's strong financial inducements may outweigh the signal. Despite the recent expansion of voluntary smoking restrictions, the market has been slow to respond to the demand for nonsmoking facilities, at least in public places such as restaurants. Nonsmoking sections represent an improvement over no restrictions but do not provide as much protection as laws banning smoking in public places, especially for employees.[11]

Fourth, allowing each individual store, restaurant, mall, school, transportation facility, and so on to impose its own policies would present conflicting messages about the need to reduce exposure to ETS. This diversity (to use Sullum's term) could dilute the general thrust of clean indoor air protections. Arguably, the attempt to permit diversity is what currently constrains enforcement of clean indoor air laws in public places. Consider, for example, airports and shopping malls that are now installing separately ventilated smoking rooms. These rooms may well protect nonsmokers against ETS but may undermine the strong message that smoking is harmful. On the other hand, smokers behind glass walls might look more pathetic and desperate than appealing to adolescents. Diversity might be defensible when there are numerous alternatives. But when there are no alternatives, such as with transportation facilities available to the public, no smoking should be the rule.

2. Recent Developments in the Enactment of Clean Indoor Air Laws

Most states and many localities have now enacted clean indoor air restrictions. Although there has been some action on the part of the federal government to reduce the amount of ETS exposure experienced by the public, most tobacco control has been accomplished at the state and local levels. As we shall see, the content of these laws varies widely, resulting in a "patchwork of smoking restrictions" (Rigotti and Pashos 1991) that apply to a large number of Americans in public places (including public and private worksites and facilities open to the public).

Laws to protect nonsmokers generally and employees in particular from ETS can be considered in terms of comprehensiveness and the strength of their individual provisions. A comprehensive law or regulation addresses smoking in all of the major places generally open to the public, does not preempt stronger local ordinances, and does not include provisions protecting smokers' rights.[12] For example, a strong, comprehensive law would include bans on smoking (or require separate ventilated systems for smoking areas) in public and private workplaces, restaurants and bars, and other enclosed public places. Lesser degrees of restriction are more frequently seen, including policies that require only a certain percentage of a facility to be smoke-free or that allow smoking in designated areas. Laws that include provisions preempting local ordinances inherently weaken protections against ETS exposure by limiting the ability of local jurisdictions to enact more stringent clean indoor air laws than exist at the state level.

Five trends capture developments in clean indoor air laws since 1989:[13] (1) a small expansion in the strength and comprehensiveness of state laws restricting smoking, (2) the continued enactment of state laws preempting stronger local ordinances, (3) a greater number and comprehensiveness of restrictions enacted at the local level, (4) the enactment of some form of nondiscrimination against smokers at the state level, and (5) the diffusion of tobacco control laws within local regions. A related development in the past few years has been an increase in voluntary workplace smoking policies. Most of the state clean indoor air laws were enacted in the late 1980s and early 1990s. Since 1993, there have been few state-level expansions in restricting smoking in private worksites or restaurants, but a greater number of local ordinances. With the exception of Califonia, antismoking policies in restaurants and private worksites have occurred either through ordinances at the local level or have emerged voluntarily.

Taken at face value, these trends appear to be somewhat contradictory. In all likelihood, the mixed legislative results are a product of the shifting balance between the tobacco industry and tobacco control proponents as various arguments (i.e., science versus individual freedoms) gain favor in the legislative debate. The trends also reflect compromises agreed to as the price of enacting legislation. For example, the only way to enact statewide clean indoor air act restrictions in Florida and Illinois was to accede to preemption (Jacobson et al. 1993).

Federal Clean Indoor Air Laws

State and local governments have assumed primary responsibility for enacting clean indoor air laws. Nevertheless, the federal government can take action to restrict smoking in its own facilities and has the authority to regulate clean indoor air to protect the public's health.[14] For example, the U.S. Postal Service eliminated smoking in all facilities in 1993, followed by the Department of Defense in 1994. The Occupational Safety and Health Administration (OSHA) has been considering rules that would essentially ban smoking in private worksites (requiring, at a minimum, separately ventilated rooms for smokers) since 1994.[15] Most important, EPA has taken the lead in disseminating research showing the harms from ETS, which has had a significant influence on the public debate over clean indoor air laws.

Federal tobacco policy is well known for its susceptibility to influence from the tobacco industry. Studies have shown a strong relationship between the level of tobacco industry contributions to individual congressional members and the probability that these members will vote against tobacco control legislation (Samuels and Glantz 1991; Bearman, Goldstein, and Bryan 1995; Siegel et al. 1997). Although its role has been minimal in enacting clean indoor air laws, Congress gradually eliminated smoking on airlines, first by banning smoking on short flights and then extending the ban to all domestic flights.

State Clean Indoor Air Laws

State statutes limiting smoking in public places were relatively rare prior to 1970 and were not revived until the comprehensive 1975 Minnesota clean indoor air law led the way. Today, every state but Alabama restricts smoking in some manner in public places.[16] These laws range from nominal restrictions (public buildings and schools in Indiana and Kentucky), to extensive restrictions (prohibitions on smoking in many public places in Vermont). Only a few states (California, Minnesota, New York, Massachusetts, and Utah) have enacted comprehensive clean indoor laws that restrict or prohibit smoking in a wide variety of public places. In table 8.1,[17] we combine published data from the Centers for Disease Control and Prevention, the Coalition on Smoking OR Health (CSOH), and the American Lung Association (ALA) to show state laws on several dimensions: clean indoor air restrictions at government worksites, private worksites, and restaurants; preemption; and nondiscrimination provisions.

A comparison across the states that have laws restricting ETS exposure in public places is quite difficult because the states define public places differently. There are also varying degrees of restrictiveness applied to the laws and regulations within the states, as noted earlier. For instance, of the 42 states[18] that have laws restricting smoking in state government and other public worksites, only 13 either prohibit smoking entirely or require designated smoking areas with separate ventilation, whereas 29 states limit smoking to designated areas (Fishman et al. 1999). Four other states allow, but

Table 8.1. State Clean Indoor Air Laws—2000

	Bars	Child care centers	Elevators	Government worksite	Gyms and sporting arenas	Health facilities	Private worksite	Public transit	Restaurant	Retail or grocery stores	Schools	Shopping centers
Alabama												
Alaska		P	P	X	X	P	X	X	X	X	X[a]	
Arizona			X	X		X		X			X[a]	
Arkansas		P		A		X					X[a]	
California	P[1]	P	P	P[1]	P[1]	P[1]	P[1]	P[1]	P[1]	P[1]	P[1]	P[1]
Colorado		P	P	P	X	X	E	X	E		P	P
Connecticut			X	X	X		X	X	X	X	X	
Delaware		P	P	X	X	P	X	P	X	X	X[a]	
Florida		P	P	X	X	X	X	P	X	X	P	
Georgia		P	P		X			P			P	
Hawaii		P	P	P	X	X		X	X	X	P	
Idaho		P	P	P	X	X		X	X	X	X	
Illinois		P		X	X	X		X	X	X	P	
Indiana		X		X		X					X	
Iowa		P	P	X	X	X	X	P	X	X	X	X
Kansas		P	P	P	X	X		P	X		P	
Kentucky				A							X	
Louisiana		P	P	X	X	X	X	P	X	X	P	
Maine		X		X	X	P	X	X	X	X	X	
Maryland		P[1]	P	P	X	P[1]	P[1]	P	X	X	P	
Massachusetts		X	P	P		X		P	X	P	X	
Michigan		P	P	P	X	P[1]		X	X	X	P	X
Minnesota		P	P	P	X	P[1]	X	X	X	X	X	
Mississippi		P		P	X	P	X	P	X	X	P	

Table 8.1. (*continued*)

State										
Missouri	X		P		X	X	X	X	X	P	X
Montana			P		P	X	X	X	P	X	
Nebraska	X	X	X		X	X	X	X	X	X	
Nevada		X	P		P	X	X	X	P	X	
New Hampshire		P	P	X	P	X	X	X	P	X	
New Jersey		P	P		X	X	X	E	P	X	X
New Mexico		X		A	X	X	X		P	P	
New York		P	P		X	X	X	X	X	X	
North Carolina		P	X		X	X	X	X		X	
North Dakota		P¹	X		X	X	X	X	X	X	
Ohio		P	X		X	X	X	X	X	X	
Oklahoma		P	P		X	X	X	P	X	X	
Oregon			X		X	X	X	P	X		X
Pennsylvania		P	P		X	X	X	P	X	X	
Rhode Island		P	X		X	X	X	P	X	X	X
South Carolina		P	P		X	X	X	P	X	X	
South Dakota		X	X		P	X	X	P	X	X	
Tennessee		X	E		X	X	X	X		P	
Texas		X	P		P	X	X	X	X	X	
Utah		P	P		P	X	X	P	P	X	P
Vermont	X	P	P		P	X	X	P	P	X	P
Virginia		X	X		X	X	X	X	X	X	
Washington		P¹	P		P¹	X	X	X	P	P	
Washington D.C.	X	X	P		X	X	X	X	P	X	X
West Virginia		X			X	X	X	P	X	X	
Wisconsin		P	X		X	P	X	X	X	P	
Wyoming			X		X	X			X		P
Total (A)			3								

219

Table 8.1. (continued)

	Bars	Child care centers	Elevators	Government worksite	Gyms and sporting arenas	Health facilities	Private worksite	Public transit	Restaurant	Retail or grocery stores	Schools	Shopping centers
Total (X)	3	9	8	33	25	34	21	19	30	25	22	5
Total (X[b])		0	0	0	0	0	0	0	0	0	3	0
Total (P)		24	28	11	3	6	0	22	2	4	19	2
Total (P[i])	1	3	0	1	1	3	3	1	1	2	1	1
Total (P[a])		0	0	0	0	0	0	0	0	0	1	0
Total (E)		0	0	1	0	0	1	0	2	0	0	0
TOTAL	4	36	38	42	29	43	25	42	35	30	46	8

A = Smoking policies and restrictions allowed, but not required.

P = Smoking Prohibited

P[i] = Enclosed, separately ventilated areas required, or smoking is banned entirely

X = Smoking restrictions required

E = Smoking restrictions encouraged

a = Does not apply to areas designated through collective bargaining agreements made prior to 8/14/90

b = Designated smoking areas are permitted only in private schools, smoking is banned entirely in public schools

Sources: State Legislated Actions on Tobacco Issues, American Lung Association, 1998; Centers for Disease Control MMWR, 1998. Some discrepancy exists between the sources in their classification of the states' restrictiveness. This is most likely due to different descriptions used to define the sites, as well as variations among states in the level of smoking restrictions required to be designated in a particular category.

do not require, smoking policies or restrictions (ALA 1998; Fishman et al. 1999).

Most states also regulate smoking in a variety of public settings: 36 states restrict smoking in child day care centers, 43 states restrict smoking in hospitals and other health facilities, 42 states have restrictions on selected forms of transportation, 30 states have laws regarding smoking in grocery stores, and 29 states have restrictions in enclosed arenas (ALA 1998). Substantial variation marks the level of restrictiveness in these state laws.

In addition, 25 states restrict smoking in private worksites. Only California's law stipulates either a complete ban on smoking or a separate ventilation system for the designated smoking areas (Fishman et al. 1999). Laws regulating smoking in restaurants are in place in 31 states, but only Utah and Vermont have laws prohibiting smoking in restaurants, whereas California's law stipulates that there must be either no smoking or separate ventilation systems for smoking areas (Fishman et al. 1999). Only a few states have laws that restrict smoking in other locations, such as bars, home-based child care centers, shopping malls, or hotels and motels.

When one views state legislative actions since the 1980s, an important pattern emerges. The movement of the battle for smoking restrictions, however glacial, appears to progress from eliminating smoking in a few public accommodations, such as elevators and public transportation. Then, smoking restrictions are gradually added to other enclosed public places, most often child care centers, schools, and government worksites. After that, some jurisdictions move to limit smoking at private worksites. That narrows the remaining legislative targets among enclosed public places to restaurants, and finally bars. Except for restrictions on smoking at outdoor stadiums, no state has attempted to eliminate smoking outdoors (although some local communities, such as Tacoma Park, Maryland, have done so).[19]

Few of the state clean indoor air laws are sufficiently comprehensive to achieve long-term changes in the cumulative risks that nonsmokers face if significant time is spent being exposed to ETS. And, as with federal level tobacco legislation, the tobacco industry has been able to impose a strong influence on public policy through lobbying state legislators (Samuels and Glantz 1991; Jacobson et al. 1993). Recently, this power has been manifested mainly in the number of state preemption laws enacted and laws prohibiting discrimination against smokers.

State Preemption Laws   In response to the increasing number of local tobacco control policies (discussed later), the tobacco industry has been successful in lobbying state legislators to enact state laws preempting local ordinances. As noted earlier, preemption laws prevent local authorities from enacting restrictions more stringent than, or at variance with, the state laws. Between

1982 and 1998, a total of 31 states enacted laws preempting local clean indoor air policies, with only Maine successfully repealing a preemptive state smoking law (Fishman et al. 1999).[20] Strategies used by the tobacco industry to get these preemptions enacted include attaching preemptive clauses to antitobacco bills and garnering support from the retail industry by convincing its members that preemption is necessary for business interests (Siegel et al. 1997).

Many preemptive laws have actually diminished the level of protections previously afforded by local regulation where the local laws were more stringent than state measures. Beyond preventing localities from enacting ordinances that address community-specific needs, preemption reduces the amount of debate over local policies (Fishman et al. 1999). A local debate helps to educate the community about the dangers of exposure to tobacco. Thus, communities lacking the ability to participate in local debates over tobacco control decisions may be less attentive to the dangers involved and less aware of ways to control tobacco use.

State Smokers' Rights Laws   Smokers' rights provisions generally prevent discrimination against smokers for engaging in a lawful activity. These provisions, depending on how they are interpreted, can potentially impede the implementation of worksite no-smoking policies. For example, a smokers' rights law could prevent an employer from refusing to hire current smokers.

Between 1989 and 1995, 30 states enacted laws prohibiting discrimination against smokers (CSOH 1995). To the best of our knowledge, there are no studies determining whether smokers have been able to use these laws to impede the implementation and enforcement of clean indoor air laws.

Local Clean Indoor Air Laws

Local antismoking ordinances and regulations are often more comprehensive and restrictive than state laws.[21] They are also more likely to have local enforcement mechanisms through a variety of agencies, including local health departments, city managers' offices, law enforcement departments, local environmental health agencies, and fire departments (Brownson et al. 1997; Jacobson and Wasserman 1999). Conformity with clean indoor air policies are most often self-enforcing (Jacobson and Wasserman 1999). As a result, local ordinances tend to achieve high rates of compliance, even though extensive resources are usually not dedicated to their enforcement.

In 1989, 397 city and county smoking ordinances were listed in NIH's *Handbook on the Major Local Smoking Ordinances*, covering a total population of nearly 52.5 million people. This included 297 localities that mandated workplace smoking policies, the majority of which required both private and public employers to have a written smoking policy. The strength of the policies, however, ranged from virtually eliminating smoking in the workplace to simply requiring the adoption of some form of smoking policy. Additionally, there were 369 cities and counties nationwide in 1989 that addressed smoking in restaurants. Again, there was a significant degree of variation in the restrictiveness of the policies, ranging from eliminating smoking in restaurants to requiring that nonsmoking sections be provided. Finally, a total of 298 local ordinances restricted smoking in other enclosed places, which included general businesses, retail stores, and other facilities open to the public.

The data for the 1999 NIH *Handbook* reveal that a substantial number of more restrictive ordinances have been enacted in the last decade that limit or eliminate smoking in public places. As of late 1998, there were 859 local clean indoor air ordinances across the country, including 645 local ordinances that restrict smoking in workplaces and 753 city and county ordinances that limit smoking in restaurants. Of those totals, only 209 and 227, respectively, require the total elimination of restaurant smoking, leaving the majority of the public with continued ETS exposure.

Unlike their state and federal counterparts, local officials are less susceptible to tobacco industry influences (Samuels and Glantz 1991; Jacobson et al. 1993). In most cases, public health advocates are more effective in local policy making than at the other governmental levels, in part because they are able to use their community connections to influence local policy (Jacobson et al. 1993). As a practical matter, there are so many towns, cities, and counties across the nation that it is not feasible for the tobacco industry to devote its resources (including campaign contributions) to fight all local tobacco control initiatives.

Diffusion

Some researchers have reported that the presence of smoking restriction policies in neighboring cities/towns/counties is an important predictor for whether a community will implement its own smoking ordinance. In a 1998 study in Massachusetts, researchers found that, on average, communities adopting a smoking limitation were surrounded by a higher percentage of towns with some form of smoking policy than the communities that did not adopt such laws (Bartosch and Pope 1999b). Similarly, towns enacting highly restrictive smoking policies were bordered by a significantly higher percentage of other highly restrictive laws than either moderately restrictive communities or those without any smoking policies (Bartosch and Pope 1999b). This clustering of towns with smoking ordinances may be due to the diffusion of policy ideas between communities in close proximity. Or neighboring communities' common characteristics may influence their decisions to enact smoking policies.

Although not systematically studied, anecdotal evidence from other states supports the hypothesis that diffusion at the local level is an important factor in explaining the enactment of local ordinances. For instance, it is reasonable to assume that the dramatic increase in local antismoking ordinances throughout California resulted from a diffusion process. Yet diffusion clearly has its limits. Beverly Hills enacted a ban on smoking in restaurants but repealed it when restaurateurs were able to show a substantial short-term decline in business, as patrons shifted to neighboring communities that had not adopted similar bans. This problem was subsequently surmounted by the enactment of a statewide law banning smoking in restaurants—one advantage of statewide laws relative to local ordinances.

Voluntary Restrictions on Smoking

As a general proposition, tobacco control advocates have had good reason not to rely on market arrangements to determine acceptable tobacco control policy. Except for a few situations, such as no-smoking rooms and floors in hotels and some airline restrictions, the market has not been very responsive to public support for smoking restrictions. For example, the traditional merchant argument used to oppose voluntary smoking restrictions is that "we accommodate our customers, many of whom smoke." Underlying this argument is the belief that smokers spend more than nonsmokers and are more vocal about their preferences. To date, nonsmokers have not sent a strong enough message to overcome many merchants' reluctance to antagonize their smoking patrons. That reluctance may be changing, as more merchants and worksites seem to be adopting voluntary smoking restrictions.

The adoption of voluntary smoking restrictions has not been studied systematically, but survey evidence and emerging anecdotal evidence suggests that some interesting changes may be occurring. First, analyses of the National Cancer Institute's Tobacco Use Supplement to the Current Population Survey (CPS) over time indicate that 46% of workers from 1992 to 1993 were covered by some variant of a no-smoking policy, up from just 3% in 1986 (Brownson et al. 1997; Gerlach, Shopland, Hartman, Gibson, and Pechacek 1997). Some of these restrictions were no doubt mandated by state or local laws. Yet Gerlach et al. (1997) concluded that because many workplaces were not covered by clean indoor laws from 1992 to 1993, "the policies reported in this survey are largely a reflection of self-imposed restrictions." In a survey conducted for the Community Intervention Trial for Smoking Cessation (COMMIT), Sorensen, Glasgow, Topor, and Corbett (1997) found that the adoption of no-smoking worksite policies was higher among non-manufacturing industries, such as service and retail businesses, those employing more female workers, and those with greater than a hundred employees. And Bergman and Falit (1997) found that 84% of all noninstitutional facilities serving the elderly in Michigan were smoke-free, with 38% of respondents indicating that the action was taken voluntarily.[22]

Even in restaurants (discussed later in greater detail), long considered a bastion of resistance to voluntary restrictions, recent news accounts suggest important changes. Although this evidence is clearly anecdotal and can at best represent a developing phenomenon, the fact that changes are occurring at all indicates how much smoking policy has changed in recent years. For example, fast food chains such as Wendy's, Burger King, and McDonald's have banned smoking. In New Hampshire, where there is no state or local ordinance banning smoking in restaurants, more than 70 restaurants have voluntarily gone smoke-free (Milkovits 1998). In Arizona, also a state with minimal smoking restrictions, Corella (1999) reported that "the Southern Arizona Restaurant Association estimates that about 627 of the 1481 restaurants in Pima County are already smoke-free. That's more than double the 300 restaurants here that had non-smoking sections in 1984."[23] In Spokane, Washington, about 50% of the country's restaurants are smoke-free, despite being exempt from the state's clean indoor air law (Cannato 2001).

Six factors primarily account for this shift. First, given the decline in adult indoor smoking, more customers are requesting no-smoking sections, hence reducing the demand and need for smoking areas. Second, the publicity surrounding ETS has encouraged restaurateurs and other businesses to rethink smoking policies. Third, the threat of litigation over ETS exposure (such as the airline attendants' case mentioned earlier) has influenced some of the fast food chains, and perhaps others, to abandon smoking sections in favor of prohibiting smoking altogether. Fourth, as discussed later, there is no systematic evidence that proprietors who choose to go smoke-free actually lose business.[24] Fifth, it is certainly possible that voluntary actions have been taken in anticipation of state or local laws. And sixth, employee preferences may be a factor, though, as shown later, bartenders have expressed mixed views about smoking bans.

The success of voluntary smoking restrictions depends on how employees respond to the changes, how the restrictions affect business, and whether competitors adopt similar measures. But the success of smoking bans in bars and restaurants may well rest primarily with nonsmokers. Because these bans likely will not be heavily enforced (Jacobson and Wasserman 1999), patronage by nonsmokers will be critical in generating owner support for smoking bans. In the following example a Pennsylvania bar owner explains why he voluntarily banned smoking but then switched back (Bruch 1998): " 'At first the nonsmokers came, and it was good,' he said. 'But after a couple of months, business started dropping off. The nonsmokers weren't patronizing us anymore.' "

The market response to tobacco control may vary across different settings. For example, there does not appear to be much of a market for nonsmoking bars, but there may be a market for landlords to ban smoking from their apartments to attract renters who would otherwise be bothered by smoke wafting into their apartments. If so, a more nuanced regulatory strategy would be appropriate, in which the government intervenes when a market response is unlikely or provides incentives to stimulate a market response.

3. Effectiveness of Laws Restricting Smoking in Public Places

It is important to evaluate the effects of clean indoor air laws to determine if they reduce nonsmokers' exposure to ETS, if they encourage smoking cessation or a reduction in smoking, and whether the laws are actually implemented and enforced. For a variety of reasons, research on the effectiveness of clean indoor air laws has lagged. Because smoking rates are determined through the complex interaction of a range of influences, including clean indoor air laws, civil norms, and public opinion, it is difficult to attribute changes to a single cause. Another challenge for researchers is the difficulty of measuring or observing actual cessation or reduction rates. Despite these challenges, emerging research suggests that these laws can be effective in reducing exposure to ETS and in promoting cessation.

Impact of Bans on ETS Exposure

Worksites Comprehensive worksite smoking bans have been shown to reduce nonsmokers' ETS exposure and to have a positive influence on the smoking habits of a significant number of employees (Siegel et al. 1997; Chapman et al. 1999; Moskowitz, Lin, and Hudes 2000). A study from California suggested that strong local smoking ordinances reduced nonsmokers' workplace exposure to tobacco smoke and decreased ambient air levels of ETS (Pierce et al. 1994). And the implementation of the Massachusetts Tobacco Control program led to an average reduction in ETS exposure across all workers from 4.5 to 2.2 hours per week (Abt Associates 1998). Likewise, CDC reported that the percentage of respondents to the Current Population Survey working in a smoke-free environment rose from 46.5% in 1992–1993 to 63.7% in 1995–1996 and continues to increase (CDC 2000).

Optimal protection from environmental tobacco smoke is best achieved through a total ban on workplace smoking, with separate ventilating systems a next-best alternative. In workplace settings that allow smoking in designated areas without also installing separate ventilation systems, substantial exposure to secondhand smoke continues (Brownson, Davis, Jackson-Thompson, and Wilkerson 1995; Brownson et al. 1997), although at lower levels of both concentration and duration of exposure (Siegel 1993). The aerosol particles from tobacco products still diffuse to all areas within the work area or nonsmoking section of a restaurant, including areas designated smoke-free. From a policy perspective, however, separate smoking and non-smoking areas may be a good first step that can be used as leverage for stronger restrictions over time.

Although the main goal of these laws is to reduce the public's exposure to ETS, a number of additional benefits will result from limitations on smoking in public places (Andrews 1983; Becker et al. 1989; Sorensen, Beder, Prible, and Pinney 1995). These benefits include a decrease in the overall prevalence of smoking, a reduction in the daily consumption of tobacco products, an increased rate of smoking cessation, a decreased number of relapses from attempts to quit, and a decreased number of people initiating smoking habits. In a longitudinal survey for the COMMIT trial, Glasgow, Cummings, and Hyland (1997) found that worksite smoking bans resulted in 25% more cessation attempts and 25% higher cessation rates than among workers not covered by smoking bans. They also found a small, but statistically significant reduction in daily use for those who did not quit. Not surprisingly, they concluded that a ban would provide greater reductions in ETS, and higher cessation rates, than designated smoking sections.[25] Increased rates of smoking cessation have also resulted when the bans were combined with other smoking cessation programs and support activities to encourage attempts to quit (Sorensen, Lando, and Pechacek 1993; Sorensen et al. 1995).

Nationwide population-based surveys have indicated that smoking bans at worksites reduce smoking prevalence by approximately 5% overall, and that average daily consumption by smokers has decreased by about 10% (Brownson et al. 1997). The percentage of smokers who reported that they considered quitting smoking was also higher in smoke-free worksites (Borland et al. 1992; Woodruff, Rosbrook, Pierce, and Glante 1993; Brownson et al. 1995; Brownson et al. 1997). Conversely, a California study found that smoking prevalence and consumption appeared to increase when workers moved from a smoke-free workplace to one that allowed work area smoking (Brownson et al. 1997). Policies restricting smoking in public places, therefore, appear to be having a positive impact on reducing the smoking habits of some smokers.

Hospitals   Prohibiting smoking in hospitals has been associated with substantial declines in both employee and customer/patient ETS exposure and cigarette consumption. The hospital industry is unique in implementing a nationwide smoking ban, based on accreditation requirements for the Joint Commission on Accreditation of Healthcare Organizations (JCAHO). Full compliance with the ban was required as of December 31, 1993. Surveys conducted two years after the ban was in place show that the policy was a success, with 95.6% of hospitals around the country in compliance with the smoking ban (Longo, Brownson, and Kruse 1995). In addition, Longo et al. (1996) compared smoking behavior among employees in hospitals after smoking bans were imposed and smokers in the corresponding communities. Five years after the hospital bans were implemented, hospital employees had a statistically significant higher cessation ratio.

Savings To Employers   There may also be cost savings to employers through the implementation of smoke-free worksite regulations. These savings represent funds associated with fire risk from tobacco products, smoke and burn damage to property and furnishings, cleaning costs, workers' compensation, disability, accidents, life insurance, absenteeism, productivity losses, and occupational risks related to the synergistic effects of tobacco smoke and other hazardous agents such as asbestos (Brownson et al. 1997). To be sure, it is exceedingly difficult to evaluate the true economic savings from smoke-free workplace policies. But an EPA analysis concluded that a national ban on smoking in the workplace would be a significantly cost-beneficial social investment, with benefits exceeding costs by approximately $39–72 billion per year (EPA 1994). These estimates assume compliance with the clean indoor air policies.

Economic Impacts of Smoke-Free Policies—
Bars and Restaurants

Along with small employers, the strongest opponents of restrictions on smoking in public places have been bar and restaurant owners. Despite such opposition, some recent state legislation and local ordinances have banned smoking in restaurants and required strict ventilation systems in bars. (In some instances, smoking has also been banned in bars.) The most prominent examples are the 1995 California law (AB 13), banning smoking in restaurants and, as of 1998, in bars, along with programs in Massachusetts (1992) and New York City (1995). Because these laws represent a key test in the continued expansion of clean indoor air laws and policies, and remain highly contentious, we treat them separately in this section.

California   After the California law banning smoking in restaurants and bars went into effect in early 1998, there was a furious and negative reaction from bar and restaurant owners who feared lost business.[26] Several news accounts interviewed patrons who promised defiance. The tobacco industry sponsored a sophisticated public relations campaign to repeal the law, and legislation to do just that was introduced in the California legislature.

But six months later (June 1998), sales tax receipt data from the California Board of Equalization showed a 1.06% increase in sales from the state's smallest bars (usually stand-alone establishments that constitute 15% of California bars), those most likely to be adversely affected by the smoking ban. We describe similar evidence for restaurants later. Just as important, a survey conducted in June 1998 by the Field Research Corporation for the California Department of Health Services found that 59% of the general public and 46% of bar patrons supported the law (with 39% opposed). The survey also found that 85% of bar patrons reported that the law would not change which bars they frequent. These results were consistent with a *Los Angeles Times* survey.

By October 1998, public support increased to 65%, and a majority of bar patrons (59%) now supported the ban. Among bar owners, however, 61.8% disapproved of the ban (33.5% approved), with 90.1% disapproval among stand-alone bar owners. Bar employees also disapproved by 69.7% to 28.4%. Overall, the survey indicated a 27.9% noncompliance rate, rising to 52.5% in stand-alone bars. By October 2000, support among bar patrons increased to 73%, and among smokers to 44%.

In contrast to these results, the National Smokers' Alliance claimed a 15% business loss. Also, the American Beverage Institute released a study in May 1998 showing that 60% of California bartenders surveyed suggested that they lost business and tips, and 30% said there were layoffs or shorter work weeks for bar employees following the start of the year.[27]

One year after initiation, the news accounts suggest mixed results. Uneven enforcement has led to increasing noncompliance rates, especially in stand-alone bars. Not surprisingly, bartenders have been slow to enforce the law, claiming that patrons don't stay as long and customer crowds are thinner. And more news stories have appeared showing instances of defiance or noncompliance. Nevertheless, the law continues to generate strong public approval and perhaps higher than expected compliance in random compliance checks (such as 70% in Sacramento and 78% in San Francisco). Sales tax revenues from restaurants and bars rose 6% during the first quarter of 1998 relative to the first quarter of 1997, with a strong expansion of tourism. Most significantly, four legislative attempts to repeal the law failed because of considerable public support. In addition, Eisner, Smith, and Blanc (1998) report improved respiratory functions among bartenders in California following implementation of the ban.

Massachusetts   Massachusetts is another state with interesting trends in local restaurant smoking policies. Following a 1992 statewide referendum that raised the state's excise tax on cigarettes by 25 cents per pack, revenues were generated for the creation of the Massachusetts Tobacco Control Program (MTCP). This program funds community initiatives for over 260 local boards of health to enact and enforce policies to protect the public from environmental tobacco smoke (Bartosch and Pope 1999b). In Massachusetts, state legislators have granted local boards of health the broad authority to "make reasonable health regulations," and they receive significant funds from the MTCP to enforce them (Bartosch and Pope 1999b). Studies examining the differences between communities that enacted local restaurant smoking policies versus those that did not indicate that places with policies are medium-sized towns with lower proportions of blue-collar workers than nonadopting communities. More importantly, Bartosch and Pope (1999a) found no statistically significant difference in sales between restaurants covered by no-smoking ordinances and those where smoking is permitted. Bartosch and Pope (1999a) also found that many of the towns and cities followed a pattern of first adopting a smoking policy and then increasing the level of protectiveness over time.

New York City   In early 1995, New York City enacted a law restricting smoking in most public facilities, including restaurant-dining areas, workplaces, and sports stadiums (Clarke, Wilson, Cummings, and Hyland 1999; Hyland, Cummings, and Wilson 1999). Under the law, smoking is specifically prohibited within indoor dining areas of restaurants with more than 35 seats. Smoking is allowed in bar areas, as long as separated by six feet from dining areas or by a ceiling to floor partition (Hyland, Cummings, and Wilson 1999).

Before this law, smoking regulations applied only to restaurants with more than 50 indoor seats. Studies examining implementation show that the new law had little impact on the dining out patterns of consumers, did not result in job losses for the city's restaurant industry, resulted in high rates of compliance, and did not have a detrimental effect on business (Hyland and Cummings 1999a, 1999b, 1999c; Hyland, Cummings, and Wilson 1999). In fact, these studies document a gain in employment, and a 2% rise in sales tax receipts relative to a 4% decrease in the rest of New York State. Interestingly, the number of restaurants in New York City rose by 6% after imposition of the law (Hyland, Cummings, and Nauenberg 1999).[28]

Summary   The initial studies of smoking bans in restaurants (and bars in California) suggest that there are no economic upheavals when smoking is banned in public places.[29] Summarizing the existing data, Glantz (1999) notes convincingly that studies of sales tax data from 81 localities in six states (67 of which are entirely smoke-free) demonstrate that ordinances restricting smoking in restaurants have no adverse effect on revenues.[30]

In an important and related finding, Glantz and Charlesworth (1999) extend Glantz's previous work to consider the effects of restaurant smoking bans on tourism, which the tobacco industry has used as another argument against smoking bans. Their study examined tourism revenues in eight locations where the tobacco industry raised the issue of reduced tourism revenue in opposing restaurant smoking bans. The authors conclude that four localities show substantial revenue increases, four show no significant changes, and one saw a slower rate of increase. According to the authors, restaurant smoking bans had no adverse impact on international or domestic tourism.

Lessons   Five lessons stand out from these experiences. First, there is consistent public support, even among bar and restaurant patrons, for these bans. Second, the primary problem is likely to be with stand-alone bars. Getting support from bartenders may be an important implementation issue. Third, these laws are not likely to be stringently enforced, but, as noted in the next section, are dependent on civil norms or public pressure to be implemented. Fourth, early research suggests that smoking bans in bars and restaurants will not result in lost income. Fifth, there is an opportunity for tobacco control advocates to educate both the nonsmoking public and restaurant owners about the advantages of voluntarily adopting no-smoking policies, regardless of what state or local laws dictate (Biener and Fitzgerald 1999).[31]

In view of the conceptual and practical problems with restricting smoking in homes or in many outdoor spaces, at this point bans on smoking in bars, restaurants, and private worksites represent the most stringent laws likely to be enacted. What is lacking is widespread diffusion of these laws across states.

Compliance with Smoking Bans

Compliance with clean indoor air laws is a critical aspect of the implementation and effectiveness of smoke-free legislation. Without compliance, anticipated health benefits from decreases in ETS exposure will not be realized, credibility of the laws themselves will be lost, and future efforts for reform will be hampered by the inability to enforce current policies. Smoking restrictions require a mechanism for monitoring the behaviors of people in smoke-free areas. They also require a means of sanctioning individuals who violate the smoking restrictions, as well as owners and staff members of smoke-free facilities who fail to enforce or abide by regulations.

As Jacobson and Wasserman (1999) demonstrate, clean indoor air laws are rarely enforced. Nevertheless, a range of potential enforcement mechanisms exist, including tracking the complaints registered against establishments regarding violations of the smoking policies, owner/manager surveys as a form of self-policing, or random site inspections to determine if restaurants, stores, and other public facilities actually comply with smoke-free policies. Each of these methods has inherent limitations in its ability to determine levels of compliance accurately.

It is reasonable to assume that the large majority of complaints regarding infractions of the policies will go unreported. Inevitably, relying on self-policing to estimate compliance will miss noncompliant establishments. Random inspections of facilities merely capture a moment in time but are the most likely mechanisms for maintaining a certain level of accountability because of the uncertainty surrounding inspection visits. In any large city, a tremendous amount of time and money would be required to consistently inspect the thousands of stores, shops, and restaurants. In reality, this type of strict governmental monitoring is unlikely to occur. To be effective, clean indoor air laws must be essentially self-enforcing (Jacobson and Wasserman 1999).

Rigotti et al. (1988, 1992, 1993, 1994) have conducted a significant amount of research regarding the compliance of businesses with antismoking laws, in particular the self-enforcement approach. Results from these studies, conducted in Cambridge, Massachusetts, indicate that awareness of the local no-smoking ordinance in workplaces declined from 92% to 73% over the two years after passage. Eighty percent of companies surveyed restricted smoking both 3 and 24 months after passage, but only half the businesses fully complied with the law at either date. Based on this work, Rigotti, Stoto, and Schelling (1994) conclude that business size is important in determining compliance, with small businesses less likely to rely on self-enforcement; that the antismoking laws led to a high level of smoking restrictions; and that reminders to business are needed to avoid erosion in compliance over time.[32]

4. Future Policy Considerations

Despite the arguments raised by opponents of clean indoor air laws, civil norms regarding smoking in public places have changed fundamentally in the past decade. The public has a much lower level of tolerance for smoking in public places than in the past. A survey by Biener and Fitzgerald (1999) showed that nearly 50% of nonsmokers reported having avoided a smoky place at some time in the past because they would be exposed to more ETS than they were willing to tolerate. The notion that people have a right to smoke wherever they want has been replaced by an increasing recognition of the public's right to breathe air free from the hazardous side effects of ETS. Current sentiment is that the individual's right to smoke in public places is not absolute. Because of the danger that ETS poses, there must be limitations to where smoking is allowed.

At least in the short term, the gains in clean indoor air laws are unlikely to be reversed. The current situation thus presents tobacco control advocates with both opportunities and challenges.

Opportunities

The first opportunity is to consolidate the gains already made. Tobacco control advocates will play a critical role in doing so. First, advocates can hold the government accountable by monitoring the implementation and enforcement of existing clean indoor air laws and publicizing results.[33] Second, advocates must organize opposition to additional state preemption laws, as noted later. Third, advocates can support voluntary restrictions by providing favorable publicity and by encouraging their members and the public to patronize nonsmoking businesses. The support of voluntary smoking restrictions would obviate the need to engage the political system and would encourage other businesses to adopt no-smoking policies. It would also counter criticism from smokers, conservatives, and libertarians because it would provide a market response to a social problem.

The second opportunity is to extend these gains. As demonstrated earlier, the number of locales enacting clean indoor air laws peaked in the mid-1990s before declining in the late 1990s. Many areas of the country remain uncovered by clean indoor air laws. In view of the public's increasing dislike for the tobacco industry and the changed civil norms regarding smoking in public places, the timing seems right to push for another wave of smoking restrictions. This wave must focus on extending the laws to include smoking restrictions in restaurants and bars.

Because laws and regulations stimulate or validate changing cultural norms, it is important not to abandon the force of law in maintaining the desired goal of reduced tobacco use. Changes in civil norms facilitate the enactment of legislation that, in turn, codifies civil norms. Given their symbolic authority, laws institutionalize nascent civil norms (Kagan and Skolnick 1993). Legislation therefore acts to express the government's public policy concern that tobacco use is dangerous to health, contributes to a social climate that discourages smoking in public places (Roemer 1986), and legitimizes attempts to bring additional public pressure to reduce cigarette consumption. Just as civil norms, without legislative support, may not last, legislation alone, without evolving civil norms that render tobacco control laws more effective, will not achieve the goal of reducing cigarette consumption, a lesson learned in the early 1900s. Tobacco control advocates must therefore promote both legislative and voluntary antismoking policies to achieve sustainable changes in tobacco use.

Challenges

Along with the opportunities, advocates must confront five major challenges. The first is the potential backlash against governmental policies if the public perceives smoking restrictions to be onerous and paternalistic. For example, it is unlikely that the public would support restrictions on smoking in the home.[34] Pushing to extend restrictions beyond public places would be counterproductive and could jeopardize the gains already made. Advocates must be sensitive to this balance so that pejorative terms like "health Nazis" do not describe the reality.

The second challenge is to reverse the preemption laws enacted during the 1990s. If, as many have argued, enacting strong local ordinances represents the best opportunity for success, preemption laws will need to be reversed. Although not easy, this should be a paramount short-term goal.

The third challenge is to make the case that government regulation is still appropriate and needed. Despite the arguments we outlined justifying governmental intervention to restrict smoking, many still believe strongly that decisions regarding smoking policies should be left to the market to resolve.

The fourth challenge is to extend the reach of voluntary smoking restrictions adopted by the private sector. An advantage of this strategy is that it is market-based, thereby depriving opponents of a primary line of attack against clean indoor air laws. Another advantage is that expanding voluntary restrictions will reinforce civil norms in opposition to smoking in public places.

A fifth challenge lies in responding to Sullum's diversity argument, especially regarding restaurants and bars. Because the current approach in most jurisdictions is to require no-smoking sections that do not provide adequate protection to third parties, a preferable alternative might be to require restaurants and bars to choose to be either a smoking or a no-smoking establishment. Such a compromise is appealing because it could achieve considerable reductions in smoking in public places. But it comes with the potential cost of diluting the argument for more restrictive clean indoor air laws.

Long-Term Considerations

Even though short-term trends appear to be positive, the history of tobacco control is replete with warning signs that success is not irreversible. The tobacco industry remains a resourceful, creative, and powerful opponent. Thus, the pressure for tobacco control efforts must be sustained over time.

Research Our review suggests several lines of research that should be conducted. First, continuing research into the effectiveness of clean indoor air laws is imperative for understanding whether these laws actually reduce nonsmokers' exposure to ETS. Second, the incipient evidence of increasing numbers of voluntary restrictions and diffusion across contiguous geographical boundaries needs to be confirmed (or refuted) by further research. Third, additional measures of regulatory stringency should be developed and tested. These measures could assist policy makers in determining what types of clean indoor air restrictions to enact.

Education Our review also suggests that additional education regarding the hazards of smoking and exposure to environmental tobacco smoke could be beneficial by increasing the number of individuals who take steps to reduce ETS. This is one aspect in the campaign for smoke-free, healthier environments that could be effective, regardless of the presence or absence of official antismoking policies.

Both states and antismoking coalitions should be involved in these efforts. States have a responsibility to continue informing people of the risks they face from tobacco and the alternative means of protection available. Coalitions can support the government by working with businesses to expand voluntary no-smoking policies.

Education alone is unlikely to lead to broad social change. But there seems little doubt that education has greatly contributed to changing civil norms regarding smoking. A broad-based antismoking education campaign has the potential to increase pressure for implementing clean indoor air restrictions. Therefore, states and advocates should continue and expand their efforts in promoting antismoking education.

ETS Exposure In the Home The home environment is another area where significant efforts need to be made regarding education and risk reduction. The major source of ETS exposure among young children is from smoking by parents or other adults in the home; estimates suggest that nearly half of the children ages 5 years and younger are exposed to ETS in the home (Brownson et al. 1997). It is certainly ironic that the home, where children's exposure to ETS is greatest, is exempt from antismoking laws and restrictions. Fundamental privacy protections limit the reach of public policy in this area. Nonetheless, many interventions could result in less smoking in the home without infringing on privacy (Gilpin, White, Farkas, and Pierce 1999).[35] These include smoking cessation programs for adolescents and adults, community-based interventions to educate parents about the dangers of ETS to children, and physician-based counseling (Ashley et al. 1998). Currently, there is little evidence regarding the effectiveness of these approaches, although both Gilpin et al. (1999) and Ashley et al. (1998) report changes over time in attitudes toward smoking in the home. Thus, these authors support additional policy intervention.

Product Regulation   Clean indoor air laws alone will not solve the smoking problem. Although it is beyond the scope of this chapter to address the scope of a comprehensive tobacco control strategy, one issue is the extent to which the content of cigarettes should be regulated. We agree with most advocates in favoring regulation of tobacco products by the FDA as a long-term strategy for tobacco control.

Conclusion

In a democracy, there is a constant tension between the right of the government to protect the public's health and the equally powerful right of the individual to determine how to live his or her own life, free from governmental interference. Striking the proper balance is never easy, particularly when the economic survival of politically powerful interests is at stake. The continued expansion of clean indoor air laws, without eliminating smokers' ability to consume a lawful product, maintains the necessary balance. Clean indoor air laws are justifiable policies, philosophically and pragmatically, because of their powerful potential to protect the public's health.

NOTES

1. Legal use of tobacco is restricted to persons over 18 years of age in all states.
2. The economic rationale is discussed later.
3. *Broin v. Philip Morris Companies, Inc.*, 641 So.2d 888 (Fla. 1994).
4. One possible reason for the involvement of libertarian scholars is that antismoking laws have become more stringent over the past decade, hence more clearly implicating personal freedom concerns to a broader audience. Libertarians are concerned both about the actual restrictions on personal freedoms with more stringent antismoking laws and with the potential implications for limits on other personal behaviors.
5. For example, a poll taken by the Eagleton Institute at Rutgers University in April 2000 concluded that 83% of New Jersey residents favor workplace smoking bans, whereas 67% favor a ban in restaurants.
6. As an aside, there is an interesting conceptual anomaly at work here. Many of the most vociferous opponents of government interference in personal decisions also

espouse a majoritarian philosophy that defers to the elected representatives to set social policy. In this instance, Sullum wants it both ways. He opposes governmental intervention but also opposes the right of the majority to define social policy.

7. A recent editorial in the *Ottawa Citizen,* "Some Choices on Smoking," 28 June 1998, supports the idea of diversity: "The nearest thing to a middle way is to require restaurants and bars to designate themselves smoking or non-smoking, unless they have a separate room for smokers, ventilated to the outside. Many owners would choose, for reasons of space or expense, to stick with one area and simply make it smoking or non-smoking. The designation would have to be displayed prominently at the door."

8. An equally damning assessment was issued by Federal District Judge William Osteen in rejecting EPA's estimates of 3,000 yearly deaths from ETS. See *Flue-Cured Tobacco Coop. Stabilization Corp. v. United States Environmental Protection Agency,* 4 F. Supp.2d 435 (M.D.N.C. 1998). As noted earlier, however, Cal. EPA (1997), using more recent studies, confirmed EPA's general analysis, if not the specific estimates. Sullum (1998, 174) argues that "contrary to the impression created by these messages, there is no evidence that occasional encounters with tobacco smoke pose a significant risk."

9. In response to Levy and Marimont (1998), Michael Eriksen, director of the Office on Smoking and Health at CDC, refuted their claims. See http:/www.tobacco.org/News/990514eriksen.html. See, also, Cal. EPA (1997).

10. We thank our colleague Harold Pollack for suggesting this phrasing.

11. An interesting question to ponder is why, in tight labor markets, employees generally (and those in restaurants and bars particularly) don't gravitate toward non-smoking environments, forcing employers to compete on that dimension.

12. There have been several attempts to develop indices to compare the stringency of laws across jurisdictions. In the past, most such indices have relied on numerical counts without adjusting for factors such as preemption, provisions protecting smokers' rights, or enforcement. Based usually on a 0 to 4 scale, these indices have provided only gross measures of stringency that have not proved very effective in analyzing stringency. Recently, Klonoff et al. (1998) developed a sophisticated assessment scale using 55 questions to compare and evaluate clean indoor air restrictions. And Alciati et al. (1998) developed a far more sophisticated methodology for evaluating state laws restricting youth access to tobacco. Either of these could prove valuable for assessing the stringency of tobacco control laws, but both are highly complex and may be difficult to interpret.

13. During the 1990s, the state legislative focus has been on enacting laws to restrict youths' access to tobacco (Jacobson and Wasserman 1999; Fishman et al. 1999).

14. For a comprehensive review of federal antismoking activity, see CDC's *TIPS: Chronological Review on Smoking, 1964–1996.*

15. 54 Fed. Reg. 15,968–16,039 (1994).

16. There is some discrepancy among sources regarding state-level clean indoor air restrictions. This is most likely due to the descriptions used to define a particular site (e.g., "gyms and sporting arenas" vs. "enclosed spaces"), as well as variations in the level of smoking restrictions required for designation in a particular category. For example, the Office on Smoking and Health (Fishman et al. 1999) lists Alabama,

Kentucky, Mississippi, and North Carolina as having no clean indoor air restrictions, while the American Lung Association (ALA 1998) lists only Alabama.

17. Table 8.1 is an updated version, using data compiled by the American Lung Association (State Legislated Actions on Tobacco Issues), from a similar table appearing in Jacobson, Wasserman, and Anderson (1997).

18. For convenience, we include the District of Columbia as a state.

19. At least one recent news story has reported that apartment and condominium residents are beginning to file complaints with local health departments about ETS exposure from neighboring apartments or condos (Tansey 1999). According to the article, apartment listings specifying "no smoking, no pets" are already common in Santa Clara, California, newspapers.

20. Not all preemption provisions are alike. Massachusetts' preemption applies only to the sale of cigarette rolling paper, whereas other states preempt local jurisdictions from enacting any clean indoor air restrictions (i.e., Florida).

21. In addition to the articles cited, the information on local tobacco control ordinances was provided by the American Nonsmokers Rights Foundation (ANRF). The authors appreciate ANRF's cooperation. Although useful, the ANR database relies on self-reporting from local jurisdictions. Therefore, the ANR information most likely understates the number of local antismoking ordinances.

22. Increasing numbers of indoor shopping malls have banned smoking.

23. Interestingly, Corella (1999) also reported that many proprietors of smoke-free restaurants opposed Tucson's proposed ordinance banning smoking in restaurants because the decision should be left to the individual business owner. The ban was enacted anyway.

24. In numerous Internet list servers posting articles on tobacco control, most proprietors report that most smokers return (though some never do) and that non-smokers are making up for any loss of smokers. At the same time, there are also reports of restaurants going smoke-free but changing when the smoking clientele abandons the business.

25. The authors also noted that designated smoking sections reduced ETS tobacco use relative to worksites without smoking restrictions.

26. This account is summarized from news articles reported on various electronic tobacco list servers.

27. These studies have not appeared in peer-reviewed publications, nor have they been analyzed or verified by independent reviewers. We include them here only to report what the industry claims, not to provide independent credence.

28. Needless to say, the industry disputes these findings. Their studies, not publicly released, show a decline in employment and a loss of business (Martin 1999). See also, Gorski (1999). One limitation of the Hyland, Cummings, and Nauenberg (1999) study is that 8,000 out of the 15,000 restaurants surveyed were small enough to allow smoking or had bars where smoking is permitted.

29. See Warner et al. (1996) for an economic analysis showing that reductions in spending on tobacco products will actually raise employment levels in nontobacco producing states.

30. In 1994, the National Restaurant Association testified before Congress that OSHA's proposed ban on workplace smoking would cost the restaurant industry $18.2 billion nationally, with an additional $913 million in lost state and local tax

revenues (National Restaurant Association 1994). Even if the overall impact of restaurant bans has not been negative, the gains will not be equally distributed. For example, a Fort Wayne, Indiana, City Council survey found that restaurant earnings declined between 5 and 24% in all but one of the 24 restaurants surveyed following that city's smoking ban (Ellick 1999). It is also unlikely that restaurant owners will take the recent research findings at face value. In Fairhaven, Connecticut, for instance, Stewardson (1999) reports that restaurant owners have begun developing "battle plans" to defeat a proposed smoking ban.

31. On the other hand, some smokers might reduce their dining out patterns if smoking is not allowed.

32. For similar conclusions in other settings and areas, see Nordstrom and DeStefano (1995); Patten et al. (1995); and Brownson et al. (1995).

33. See Jacobson and Wasserman (1999) for more detail on this point.

34. In some cases, family law judges have taken smoking into account in awarding custody and conditioning visitation rights. So far, these are random decisions that do not indicate broad public support for overcoming what most Americans view as the right to conduct their home life with considerable freedom from governmental interference.

35. See, for example, the EPA's Campaign to Reduce Children's Exposure. Nonetheless, smoking has occasionally been an issue in child custody proceedings and some advocates have suggested that smoking in the home be treated as child abuse. An aggressive campaign to enact laws prohibiting smoking in the home could be counterproductive. A better strategy would be to focus on voluntary restrictions and smoking cessation programs.

REFERENCES

Abt Associates, Inc. 1998. *Independent Evaluation of the Massachusetts Tobacco Control Program: Fourth Annual Report*. Boston, Mass.

Alciati, M. H., M. Frosh, S. B. Green, et al. 1998. State laws on youth access to tobacco in the United States: Measuring their extensiveness with a new rating system. *Tobacco Control* 7:345–52.

American Lung Association (ALA). 1998. *State Legislated Actions on Tobacco Issues*. Washington, DC: ALA.

Andrews, J. L., Jr. 1983. Reducing smoking in the hospital: An effective model program. *CHEST* 84:206–9.

Arno, P. S., A. M. Brandt, L. O. Gostin, and J. Morgan. 1996. Special communication: Tobacco industry strategies to oppose federal regulation. *JAMA* 275 (16):258–1262.

Ashley, M. J., J. Cohen, R. Ferrence, S. Bull, S. Bondy, B. Poland, and L. Pederson. 1998. Smoking in the home: Changing attitudes and current practices. *American Journal of Public Health* 88:797–800.

Bartosch, W. J., and G. C. Pope. 1999a. The economic effect of smoke-free restaurant policies on restaurant business in Massachusetts. *Journal of Public Health Management Practice* 5:53–62.

———. 1999b. Local restaurant smoking policy enactment in Massachusetts. *Journal of Public Health Management Practice* 5:63–73.

Bearman, N. S., A. O. Goldstein, and D. C. Bryan. 1995. Legislating clean air: Politics, preemption, and the health of the public. *North Carolina Medical Journal* 56:14–19.

Becker, D. M., H. F. Conner, H. R. Waranch, F. Stillman, L. Pennington, P. S. Lees, and F. Oski. 1989. The impact of a total ban on smoking in The Johns Hopkins Children's Center. *JAMA* 262:799–802.

Bergman, J. A., and J. L. Falit. 1997. Non-smoking policies, tobacco education, and smoking cessation programmes in facilities serving the elderly in Michigan, United States. *Tobacco Control* 6:194–8.

Biener, L., and G. Fitzgerald. 1999. Smoky bars and restaurants: Who avoids them and why? *Journal of Public Health Management Practice* 5:74–8.

Bonita, R., J. Duncan, T. Truelsena, et al. 1999. Passive smoking as well as active smoking increases the risk of acute stroke. *Tobacco Control* 8:156–60.

Borland, R., J. P. Pierce, D. M. Burns, E. Gilpin, M. Johnson, and D. Bal. 1992. Protection from environmental tobacco smoke in California: The case for a smoke-free workplace. *JAMA* 268:749–52.

Brownson, R. C., J. R. Davis, J. Jackson-Thompson, and J. C. Wilkerson. 1995. Environmental tobacco smoke awareness and exposure: Impact of a statewide clean indoor air law and the report of the US Environmental Protection Agency. *Tobacco Control* 4:132–8.

Brownson, R. C., M. P. Eriksen, R. M. Davis, and K. E. Warner. 1997. Environmental tobacco smoke: Health effects and policies to reduce exposure. *Annual Review of Public Health* 18:163–85.

Bruch, L. J. 1998. Chestnut Hill Bar goes smoke free. *Philadelphia Inquirer,* 13 October.

Burns, D. M., R. Axelrad, D. Bal, J. Carol, R. M. Davis, M. L. Myers, J. M. Pinney, N. A. Rigotti, and D. R. Shopland. 1992. Report of the Tobacco Policy Research Study Group on smoke-free indoor air policies. *Tobacco Control* 1 (suppl.):S14–8.

California Environmental Protection Agency. 1997. Health effects of exposure to environmental tobacco smoke. *Tobacco Control* 6:346–53.

Cannata, A. 2001. Clearing the air: Longtime smoker-friendly restaurants begin to ban smoking. The Spokesman-Review.com.

CDC. 2000. Scate-specific prevalence of current cigarette smoking among adults and the proportion of adults who work in a smoke-free environment—United States, 1999. MMWR 49:978–82.

Chapman, S., R. Borland, M. Scollo, R. C. Brownson, A. Dominello, and S. Woodward. 1999. The impact of smoke-free workplaces on declining cigarette consumption in Australia and the United States. *American Journal of Public Health* 89:1018–23.

Clarke, H., M. P. Wilson, K. M. Cummings, and A. Hyland. 1999. The campaign to enact New York City's Smoke-Free Air Act. *Journal of Public Health Management Practice* 5:1–13.

Coalition on Smoking OR Health (CSOH). 1995. *State Legislative Actions on Tobacco Issues.* Edited by Jessica Bartelt. Washington, DC: CSOH.

Corella, H. R. 1999. Eateries—Even smokeless ones—Oppose ban. *Arizona Daily Star,* 13 April.

Davis, R. M., G. Boyd, and C. A. Schoenborn. 1990. "Common courtesy" and the elimination of passive smoking: Results of the 1987 Health Interview Survey. *JAMA* 263:2208–2210.

Eisner, M. D., A. K. Smith, and P. D. Blanc. 1998. Bartenders' respiratory health after establishment of smoke-free bars and taverns. *JAMA* 280:1909–14.

Ellick, A. B. 1999. Anti-Smoking Law has many choked with anger. *Indianapolis Star-News,* 6 July.

Environmental Protection Agency (EPA). 1992. *Statement—Respiratory Health Effects of Passive Smoking: Lung Cancer and Other Disorders.* EPA/600/6–90/006F. Washington, DC: EPA.

———. 1993. *Fact Sheet—Respiratory Health Effects of Passive Smoking.* EPA-43-F-93–003. Washington, DC: EPA.

———. 1994. Setting the Record Straight: Secondhand smoke is a Preventable Health Risk. (EPA-402-F-94-005. Washington, DC: EPA.

Feinberg, J. 1989. *Harm to Self.* Oxford: Oxford University Press.

Fishman, J. A., H. Allison, S. B. Knowles, B. A. Fishburn, T. A. Woollery, W. T. Marx, D. M. Shelton, C. G. Husten, and M. P. Erikson. 1999. State laws on tobacco control—United States, 1998. *Morbidity and Mortality Weekly Report Surveillance Summaries* 48(SS03):21–62.

Gerlach, K. K., D. R. Shopland, A. M. Hartman, J. T. Gibson, and T. F. Pechacek. 1997. Workplace smoking policies in the United States: Results from a national survey of more than 100,000 workers. *Tobacco Control* 6:199–206.

Gilpin, E. A., M. A. White, A. J. Farkas, and J. P. Pierce. 1999. Home smoking restrictions: Which smokers have them and how they are associated with smoking behavior. *Nicotine & Tobacco Research* 1:153–62.

Glantz, S. A. 1999. Smoke-free restaurant ordinances do not affect restaurant business. Period. *Journal of Public Health Management Practice* 5:vi–ix.

Glantz, S. A., and A. Charlesworth. 1999. Tourism and hotel revenues before and after passage of smoke-free restaurant ordinances. *JAMA* 281 (20):1911–18.

Glasgow, R. E., K. M. Cummings, and A. Hyland. 1997. Relationship of worksite smoking policy to changes in employee tobacco use: Findings from COMMIT. *Tobacco Control* 6 (suppl. 2):S44–8.

Gori, G. B., and J. C. Luik. 1999. *Passive smoke: The EPA's betrayal of science and policy.* Vancouver: The Fraser Institute.

Gorski, M. 1999. Chasing our customers away. Letter to the *Washington Post,* 20 July.

Hyland, A., and K. M. Cummings. 1999a. Consumer response to the New York City Smoke-Free Air Act. *Journal of Public Health Management Practice* 5:28–36.

———. 1999b. Restaurant employment before and after the New York City Smoke-Free Air Act. *Journal of Public Health Management Practice* 5:22–7.

———. 1999c. Restaurateur reports of the economic impact of the New York City Smoke-Free Air Act. *Journal of Public Health Management Practice* 5:37–42.

Hyland, A., K. M. Cummings, and E. Nauenberg. 1999. Analysis of taxable sales receipts: Was New York City's Smoke-Free Air Act bad for restaurant business? *Journal of Public Health Management Practice* 5:14–21.

Hyland, A., K. M. Cummings, and M. P. Wilson. 1999. Compliance with the New York City Smoke-Free Air Act. *Journal of Public Health Management Practice* 5:43–52.

Jacobson, P. D., and J. Wasserman. 1999. The implementation and enforcement of tobacco control laws: Policy implications for activists and the industry. *Journal of Health Politics, Policy, and Law* 24:567–98.

Jacobson, P. D., J. Wasserman, and J. R. Anderson. 1997. Historical overview of tobacco legislation and regulation. *Journal of Social Issues* 53(1):75–95.

Jacobson, P. D., J. Wasserman, and K. Raube. 1993. The politics of anti-smoking legislation: Lessons from six states. *Journal of Health Politics, Policy, and Law* 18: 787–819.

Kagan, R. A., and J. H. Skolnick. 1993. Banning smoking: Compliance without enforcement. In *Smoking Policy: Law, Politics, and Culture.* Edited by R. L. Rabin and S. D. Sugarman, 22–48. New York: Oxford University Press.

Klonoff, E. A., H. Landrine, R. Alcaraz, R. R. Campbell, D. L. Lang, K. L. McSwan, B. Parekh, and G. Norton-Perry. 1998. An instrument for assessing the quality of tobacco-control policies: The ACT-L scale. *Preventive Medicine* 27:808–14. Article No. PM 980363.

Levy, R. A., and R. B. Marimont. 1998. Lies, damed lies, & 400,000 smoking-related deaths.*Regulation* 21:24–9.

Longo, D. R., R. C. Brownson, J. C. Johnson, J. E. Hewett, R. L. Kruse, T. E. Novotny, and R. A. Logan. 1996. Hospital smoking bans and employee smoking behavior: Results of a national survey. *JAMA* 275:1252–7.

Longo, D. R., R. C. Brownson, and R. L. Kruse. 1995. Smoking bans in US hospitals: Results of a national survey. *JAMA* 274:488–91.

Mannino, D. M., M. Siegel, D. Rose, J. Nkuchia, and R. Etzel. 1997. Environmental tobacco smoke exposure in the home and worksite and health effects in adults: Results from the 1991 National Health Interview Survey. *Tobacco Control* 6:296–305.

Martin, D. 1999. Smoking ban has not hurt restaurants, analysts say. *New York Times,* January 12.

Milkovits, A. 1998. Diners told to butt out. *Foster's Daily Democrat* (Dover, NH), 19 July.

Moskowitz, J. M., Z. Lin, and E. S. Hudes. 2000. The impact of workplace smoking ordinances in California on smoking cessation. *American Journal of Public Health* 90:757–61.

National Restaurant Association. 1994. *Press Release: Economic Impact of OSHA-Imposed Smoking Ban Would Be Staggering, Restaurant Industry Testifies.* 24 October.

Nordstrom, D. L., and F. DeStefano. 1995. Evaluation of Wisconsin legislation on smoking in restaurants. *Tobacco Control* 4:125–8.

Patten, C. A., J. P. Pierce, S. W. Calfin, C. C. Berry, and R. M. Kaplan. 1995. Progress in protecting non-smokers from environmental tobacco smoke in California workplaces. *Tobacco Control* 4:139–144.

Pierce, J. P., T. G. Shanks, M. Pertschuk, E. Gilpin, D. Shopland, M. Johnson, and D. Bal. 1994. Do smoking ordinances protect non-smokers from environmental tobacco smoke at work? *Tobacco Control* 3:15–20.

Rigotti, N. A., D. Bourne, A. Rosen, J. A. Locke, and T. Schelling. 1992. Workplace compliance with a no-smoking law: A randomized community intervention trial. *American Journal of Public Health* 82:229–35.

Rigotti, N. A., and C. L. Pashos. 1991. No-smoking laws in the United States: An analysis of state and city actions to limit smoking in public places and workplaces. *JAMA* 266:3162–7.

Rigotti, N. A., M. A. Stoto, M. F. Brier, A. Rosen, and T. Schelling. 1993. Retail stores compliance with a city no-smoking law. *American Journal of Public Health* 83:227–56.

Rigotti, N. A., M. A. Stoto, M. Kleiman, and T. Schelling. 1988. *Implementation and Impact of a City's Regulation of Smoking in Public Places and the Workplace: The Experience of Cambridge, Massachusetts.* Cambridge, MA: Institute for the Study of Smoking Behavior and Policy, JFK School of Government, Harvard University. Publication No. S-88–17.

Rigotti, N. A., M. A. Stoto, and T. Schelling. 1994. Do businesses comply with a no-smoking law? Assessing the self-enforcement approach. *Preventive Medicine* 23: 223–9.

Roemer, R. 1986. Legislation to control smoking: Leverage for effective policy. *Cancer Detection & Prevention* 9:99–112.

Saad, L. 2000. Smoking in restaurants frowned on by many Americans. Gollup News Services. Princeton N.J.

Samuels, B. E., and S. A. Glantz. 1991. The politics of local tobacco control. *JAMA* 266:2110–7.

Scanlon, T. 1999. *What We Owe Each Other.* Cambridge, MA: Harvard University Press.

Siegel, M. 1993. Involuntary smoking in the restaurant workplace: A review of employee exposure and health effects. *JAMA* 270:490–3.

Siegel, M., J. Carol, J. Jordan, R. Hobart, S. Schoenmarklin, F. DuMelle, and P. Fisher. 1997. Preemption in tobacco control: Review of an emerging public health problem. *JAMA* 278:858–63.

Sorensen, G., B. Beder, C. R. Prible, and J. Pinney. 1995. Reducing smoking at the workplace: Implementing a smoking ban and hypnotherapy. *Journal of Occupational & Environmental Medicine* 37:453–60.

Sorensen, G., R. E. Glasgow, M. Topor, and K. Corbett. 1997. Worksite characteristics and changes in worksite tobacco-control initiatives: Results from the COMMIT study. *Journal of Occupational & Environmental Medicine* 39:520–6.

Sorensen, G., H. Lando, and T. F. Pechacek. 1993. Promoting smoking cessation at the workplace: Results of a randomized controlled intervention study. *Journal of Medicine* 35:121–6.

Sorensen, G., N. Rigotti, A. Rosen, J. Pinney, and R. Prible. 1991. Effects of a worksite nonsmoking policy: Evidence for increased cessation. *American Journal of Public Health* 81:202–4.

Stewardson, J. 1999. Restaurateurs rebel against smoking bans. *Standard Times* (New Bedford, Conn.), 2 July.

Sullum, J. 1998. *For Your Own Good: The Anti-Smoking Crusade and the Tyranny of Public Health.* New York: Free Press.

Tansey, B. 1999. In pursuit of smoke-free living space—Apartment dwellers fear health risks from neighbors' cigarettes. *San Francisco Chronicle*, 28 June.

Tollison, R. D., and R. E. Wagner. 1991. Self-interest, public interest, and public health. *Public Choice* 69:323–43.

U.S. Department of Health and Human Services (USDHHS). 1986. *The Health Consequences of Involuntary Smoking. A Report of the Surgeon General.* Rockville, MD: U.S. Department of Health and Human Services, No. 87–8309.

Warner, K. E., G. A. Fulton, P. Nicolas, and D. R. Grimes. 1996. Employment implications of declining tobacco product sales for the regional economies of the United States. *JAMA* 275:1241–6.

Woodruff, T. J., B. Rosbrook, J. Pierce, and S. A. Glantz. 1993. Lower levels of cigarette consumption found in smoke-free workplaces in California. *Archives of Internal Medicine* 153:1485–93.

9

International Aspects of Tobacco Control and the Proposed WHO Treaty

Stephen D. Sugarman

In the past, national and local governments have been the primary sources of official policies aimed at tobacco control. Global and regional organizations have mainly served in advisory capacities. But changing perceptions of the "tobacco problem" have resulted in calls for the formal regulation of tobacco on a worldwide basis. Most significantly, the World Health Organization (WHO) has launched a major effort intended to culminate in the adoption of an international tobacco control treaty.

Section 1 of this chapter describes three global tobacco problems that together have prompted the proposed treaty: (1) the growing worldwide epidemic of tobacco-related diseases, (2) the growing economic and political power of the international tobacco companies, and (3) the growing "cross-border" tobacco peril, as exemplified by cigarette smuggling.

Section 2 examines the proposed treaty as a policy response to these problems. First, I consider the prospects for global tobacco control absent a treaty. Then I review the specifics of the proposed treaty and present optimistic scenarios that explore the ways in which the treaty could lead to the imposition of worldwide tobacco controls that nations acting without a treaty could not, or would not, otherwise achieve. That optimistic picture is followed by some cautionary scenarios that explore how the proposed treaty might fail. The chapter closes with a discussion of how much impact the proposed treaty, if widely adopted, might have on the global tobacco epidemic.

1. Three Global Tobacco Problems

Tobacco-Related Disease: An Enormous and Growing
Worldwide Public Health Problem

Tobacco is currently a huge public health problem nearly everywhere in the world (WHO 1997; Abedian, van der Merwe, Wilkins, and Jha 1998; World Bank 1999; ASH 2000; Campaign for Tobacco-Free Kids 2000; UICC 2000). Epidemiologists estimate that as many as 4 million people a year now die from smoking-related diseases. Moreover, because of the typically long latency period between the initiation of smoking and death from tobacco-related diseases, future estimates are possible based on the expected trajectory of today's smokers. On that basis, that the annual global death count is now projected to reach more than 8 million by the year 2020, and perhaps 10 million by 2030. Furthermore, because of changing patterns of tobacco use, the incidence of mortality is shifting from richer, industrialized nations to poorer countries. For example, whereas about two-thirds of the tobacco-related deaths during the 1990s occurred in so-called developed nations, by 2030 an estimated two-thirds of the deaths from tobacco-related disease will occur in developing countries.

The following numbers describe the coming shift from a slightly different perspective. In the United States during the 1990s, the more than 400,000 annual tobacco-related deaths accounted for about 20% of all U.S. deaths in that period. In 1995, in developed nations as a whole, tobacco use accounted for about 17% of deaths. By contrast, the 3 million annual deaths worldwide from smoking-related diseases in the early 1990s amounted to "only" around 6% of all deaths. By the year 2020, however, the expected 8.4 million tobacco-related deaths worldwide would amount to roughly 12% of all projected deaths in that year, and 10 million tobacco-related deaths in 2030 would account for approximately 1 of every 6 deaths around the world that year.

This huge predicted growth in the future death toll is only partially attributable to the recent large increase in world population. During the past 30 years, smoking prevalence in the developing nations taken as a whole has sharply increased. Between 1970 and 1990, for example, cigarette consumption per person over the age of 15 in developing countries grew from 860 a year to 1,410 a year. By contrast, smoking in the more developed countries has actually declined somewhat, especially during the 1980s, with consumption of cigarettes per person over the age of 15 having dropped from 2,980 in 1980 to 2,590 in 1990.

China and India, the world's two most populous nations, together will account for a large share of the projected increase in tobacco deaths in the coming two or three decades. From around 1970 to 1990, the estimated number of cigarettes smoked per adult in China increased by more than 250%, and tobacco consumption is up in India as well. By 2020 or 2030, China and India together are expected to account for somewhere between 30% and 45% of all deaths worldwide from tobacco use.[1]

Of course, in principle some revolutionary medical or technological break-through could foil this bleak picture. But one should not be optimistic. Cures for lung cancer, heart disease, or emphysema, and so on are unlikely to emerge in the near term. Besides—short of some miracle vaccine—such a cure might well be too expensive or technologically sophisticated for the health care systems of poorer nations. For example, recent reports suggest that regular CAT scans could allow for the detection of lung cancer from smoking at its earliest stages, thereby potentially leading to medical treatment that might significantly extend a patient's life. But a full-scale, nationwide lung cancer "screening and treatment" strategy is probably implausibly ex-pensive for most countries and surely out of the question for the poorer ones.

A technological fix would mean the creation of safe substitutes for today's tobacco products. These prospects are addressed in the chapter by Kenneth Warner. It is worth noting here that alternative nicotine delivery systems (ANDS) would probably raise similar financial constraints for smokers in poor countries, at least in the medium term. The prospects for the creation and public acceptance of inexpensive safer cigarettes or pseudo-cigarettes remain highly uncertain.

Of course, the projected future worldwide tobacco death toll could be significantly reduced by dramatic increases in cessation rates, as well as by dramatic decreases in start-up rates. But because of past experience with smoking patterns in richer countries, it is difficult to be optimistic for the medium term, given today's political, economic, and social climate. In the first place, in lower income nations today, few current smokers quit each year, or even say that they would like to do so. Moreover, many poorer countries are now at a much earlier stage in the national smoking and tobacco-related death cycle, which the richer Western nations have generally passed through, so that in 20 years, other things equal, they are likely to have proportionately more (rather than fewer) smokers than they have today.

Gender differences are especially noteworthy. As indicated earlier, the av-erage number of cigarettes consumed per person in the developing countries, although rapidly increasing, is still well below the average for the developed countries. One important reason is that women's smoking rate in many coun-tries remains low. For example, in Malaysia, Iraq, and Egypt, around 40% of men, but less than 5% of women, smoke; in the Philippines, Latvia, and Nigeria, men smoke at more than four times the rate of women. In some wealthier Asian nations, the gender imbalance is even more pronounced; in

Taiwan today, for example, an estimated 47% of adult men, but only 5% of adult women, are smokers, and in Korea the comparable numbers are estimated to be 68% and 7%.

Worldwide, during the 1990s, it was estimated that, whereas 47% of men smoked, only 12% of women smoked. In earlier times, this pattern held for the United States and Western Europe as well. But for many years now, women in these countries have been smoking at nearly the same rate as, and occasionally (e.g., in Sweden) at an even higher rate than, men. Hence, if these historical trends continue, large increases in women's smoking rates in other countries are to be expected—particularly as the countries get wealthier and as women's roles change.

Japan is an interesting case (Sasamoto n.d.; Watanabe 1997; Osaki, Kawaminami, and Minowa forthcoming). During World War II and in the years immediately following, the overall smoking rate was rather low—at first because cigarettes were largely unobtainable and later because most Japanese were so poor. But as Japan recovered economically, the percentage of adult men who said they smoked skyrocketed, quickly exceeding prewar levels and reaching an astounding nearly 85% in the mid-1960s. Since then, the men's smoking rate has been slowly, but steadily, declining, although most of the reduction occurred by 1986. Nevertheless, as of the late 1990s, the daily men's smoking rate was still very high, over 55%.

Meanwhile the women's smoking rate in Japan between 1965 and 1995 remained essentially constant at around 15%. But this plateau may be just a temporary phenomenon. Women's roles in Japan are changing quickly. Japanese women now marry later and remain in the work force longer (rather than becoming stay-at-home mothers shortly after finishing their schooling, which was the strong pattern in the past). Hence, it is perhaps not surprising that recent studies have found that 40% of single Japanese female shop workers in their twenties were smokers.

Put differently, there is an enormous potential market in female smokers in a large portion of the world. Consider, for example, that in the early 1990s, women over age 15 smoked at a 30% rate or more in Denmark, Norway, the Czech Republic, Israel, and Russia—all countries known for greater gender equality. Although traditional Asian cultural patterns and Islamic religious beliefs might prevent or long delay women's substantial uptake of smoking in some nations, surely the tobacco companies have their eyes on those potential customers.

The upshot is that realistic advocates who seek a large reduction in the worldwide rate of death and illness from tobacco products need to take a long-term perspective on their work. For example, a recent World Bank study suggests that even if worldwide adult smoking were cut back sharply so that consumption in 2020 was half of what it is today, the cumulative number of smoking-related deaths since 1950 would be cut by less than 15% as of 2025. By 2050, however, the cumulative number of smoking-related deaths since 1950 could be cut by nearly 40% if adult consumption were to be halved by 2020 (World Bank 1999).

Some naysayers claim that tobacco-related diseases are largely a problem of old age and emphasize that the average lifetime smoker in the United States is statistically at risk of losing "only" around 6 years of life because of smoking (Levy and Marimont 1998). Hence, they say, poorer countries especially should instead worry much more about other health problems, such as communicable diseases. But this inappropriately minimizes the harm from tobacco products (Lukachko and Whelan 1999; Peto et al. 1992, 1996). Additional statistics provide a fuller picture. For example, U.S. data show that smokers who actually die from smoking-related diseases lose 12–13 years of life on average. Moreover, around 40% of those who die from smoking do so before the age at which the typical American retires from work, and those smokers lose more than 20 years of life on average.

It is not surprising then that Gro Harlem Brundtland, Norway's former prime minister and the head of WHO, has deemed tobacco and malaria as the two most serious global health problems.

Increasing Global Sales Dominance by the Giant Transnational Tobacco Companies

For much of the twentieth century, many countries throughout the world maintained a local monopoly, or near monopoly, on tobacco sales inside their national market. Often this was achieved through nationally owned and operated tobacco product manufacturing companies and sometimes through exclusively licensed national monopolies. Imported retail tobacco products were either banned or subjected to ruinous tariffs.

This strategy was adopted far more from a revenue-producing perspective than from a health perspective. Maintaining exclusive and close oversight over the tobacco product market seemed, especially in earlier years, to best assure successful excise (and related) tax collection (to say nothing of allowing the government to gain revenues from the profits generated by the sale of tobacco products). And, in strongly socialized economies, state-owned tobacco industries were the norm just as state ownership prevailed in other key sectors of the economy.

Until quite recently, local monopoly was the strong pattern throughout Asia and Eastern Europe. This remains largely the case in China, for example, where the state tobacco company still controls more than 95% of the national market and, as a result, accounts for an estimated 30% of all cigarette sales worldwide—making it the world's largest tobacco enterprise.

But now, outside of China, the international tobacco companies have achieved considerable penetration into both of these geographic areas (Holzman 1997; Bloom 1998; Hammond 1998; Weissman and Hammond 1998). In East Asia, market entry has been accomplished by aggressive assertion of free trade rights—and with the strong assistance of the U.S. trade representative during the Reagan administration. In Eastern Europe, market entry has been achieved in the aftermath of the disintegration of the communist economic system through outsiders' widespread purchase of formerly state-owned tobacco companies or their facilities.

A further, quite recent development has been a restructuring among the transnational tobacco giants themselves. Now there are but three big worldwide players. Philip Morris is the U.S.-based giant and the largest of the international firms with about 16% of the worldwide market. British-American Tobacco (BAT), operating in the United States through its subsidiary Brown & Williamson, recently took over most of Rothman's, formerly the fourth largest international firm, making BAT now nearly as large as Philip Morris. Japan Tobacco, which recently purchased nearly all of R. J. Reynolds's operations outside of the United States, now controls nearly 10% of the world market. At least one and often all three of these firms operate in most countries with any significant tobacco demand, and together they account for more than half of the cigarettes sold worldwide outside of China.

This does not mean that the giant international firms dominate sales in all countries. Local manufacturers still have a large share of the French and Spanish markets, for example, but although these firms are substantial enterprises and themselves have some sales abroad, they are not among the international giants. Nevertheless, the increasing importance in the worldwide tobacco market of a few giant companies (all broadly transnational, apart from the Chinese monopoly) is itself seen by many as a reason to view smoking and its control no longer merely as a series of separate national problems, but rather a global one.

Put simply, the concern is that the tobacco giants have the potential to exercise both strong economic and political power in country after country (Yach and Bettcher 2000). On the political side, this claim is not always convincing. In Japan, Taiwan, and Korea, for example, where outside transnational companies have become fairly strong competitors with the former national monopoly, it is difficult to see how those international giants will have *more* clout with the government than the local monopolists have had in the past (Levin 1997). The picture is perhaps a bit different in places like Australia, New Zealand, Canada, and South Africa, where the BAT-Rothman's merger will give the new BAT enterprise more than half, and sometimes more than 90%, of the market in each of those countries. In these cases, the new giant may have more reason to invest in political influence and so could have more political might than the sum of several competitors had before.

It is perhaps more convincing to put the concern about the tobacco giants' political power this way: when a government's tight connection with its local monopoly is severed, an opening for the introduction of strong new public health–oriented tobacco control policies might emerge. Yet this opportunity might well be blocked by the political muscle of the international firms. In Eastern Europe, for example, after the fall of communism, new governments generally welcomed the international tobacco companies, and some implicitly (perhaps explicitly) promised them a regulation-friendly place to do business.

The economic concern is that tobacco product sales will significantly increase in countries that experience market penetration by the international firms (Taylor, Chaloupka, Guindon, and Corbett 2000; but see Tren and High 2000). There are several ways in which this might come about. First, these firms may simply offer "better" products because their cigarettes are more flavorful, or more consistent from pack to pack, or less bitter or burning in their taste (perhaps because different sorts of tobacco leaves are used, or nicotine levels are better controlled), and so on. It is also possible that cigarettes made by the international giants are more addictive. In addition, international (especially American) brands might be more attractive to some consumers simply because of the status associated with consuming a foreign import. Whatever the reason, if the imported product is more "desirable" to consumers than the old home-made brands, national consumption could increase.

Second, in most countries local monopolies in the past traditionally engaged in little advertising and promotion. By contrast, glamorous widespread marketing campaigns are the hallmark of the international tobacco companies everywhere. Although this may be necessary for the international firms to steal away some of the market share of their local competitors, many believe that these campaigns also increase demand for tobacco products and hence boost tobacco sales overall. Research from Southeast Asia suggests this is just what happened. Moreover, transnational firms are also thought to have the advantage of learning from their own experience as to what sorts of marketing efforts work in some countries—experience that they can try out in other countries as well. Especially important may be promotional gimmicks that the stodgier local monopolies might have ignored or been unaware of in the past.

Third, the entry of the international brands into new markets may create price competition that did not occur in the previously monopolized market. This is a standard economic axiom for what happens when free trade comes to formerly protected markets. Although the price of imported tobacco products may decline simply because tariffs are eliminated, the international firms themselves have not generally tried to bring in products that underprice the local ones (Council on Scientific Affairs 1990). That sort of competitive behavior may occur with steel or clothing, but rarely for tobacco products. Rather, economic analysis predicts that the local brands themselves will cut their prices to try to ward off their new international competitors, thereby also causing an increase in sales overall. There is evidence that this defensive response, resulting in increased overall sales, is exactly what has happened in nations such as Korea and Taiwan (Chaloupka and Laixuthai 1996).

Yet another worry about international dominance is that these corporate behemoths are increasingly entering countries with no tradition of tobacco control efforts (their tobacco taxes having been motived solely by revenue concerns) and little structural capacity within the government to embrace such measures. Many African and Latin American nations and some Asian nations are in this situation. For example, the health and welfare ministry may have no, or few, professionals responsible for tobacco matters, little data may be collected about tobacco use and tobacco-related disease, the public health community may be small or focused on other diseases, public awareness of the dangers of tobacco products may be low, and so forth. In such settings, the willingness and ability of public officials to battle the international tobacco companies may be minimal, especially if the country has not yet experienced the enormous tobacco-related death count that others have. Yet, for the tobacco companies, these countries are good targets for increased cigarette sales.

Expanding Cross-Border Tobacco Problems

Smuggling   Although the taxation of tobacco products has been government policy around the world for decades, only recently has this policy been embraced as a tobacco control strategy. Before, tobacco was seen as a product for which there was strong demand and from which a public revenue stream could be exacted without too much political opposition. Even in places where tobacco use is popular, it is still often a politically attractive candidate for taxation because of its cultural connection with pleasure or "sin" (along with alcohol products and other "luxuries" or indulgences). Now, as economists have shown how demand for tobacco products is influenced by their price (especially among younger people), many tobacco control advocates see high tobacco taxation as the single most important regulatory device for countries to adopt.

But tobacco tax policy (whether motivated for revenue-production or demand-reduction reasons) is undermined if the tax is evaded and tobacco products are available to smokers at a lower price. In fact, this now happens to a moderate, and apparently growing, extent as a result of a variety of activities, the most important of which is "smuggling" (Joossens and Raw 1995; Galbraith and Kaiserman 1997; WHO 1997; Joossens 1998; World Bank 1999).

About 17% of the world's cigarettes are exported from the country of manufacture. Some have estimated that as many as 30% of those exported cigarettes (around 300 billion a year) are smuggled into other countries (or back into the country of origin)—that is, approximately 5% of all cigarettes. Of course, the incidence of smuggled cigarettes varies considerably from nation to nation. During the height of Canada's smuggling problem in 1993, one study estimated that untaxed cigarettes accounted for 30% of the market. In Sweden recently the problem seemed to many to be getting out of control, as criminal smuggling more than doubled its market share between 1996 and 1998, from 2% to 5%. The smuggling rate has been estimated at 4% in Russia and a bit lower in China, but perhaps 40% in Hong Kong, where many of the seemingly smuggled foreign brands are actually counterfeit. Italy has long had substantial smuggling problems, and recently, smuggling has become a substantial concern in Great Britain, where it is now estimated that smuggling suddenly accounts for 20% of cigarette sales.

The tobacco industry is quick to point out the smuggling problem in its opposition to higher tobacco taxes (British American Tobacco 2000a), and their allies, the "legitimate" retailers of their products, are plainly concerned about the problem. The picture typically portrayed by the industry goes something like this example. If tobacco taxes are low in Germany but high in Denmark, then, it is argued, cigarettes will be "smuggled" from Germany into Denmark.

At the simplest level, individual Danish smokers will go to Germany, stock up on cigarettes purchased from German retailers, and sneak them back into Denmark (avoiding the Danish tax). In this scenario, such "cross-border shopping" (or "bootlegging") clearly hurts Danish retailers, deprives the Danish government of revenues, and undermines Danish policy to discourage smoking through higher prices. In the United States, this sort of problem occurs between certain states with different tax policies, such as Massachusetts residents shopping in low-taxing New Hampshire.

However, although some of this cross-border trafficking clearly occurs, it appears to be a relatively limited phenomenon, constituting a small share of the international smuggling problem. Indeed, within the European Union (as in the Danish-German example), this sort of individual purchase for import to and consumption in one's home country is now generally no longer illegal.

A potentially bigger problem is that of organized criminal elements buying truckloads of cigarettes in Germany and clandestinely carting them into Denmark for distribution through either corrupt retailers or other black market sellers. But people in this sort of business quickly realize that there would be much more profit to be made if the cigarettes they obtained were not fully taxed in Germany, but instead were acquired elsewhere entirely without tax. Whereas this could be from within a nation that has no domestic tax, these are hard to find. And a much simpler solution is available.

Smugglers buy tobacco products, for example, from bonded warehouses in Belgium and designate them for export to Russia or Cyprus so they are free from Belgian taxes—on the understanding that an appropriate tax will be imposed by the destination country. But then, once the products are on the move, the smugglers divert them from the pretended market to the secretly intended one, say, Spain or Italy. Now the smugglers have their tobacco products in hand and so far entirely free from tax.

At this point, the tobacco industry's typical story about smuggling patterns breaks down. Industry claims notwithstanding, Denmark and other countries with especially high tax rates are not necessarily the best market for smuggled tobacco products. High Danish prices in the legitimate market make it potentially possible for smugglers of untaxed cigarettes to reap handsome profits from Danish consumers (even if the smuggled cigarettes are sold at a price that is discounted from what legitimate retailers demand). But this requires getting the products into Denmark and into the hands of Danish smokers. Yet getting traditionally honest and well-monitored Danish retailers to participate might be difficult, and using small-time street sellers may not work well, especially because reasonably well-paid Danish police and customs officials might be vigilant against this danger and relatively unsusceptible to bribes.

Better then for the smugglers to sell the cigarettes in countries where weak law enforcement or corrupt retailers give the smugglers ready access to a wide distribution network—perhaps Italy or Spain, for example, even if those countries, as compared to Denmark, have lower taxes and somewhat lower retail tobacco prices in ordinary shops. Moreover, countries such as Italy and Spain may be especially vulnerable to this sort of trade because of their long seacoasts, thereby making them fairly easy targets for fast boat deliveries from, say, Cyprus or portions of former Yugoslavia.

In the United States and Canada, the story has been somewhat different. High new taxes adopted in the late 1980s in Canada prompted the pretended export of Canadian cigarettes to, say, the United States or to Russia free of Canadian tax, often through the reservation lands of Native American tribes that straddle the U.S.-Canadian border. But instead of actually going from the reservation into the export market, these cigarettes were brought right back from the reservation into the Canadian market where they could be sold for well under the newly increased Canadian retail price in conventional retail outlets. Notice that U.S. prices and U.S. taxes were irrelevant under

this scheme, because neither U.S. smokers nor U.S. cigarettes were significantly involved. (Apparently Canadians prefer products made in Canada—
perhaps because of differences in Canadian-grown tobacco or the additives
used in the products made in the two countries.) In this case, the smugglers
took advantage of the Canadian police force's inability or unwillingness to
do sufficient battle with the Native Americans; perhaps the authorities were
also taken by surprise by the rapid involvement of organized criminal groups
in this activity. The number of cigarettes sold in Quebec through this scheme
became so large that Quebec retailers grew angry, and some of them, in
rebellion, openly joined in the illegal trade. The political fallout was a significant reduction in the Canadian tax rate (at both the national level and in
Quebec). Internal cross-border problems, then, caused the tax reduction at
the Province level to ripple from Quebec to Ontario as well. Recently, the
Canadians have decided that they now know how to fight smuggling more
effectively and have once more imposed significant new tobacco taxes. This
time the new domestic taxes are accompanied by significant export taxes that
should discourage the illegal re-import of exported Canadian cigarettes.
Whether this will cause an increase in smuggling of foreign brands is uncertain.

The smuggling problem is by no means clearly contrary to the interests
of the international tobacco companies, even though they emphasize its dangers in opposing higher tobacco taxes. After all, so long as smuggled cigarettes
are not stolen from them, they make their regular profits on sales to whole-
salers. Further, to the extent that smuggling keeps the street price down, total
sales increase. And, if customs or other police officials do manage to confis-
cate some smuggled cigarettes without disrupting the smuggling business
completely, that translates into even more sales for the industry as the smugglers' stocks are replenished. Furthermore, smuggling can be a good way for
the international firms to break first into national markets that are otherwise
closed to them, because of official trade barriers, for example. And smuggled
cigarettes sold at discounted prices may serve as something of a "loss leader"
to introduce their product to new buyers. It is primarily to placate their
ordinary retailers that tobacco companies have a financial interest in opposing
smuggling.

Moreover, although tobacco company spokesmen loudly proclaim that it
is clearly against firm policy to have anything to do with the smuggling trade,
it has not gone without comment in the antismoking community that, on
several recent occasions, individuals connected to the tobacco industry have
been accused of knowing participation in smuggling operations (International
Consortium of Investigative Journalists 2001). For example, in February
1999, a former R. J. Reynolds marketing executive was arrested and charged
with assisting smugglers operating through the St. Regis Mohawk Reservation

in upstate New York, who had sold more than $700 million in cigarettes on the Canadian black market. National Brands International, an R. J. Reynolds subsidiary, had already admitted participation in the ring and paid $15 million in fines and forfeitures for its role. Earlier, employees of BAT or its subsidiaries were found guilty of involvement in smuggling operations in both Canada and Hong Kong. Claims have been made in both Colombia and South Africa that Philip Morris has encouraged or knowingly tolerated the smuggling of its cigarettes in from neighboring countries, and several Colombian state governments have recently brought civil racketeering charges against Philip Morris in American courts. Perhaps most significantly, the EU, together with nine member nations, have brought legal actions against Phillip Morris, R. J. Reynolds, and Japan Tobacco that accuse the international giants of scheming to smuggle cigarettes on a worldwide basis, a charge the defendants have denied.

Apart from smuggling concerns, cross-border transportation of "duty-free" cigarettes should be briefly mentioned. A modest share of untaxed, imported cigarettes is legally carried home from abroad by returning citizens, or into foreign nations by travelers as gifts or for personal consumption. These cigarettes are obtained duty free at special shops that have been set up for the purpose of arranging the sale of certain typically "luxury" items, including tobacco products, without certain taxes or customs duties and therefore at a lower price than that in the market where they are consumed.

Although a complete and effective end to duty-free shopping for tobacco products would have a relatively minor public health impact, it is understandably galling to tobacco control advocates that governments, in effect, deliberately encourage more tobacco consumption by including tobacco products in the duty-free industry and eagerly rent retail outlet space to duty-free shops located in public airports and other public facilities. Ending duty-free tobacco shopping would at least have a positive symbolic benefit for public health. (Interestingly enough, within the European Union, duty-free shopping in general is now being eliminated as tariffs at national borders are ending and national pricing and internal excises on tobacco and other products are being brought into line. In the future, it will pay for the English, for example, to bring back cigarettes from France only if the French hypermarkets are able to charge lower regular retail prices than those of their British counterparts.)

Leakage Around Advertising Controls   Several nations have tried to sharply restrict tobacco product advertising within their borders, but sometimes advertising leaks in from outside.

Perhaps most important today is leakage through television. These days, in more and more countries, local citizens are able to watch foreign television broadcasts, often through satellite dishes and the like. So tobacco companies effectively promote their products on television even in countries where such ads are supposedly banned.

A second strategy is to engage in sponsorship of activities, especially sporting activities, outside of a country, knowing that the sporting event and its association with tobacco products will be seen inside the target country when the event is broadcast there. For example, a tobacco company can sponsor racing car events in exotic locales, attaching its name to the event itself or to at least one of the entered vehicles (with appropriate brand logos affixed), and it can post billboards or other signs promoting its products at the raceway in locations visible to the television cameras as they cover the event. As proof of the extent that deliberate cross-border advertising of this sort occurs, antitobacco advocates have pointed to marketing campaigns attached to sports events that have little or nothing to do with the locale where the race takes place—for example, auto races in the Middle East carrying advertising of tobacco brands not sold there but rather sold, say, in Japan.

This sort of sponsorship might well be illegal in target nation(s), but if the event can be broadcast there, those controls are evaded. Nations might try to prevent local television broadcasters from carrying such programs. But local regulation might well not go that far, and the prospect of offshore and satellite broadcasting in several markets threatens to undermine any attempt at such domestic regulation.

Although television is probably the main source of ad leakage, print and Internet media are also relevant, and the latter may become increasingly important. To the extent that smokers and future smokers surf the Internet in search for fun or for specific information about tobacco products, placing ads on "offshore" websites makes it possible for tobacco advertisers to penetrate nations that otherwise seek to ban such advertising. Magazines (and other print media) also present a threat, as local citizens read tobacco ads that appear in foreign magazines. Unlike the Internet problem, magazines containing such ads might simply be banned. Still, having the political will to adopt such controls and organizing sufficiently large enforcement agencies to deal with violations are likely to involve considerable costs, especially because, as a practical matter, such magazine bans likely deprive local citizens of access to other information as well.

Free Trade Pressures   Some nations have viewed imported tobacco products in the way U.S. government policy views imported illegal drugs such as cocaine and heroin. These are evil substances ruining "our" people, and an all-out war to block their entry (and to curtail their production at the source) should be waged. Other nations don't have such moral or health-related reasons for strongly opposing the import of tobacco products. Instead, their interest is purely economic: they simply want to have all the profits from domestic tobacco sales go to the local monopoly.

During the 1980s in particular, the United States took a position on tobacco products that dramatically opposed its position on other drugs. The "war on drugs" that sought to keep other nations' products out of the United States was matched by an equally strong war to force other countries to open up their markets to our tobacco products (Hammond 1998).

This was especially important to the U.S. companies, for the United States is not only one of the world's largest producers and exporters of tobacco leaf but also the largest exporter of finished tobacco products. But for years U.S. tobacco companies' products were being officially denied entry by many countries with strong domestic tobacco markets. The U.S. trade representative under President Ronald Reagan engaged in a vigorous campaign to break down these trade barriers.

Some other countries claimed that they were restricting trade for health reasons. This is the basis on which the United States keeps some foreign-made pharmaceutical drugs out of the U.S. market: they have yet to be proven safe and effective to the satisfaction of the FDA. But parallel foreign nation claims about cigarettes were scoffed at as disguised protectionism, which in many cases was true.

Breaking down simple import barriers was not enough for many of the transnational tobacco companies, however. They wanted also to be able to advertise in their accustomed manner. When other governments claimed that their ad controls were motivated by health concerns or desires to prevent youths from smoking, U.S. authorities viewed these claims too as hidden and illegal trade barriers. Eventually, Japan, Korea, and Taiwan capitulated, with the result in Japan, for example, that high visibility tobacco advertising increased dramatically—both by the imported brands and, in response, by Japan Tobacco, which controls the Japanese brands. (After a dozen years or so, imported brands captured nearly a quarter of the Japanese market.)

Thailand, however, resisted the U.S. pressure with respect to ads, and the dispute eventually went to the World Trade Organization (WTO). The WTO decision called for a level playing field, requiring Thailand to provide access to imported goods but discounting the objections of the importers, who claimed that uniform treatment (ad bans on all tobacco companies) gave de facto advantage to the entrenched local brands. Moreover, during the Clinton administration, the United States backed off its position of especially supporting American tobacco exports.

Nevertheless, the broader point is that many countries around the world are increasingly committed to free trade—either by a genuine conviction on the part of the nation's policy leaders or as a result of pressures brought upon the nation by the WTO, the International Monetary Fund, the United States or other G-8 countries. But worldwide free trade principles and general international free trade organizations are seen by many in the tobacco control movement as obstacles that may prevent individual nations from adopting and enforcing the health-motivated tobacco control policies they desire (or might later desire). These concerns recently emerged in the debate that took place when the U.S. Congress granted "most favored nation" trading status to China. Although most opponents of the measure were concerned about international human rights in China and jobs of American workers, the main worry of public health officials was that increased trade with China would result in even more Chinese smokers.

2. International Tobacco Control through an International Treaty?

The World Health Assembly (WHA) is the governing body of the World Health Organization, to which nearly 200 nations belong. At its May 1996 meeting, the WHA requested that the director general of WHO initiate the development of a tobacco control treaty. And at its May 1999 meeting the WHA gave its unanimous "go ahead" to the project (WHA 1998). This is the first time that WHO is using its constitutional authority to try to facilitate the creation of such an international agreement (Yach 1995: Taylor 1996; Fidler 1998).

Global Tobacco Control Absent a Tobacco Treaty

Although many tobacco control advocates worldwide have strongly endorsed the proposed WHO treaty, before discussing the planned treaty, it is worth giving some attention to ways in which progress on international tobacco issues can be, and has been, made without a treaty. This inquiry may also help to identify more clearly the additional role(s) that the treaty could play (Ad Hoc Inter-Agency Task Force on Tobacco Control 2000).

WHO Dissemination of Information and Policy Recommendations   The WHO director general has increased the importance of tobacco control within WHO, has pushed hard to get the tobacco control treaty-making process under way, and has increased substantially WHO staff capacity in the tobacco control arena. But WHO's campaign against tobacco-related disease is hardly brand new.

Over the past decade, WHO published several books and papers that document the extent of the tobacco problem around the world, identify various tobacco control strategies that some countries have adopted, and urge a specific tobacco-control agenda (e.g., Roemer 1993; Chollat-Traquet 1996; WHO Fact Sheets 1996, 1998a, 1998b, 1998c; WHO 1998). Also, WHO helps sponsor meetings and conferences where research, policy ideas, and political strategies about tobacco control are discussed. For example, a WHO-sponsored conference devoted to tobacco issues concerning women and children was held in Kobe, Japan, in fall 1999 and drew a large audience.

Moreover, the WHA, WHO's legislative arm, has adopted many tobacco control resolutions over the past several years. And, many nations substantially increased their tobacco control regimes during the 1990s—although not necessarily in response to WHA's urging. Nevertheless, worldwide tobacco controls fall way short of what WHA has endorsed, demonstrating to many people the ineffectiveness of mere resolutions. The WHO treaty, by contrast, envisions that nations of the world acting collectively will be able to persuade each other to do more for tobacco control than they as a group have so far been willing or able to do by acting individually in response to WHA recommendations.

Learning from Others Through Conferences, Journals, and Other International Networks   By no means is WHO the only forum or organization promoting the international exchange of information about tobacco control. For example, an international journal called *Tobacco Control* has been created to carry scholarly research, timely information, and policy advocacy about tobacco control around the world. It is widely read in the international tobacco control community (Tobacco Control 2000).

The Internet has also become a splendid way for tobacco control advocates around the world to communicate with each other. Probably most important, a special closed network for those interested in tobacco control, called Globalink, has been created. It provides a forum for discussions among tobacco control activists and experts; it is a current source of information about worldwide developments related to tobacco; it serves as a mechanism for those in far-flung countries seeking information and advice from colleagues elsewhere to ask for and readily obtain it; and Globalink (http://www.uicc.ch) is an easy vehicle for members to use to connect to the many active Worldwide Web-sites that post information about tobacco control from both national and international perspectives.

International tobacco control conferences seem to be growing in number and provide additional occasions for public officials, advocates, and scholars from many places to share their ideas and findings. A conference held in South Africa in 1998 yielded the book *The Economics of Tobacco Control*, a multi-authored volume with multinational contributors (Abedian et al. 1998). A conference in the Canary Islands in early 1999 drew more than two thousand participants from around the world. More than 30 nations sent representatives to an "International Policy Conference on Children & Tobacco" held in Washington in early 1999 that was sponsored by leading American politicians and national organizations involved in tobacco control. And there were thousands of participants at the international conference on smoking and health held in Chicago in summer 2000.

Through these exchanges, tobacco control advocates everywhere can find out about several important matters, including (1) how to discover, track, and report data about the prevalence of smoking and the health effects of smoking in their country in ways consistent with the best data collection efforts elsewhere; (2) what the tobacco industry is doing elsewhere; (3) what other countries are doing about tobacco control; and (4) what research says about the impact, or likely impact, of various tobacco control strategies. All of this information, in turn, may pave the way for the adoption of new national tobacco control policies.

Participants in the tobacco control movement worldwide have informally ranked countries according to the strength of their regime of tobacco regulation. For example, it is now generally agreed that nations such as Australia, Canada, New Zealand, Finland, Norway, Poland, Singapore, and Thailand have reasonably strong and comprehensive tobacco control programs. This generally means that the country has adopted national regulation that includes all (or most) of the following: (1) broad restrictions on tobacco advertising and promotion; (2) high tobacco taxes; (3) strong warnings on tobacco packaging; (4) strict limits on smoking in public places and workplaces; (5) tight controls on sales to minors; (6) organized antismoking efforts such as antismoking ads, school-based antismoking education, and widespread availability of tobacco cessation and use reduction assistance; and (7) a well-funded tobacco control infrastructure to monitor and enforce the tobacco control regime. By identifying such countries and their tobacco control packages, advocates can provide ready examples for political leaders urging changes inside their own nations.

In sum, access to all of this information puts those seeking domestic changes in tobacco policy in a better position than they were in the past. For example, when local doubters say that X or Y or Z tobacco controls won't work or will be unenforceable or economically detrimental, advocates can often point to experience elsewhere in the world that belies these fears. However, those seeking a treaty have concluded that good arguments by themselves are not enough and that formal international agreements will achieve more.

Efforts of the World Bank and Other International and Regional Organizations
Some people believe that misunderstandings about economic issues prevent

governments from adopting tobacco control policies. For example, governments may fear that higher taxes will yield lower revenues because of reduced demand and increased smuggling (when in fact higher tobacco taxes will almost always yield higher revenues), or that tobacco control will lead to massive job losses (which it usually won't). When these misjudgments are a genuine factor inhibiting national policy reforms, distinguished international bodies may help persuade national leaders that these fears are erroneous (at least for most countries) merely by publishing careful studies. The World Bank has undertaken precisely this sort of effort as part of a recent book it released called *Curbing the Epidemic* (World Bank 1999). Groups like the World Bank can play other roles as well, for example, by refusing to lend money to nations for the purpose of increasing tobacco farming (which has been World Bank policy for several years).

Those behind the framework convention believe, however, not only that groups like the World Bank, the International Monetary Fund, and regional organizations are unable to sufficiently prompt the adoption of adequate worldwide tobacco control measures on their own but also that other international groups, like the WTO, are actually undermining international tobacco control efforts. Indeed, many think that an international tobacco treaty is necessary to turn certain WTO pressures around.

Export Controls   In principle, countries that are home to international tobacco companies could regulate the conduct of those companies in other nations. For example, where warnings are stronger in the home country, a nation could force its companies to include similar warnings on the packages of cigarettes they sell elsewhere. The same policy could be applied to the disclosure of the ingredients contained in tobacco products.

But, so far, most countries have been reluctant to impose health-related requirements designed to benefit other nations' citizens. In some places this is seen as inappropriately intrusive in the internal affairs of other countries—although this concern didn't stop the U.S. trade representative during the Reagan presidency from pushing other countries to abandon their internal advertising controls. More likely, tobacco product exporting nations have been politically more responsive to their own tobacco companies than to the public health concerns of other nations. In the United States, several members of Congress have been trying, with limited success, to rein in American efforts on behalf of U.S. tobacco companies abroad, both by curtailing the pro-tobacco work of the U.S. trade representative and by trying to eliminate tax and other benefits tobacco companies obtain from general legislation designed to promote American exports; as noted earlier, the Clinton administration had not supported tobacco exporting the way its Republican predecessors had.

Nonetheless, even if some governments were persuaded to impose strong export restrictions, tobacco control leaders fear that tobacco companies would respond by shifting their base of operations, or at least by shifting the supply base for international shipments, to offshore affiliated companies likely beyond the regulatory reach of individual export-controlling nations.

Treaty supporters believe that here, too, through international agreement on standards (concerning, say, warnings, testing, and ingredients), tobacco control policy gains can be achieved that individual nations have been unwilling, or unable, to adopt on their own.

Bilateral Arrangements   Countries might agree to cooperate on a bilateral basis to deal with some of the cross-border problems discussed here, such as smuggling or the leakage of television advertising. But, all too often, the country that is the source of the problem may not be eager to cooperate. Belgium, for example, is probably eager to maintain the economic benefits that many think come from its huge tobacco warehouse business, and would be understandably worried that imposing strong regulations on that business could cause a shift of the warehouse trade to a friendlier nation. The same goes for a country that hosts a tobacco industry—sponsored auto racing event broadcast into other nations.

Although advocates of the WHO effort are counting on an international agreement to overcome these problems, the "selfishness" factor now facing those wanting to solve their cross-border problems on a bilateral basis should also serve as a warning about difficulties that may also confront a multinational effort.

Background on the Proposed Treaty

Structure and Process   Currently, WHO's intention is to structure this treaty as a "framework convention with protocols." In today's world of international law, a framework convention is usually envisioned as a largely aspirational document containing few, if any, serious binding commitments, apart from reporting requirements. The protocols to a framework convention are meant to contain more seriously binding obligations. The typical strategy behind this approach is to seek prompt and widespread adoption of the framework convention. The protocols generally come later, and the adoption of each of them would probably be individually pursued (Bodansky 1998; Joossens 1998; Taylor and Bodansky 1998).

For example, the framework convention might ask signatories to agree that tobacco is a significant worldwide problem, to pledge to work toward its solution, and to report regularly both national data about tobacco use and what actions the country has taken and what progress it has made in achiev-

ing the goals of the convention. By contrast, a protocol might require a signatory country to ban all tobacco advertising and promotion or to agree to
take certain steps to help combat international smuggling of tobacco products.

Nations signing the framework convention would probably not be required to adopt all, or even any, of the protocols. But the architects of this
strategy plainly hope that, in due course, there would be nearly as widespread
adoption of the protocols as of the framework convention itself.

There is nothing magic about this allocation of roles to the framework
convention and the protocols, however. Hence, some tobacco control advocates are urging that the framework convention itself contain several strong
binding conditions on its signatories; others are urging that a weaker framework convention and several tough protocols be forwarded together as an
initial package that nations would be urged to adopt (possibly even requiring
that those adopting the framework convention also adopt one or more designated protocols). Although the "framework convention with protocols" approach is not the only treaty strategy that WHO might have pursued, international experience with this approach convinced the WHA in 1996 that this
route is the most promising.

Seeking worldwide adoption of a weak framework convention without
any binding protocols would have been an alternative strategy. But this approach would probably achieve little or nothing more than what WHO's
already published policy recommendations on smoking policy can accomplish. Clearly, WHO strategists believe that a stronger product is both necessary and possible to achieve.

At the other extreme, WHO could have pushed for a fully binding comprehensive treaty as the first document nations would be asked to ratify. But
many fear that this approach would either doom the venture to failure or
yield, in the end, a vapid document.

Perhaps most important, the framework convention with protocols approach should be viewed as a dynamic (rather than one-time) process by
which international consensus is forged over time, binding agreements are
put into place as sufficient support develops, dissenting nations can participate substantially in the treaty even if not fully, and some of the most contentious issues can perhaps be delayed.

In the years since the WHA's 1996 resolution, WHO has begun its work
and now has a timetable in place, with the year 2003 targeted for the final-
ization and adoption of the framework convention (and perhaps several protocols) (Bettcher 1998).

Procedurally, WHO created a working group on the framework convention that was charged with suggesting possible treaty provisions by the start
of the year 2000. The working group formally met not only with represen-

tatives of many nations (WHO 1999a, 1999b, 2000a and b, 2000e) but also with representatives of certain recognized nongovernmental organizations (NGOs) as it developed its suggested provisions (INFACT 1998). The efforts of the working group, discussed further on, were reported to the WHA in May 2000. An intergovernmental negotiating body has been established and charged with drawing on the efforts of the working group and creating the text of both a convention and at least some protocols that the world community is likely to support. This negotiating process among nations is scheduled to be completed in less than three years. As of this writing the negotiating body had met once (in October 2000) and a chair's draft text had been released. Important differences between the working group's text and the chair's draft are noted in the discussion that follows.

Justifications   In fact, WHO has justified the need for an international treaty in ways that invoke each of the three global problems described in section 1. First, it is said that the treaty will "promote international cooperation in areas that transcend national boundaries." Second, the supporters of an international regime note the weakness of domestic regimes, especially in developing countries. A third justification is based upon the "enormity and gravity" of the problem, combined with the "global interdependence of tobacco markets and regulatory activities." Most generally Derek Yach, who heads WHO's efforts on behalf of the convention has said, "Tobacco is a global problem. The tobacco industry acts as a global force—countries need to act together to counter this threat to public health" (Tobacco Free Initiative 1998).

For many tobacco control advocates, the global public health problem caused by tobacco consumption speaks for itself. In light of the spreading epidemical described, it is certainly understandable that WHO professionals would sense the urgency of "doing something" about the problem. So, too, public health leaders in the richer nations understandably want to help find solutions for the poorer countries, not only because this is generally what "do gooders" from richer nations try to do but also because the richer nations are ahead of the poorer ones in experiencing the enormity of the death toll from smoking, and the purveyors of death in poorer nations are, more and more, enterprises based in the richer ones.

And, yet, it does not obviously follow that an international treaty is an appropriate response to this public health epidemic. That is, what might such a treaty be able to accomplish? More precisely, what might collective action by the nations of the world be able to achieve that nations can't (or won't) achieve on their own or bi-laterally? The remainder of this chapter explores that question in some detail.

*Proposed Provisions of the WHO Framework Convention
and Its Protocols*

Competing Visions   Although it is too soon to know whether the WHO treaty
will ever be adopted and, if so, what it will actually say, we now know what
elements WHO's working group has in mind, as influenced by positions
taken both by national representatives and NGO representatives at large multinational meetings held in October, 1999 and March, 2000 in Geneva (WHO
2000b, 2000f). We also see that the chair's draft had already modified and
somewhat weakened the working group's version.

Indeed, it became clear at the two meetings of the working group that key
nations have taken quite different initial positions as to what matters should
be included in the framework convention. As the working group notes emphasize, countries including the United States, Japan, Germany, and China
have argued for including only "principles, general objectives and guidelines,"
whereas other nations, including Canada, Australia, Norway, and Singapore,
"insisted that the body of the convention in itself should already contain
strong provisions and obligations." (WHO 2000d).

The former group of countries based its position on the desirability of
obtaining "a maximum of member states to sign the convention," and perhaps
some of those countries are already signaling their potential (or likely) refusal
to sign a treaty containing many (or certain) binding restrictions. The latter
group, by contrast, expressed fears that a weak framework convention might
be all that the nations of the world would sign and that would mean that the
WHO process would have amounted to rather little. The European Union
was reported to occupy an in-between position, which presumably means
getting as many as possible real obligations into the initial framework convention itself—those for which there is widespread support—and leaving
other obligations to be worked out over time in subsequent protocols.

The working group's work product appears to reflect the Canadian, Aus-
tralian, et al. position, for it includes many strong provisions in the document
it released. However, not a great deal should be made of this, because these
various obligations could readily be placed instead in individual or multitopic
protocols if the negotiating body so desires, and indeed the negotiating body
appears to be moving in that direction.

Before turning to the specifics of the working group's effort, I will discuss
one additional initial skirmish. Within the international community of nongovernmental tobacco control, activist factions are also emerging over the
content of the WHO treaty (Smoking and Health Action Foundation 2000).
One group has emphasized the desirability of focusing on matters that truly
require international cooperation, such as controls on smuggling and international advertising. Three quite different reasons lie behind this position.

The first is that these issues should have the highest priority because they require collective action; therefore, provisions concerning these problems promise to give countries benefits they could not obtain on their own. A second reason is that an agreement focused on these truly international control measures is more likely to be achieved—both because many countries see themselves in need of cooperative help from others in this area and because the specific controls envisioned are probably not too controversial for key nations involved. And third, people in this group fear that if the WHO treaty tries to deal with important domestic tobacco policy issues, it is likely to impose only modest obligations. Not only will modest obligations do little to combat the public health problem but such requirements cast as regulatory "floors" may have a way of becoming de facto "ceilings," thereby possibly even setting back domestic tobacco control efforts. Not surprisingly, many of the advocates in this group come from nations such as Canada, which already have domestic controls that are, in nearly all cases, stronger than what many consider possible for the WHO agreement.

On the other side of this debate are those who, though conceding that matters necessarily requiring international cooperation are important, believe that strong domestic tobacco control policies are far more important. They hope that the WHO treaty will be the mechanism through which world opinion on wise tobacco control measures will be converted into mutually agreed upon worldwide action on the tobacco epidemic.

In short, the competing camps have different conceptions of the "global" tobacco problems, as well as different expectations as to how far international agreement might go. Some see the tobacco problem as most analogous to problems such as ocean resources and global warming for which issues of "externalities" and "commons" have been targeted through international agreements. Others, however, see the tobacco problem as more analogous to problems such as international human rights or children's rights. Although treaties dealing with these latter issues address some important cross-national matters, they are most significantly about how governments are to treat their own people.

The working group dealt with this difference of opinion by trying to minimize it—by defining broadly those matters said to have an important international aspect. Tobacco tax policy is perhaps the best example. As noted earlier, for many tobacco control advocates, the single most important domestic policy a government can have is a high tax on tobacco products because of the ultimate price impact of this tax on tobacco consumption, especially by youths. The working group, however, released a document that talks about coordinated, relatively uniform tax rates from nation to nation in international terms by emphasizing the "bootleg" problem. Whatever its importance, dealing with the bootleg problem through coordinated taxes would surely be only frosting on the cake. Moreover, coordination of tax rates could mean coordination around low rates. Indeed, that by itself would reduce substantially the cross-border problem. But, of course, the working group would be totally opposed to that sort of coordination. In short, coordinated *high* taxes are desirable because they are means of reducing internal demand through market forces. This is a perfectly appropriate explanation if strong domestic obligations are to be part of the treaty. But to justify this provision as a remedy to an important cross-border problem is simply not convincing.

In fact, the largest controversy among tobacco control advocates erupted not over taxes but over clean indoor air. Initially, the working group apparently could not find any way of viewing clean indoor air provisions as a cross-border issue, and so it did not include them in the documents it initially released. After all, tobacco smoke is not like acid rain that significantly travels from one country to another (smoking on international airplane flights aside). But many supporters of clean air policies find them to be a vital national policy. They not only protect third parties from the dangers of passive smoking and help those smokers who want to quit to do so but also they prod some smokers to quit somewhat involuntarily and send a strong signal to the rest of the society, including to youths, that smoking in public is not a "normal" activity. Hence, these advocates are eager to have the obligation for clean indoor air policies in the treaty, and, as emphasized before, they are by no means persuaded by those who envision a narrower truly cross-border focus to the treaty. And in the work products presented by the working group to the WHA, clean indoor air requirements were included.

Working Group Proposed Provisions as of May 2000   I have identified 10 substantive tobacco control policies that the working group presented to the WHA in May 2000—provisions that signatory nations would be required to enact, *if* the working group's provisions were eventually included in the treaty by the negotiating body (WHO 2000c). The working group envisions an approach that would expressly provide that signatory nations may adopt strong tobacco control measures that go beyond these requirements as long as they are not inconsistent with the treaty (the "floor" and "ceiling" issue already discussed). Some of the working group's proposals envision early adoption of supplementary protocols, yet, as already noted, placement of a policy in the framework convention, in a protocol, or both is not important for now, since the negotiating body might, for example, place all of these topics in the protocols:

- Tobacco taxes: countries would agree to impose excise taxes that would be maintained at two-thirds or more of the retail price of all tobacco products and to ban duty free and other tax free sales.

- Tobacco sales to youths: countries would agree to prohibit sales to youths, ban vending machines, and require retailers to obtain evidence of age from buyers.
- Environmental tobacco smoke: countries would agree to protect their citizens from passive smoking, and in the working group's more detailed option, they would agree to prohibit smoking in a long list of specific locations, including workplaces, public transport vehicles, restaurants, and bars.
- Tobacco product content and disclosure: countries would agree to adopt standards governing the testing, design, manufacturing, and processing of tobacco products (although the document is silent about what those standards might be) and to require disclosures concerning the ingredients and additives in tobacco products (perhaps based upon WHO-approved testing methods).
- Tobacco education: countries would agree to develop educational and public awareness programs on the health risks of tobacco use and exposure to tobacco smoke, especially ensuring that children and youths are well informed of these dangers.
- Tobacco packaging and warnings: countries would agree to require cigarettes to be sold only in packages of 20 or more, to prohibit the use of words like "light" or "low tar" on the packages, and to require packages to carry strong warnings (probably both pictures and words) as to the harmful consequences of tobacco consumption. A further protocol on packaging and warning is envisioned.
- Tobacco marketing: countries would agree to prohibit (or, in the weaker optional version, merely "impose appropriate restrictions on") advertising, promotion, and sponsorship aimed at children and youths, to regulate (in an undisclosed manner) other tobacco marketing, and to require tobacco companies to disclose their expenditures on marketing. A further protocol on marketing is envisioned.
- Tobacco dependence treatment: countries would agree to encourage tobacco cessation and to provide treatment programs for those dependent on tobacco (as well as integrating tobacco dependence treatment into reproductive health programs). A further protocol on dependence treatment is envisioned.
- Tobacco liability and compensation: countries would agree to open their legal processes and forums to those seeking compensation from damages caused by tobacco products (although the working group is vague as to whether this calls for some internationally agreed upon basis for liability); the working group also appears to envision a role for international law in this process, although that role is undefined in the working group's document.

- Tobacco smuggling: countries would agree to require products made in their jurisdiction to contain a label identifying the single nation in which they are to be legally sold and to otherwise further cooperate (in undefined ways) with each other in preventing and combating smuggling. A further protocol on smuggling is envisioned.

In my opinion, only the provision on smuggling deals centrally with cross-border issues. The marketing provision (which itself is not strong) does not address the advertising leakage problem.

The working group's presentation to the WHA also contains several provisions aimed generally at international cooperation, information coordination, and the building of tobacco control capacity in all nations. I have grouped them into seven topics:

- Tobacco control funding: countries would agree to allocate a certain (as yet undesignated) proportion of tobacco tax revenue for tobacco control efforts. The working group document also suggests that "countries that export manufactured tobacco products have a special responsibility to provide technical support to developing countries to strengthen their national tobacco control programmes" and that developed countries may also provide financial support to developing countries through various channels.
- Tobacco control surveillance: countries would agree to gather and regularly report on relevant national tobacco statistics including tobacco prevalence, tobacco tax and price structures, knowledge of the health risks of tobacco, mortality and morbidity associated with tobacco use, youth access, and so on.
- Tobacco control information sharing: countries would agree to assure public access to information about the tobacco industry and to exchange with each other relevant scientific, technical, socioeconomic, commercial, and legal information, including information about tobacco industry practices.
- Tobacco control research: countries would agree to sponsor research relevant to reducing tobacco consumption and to coordinate their research efforts with those of other nations.
- Tobacco control training: countries would agree to put in place relevant programs to train a wide range of professionals in the techniques of tobacco control.
- Tobacco control participation: countries would agree to promote the participation of various public bodies and NGOs in their tobacco control efforts.
- Tobacco control technology sharing (scientific, technical, and legal): countries would agree to share with each other both expertise on to-

bacco control and any equipment or technology needed for effective tobacco control that they develop.

These sorts of provisions, though mild-sounding to some, could be key to the treaty's success. If implemented even approximately as envisioned by the working group, they would assure that nearly all countries around the globe have active, well-informed, and reasonably well-funded tobacco control experts both inside and outside government. These experts would be in constant contact with counterparts elsewhere. Successful tobacco control strategies would be quickly identified and transmitted worldwide. Nations that failed to keep pace would be targeted for attention, and tobacco control activists in those nations would be able to call on outsiders for support. This infrastructure could assist many nations in battles with both their internal tobacco companies and the international giants. At least, that is the aspiration of the working group.

The remainder of the working group's document primarily addresses important structural and procedural matters that won't be discussed here—for example, the creation of the conference of the parties that would oversee the implementation of the framework convention and the process of creating and adopting subsequent protocols; the creation of a secretariat and other bodies that serve the conference; rules about reporting, settlement of disputes, adoption of new provisions, entry into force of the convention and later protocols; and so on. Some of these are routine matters applicable to all treaties. However, the working group's approach envisions a strong and active secretariat and conference as central to its view of the proposed framework convention and protocols as an ongoing dynamic process in furtherance of global tobacco control.

Intergovernmental Negotiating Body Chair's Draft Text as of January 2001   The draft text of the framework convention was released in January 2001 by the negotiating body's chair, with the expectation that this version would be the subject of further discussion at the negotiating body's next session in Geneva in May 2001, after this chapter was completed (WHO 2001).

Although the working group's text has been substantially reorganized, the major topics have remained largely the same. However, there are some significant differences between the two texts. For example, on tobacco taxation, whereas the working group called for taxes to be set equal to at least two-thirds the retail price, the chair's text calls for harmonized tax policies "so as to achieve a stable and continuous reduction in tobacco consumption" with no indication as to what the negotiating body believes is necessary by way of tax policy to achieve that result. Moreover, it is not clear that the two themes of the chair's draft on taxes are compatible with each other. Harmonization implies having today's highly divergent level of taxes converge; but to achieve a continuous reduction in consumption would seemingly require even today's higher taxing nations to regularly boost their rates, which seems counter to an international movement toward harmonization. To be sure, lower taxing nations could dramatically increase their rates so as to catch up with the others, but that seems inconsistent with the call for a "stable . . . reduction" in consumption.

As another example, the chair's draft on advertising controls seems especially directed toward youths, whereas the working group's text seemed to envision greater regulation of advertising and promotion in general. At the same time, whereas the working group, as noted earlier, seemed to ignore the cross-border advertising issue, this concern is specifically dealt with in the chair's draft. In any case, this plank of the convention has already drawn harsh criticism as being far too weak from the tobacco control community, which seeks a total worldwide ban on all advertising and promotion (e.g., American Lung Association 2001; Framework Convention Alliance 2001).

As a third example, while the working group called for opening up the legal processes of each nation to claims for compensation for injury from tobacco products, the chair's draft is deliberately silent on this issue, identifying it as something to be taken up by the negotiating body at a latter session. Already concerns have been raised in the tobacco control community that the industry will seek to use the framework convention as a device for buying it legal immunity worldwide—an expanded solution of the sort that the industry tried and failed to get in the United States.

As a fourth example, the chair's draft actually seems to be stronger and more specific in terms of strategies for dealing with smuggling. Yet here too critics have already complained that even better and more effective approaches to smuggling are available, based in particular upon a recently adopted Basel Convention dealing with the disposal of hazardous waste, which imposes an obligation on initial suppliers to take responsibility for products even after they have left their hands (ASH 2001).

Finally, the chair's draft includes as one of its guiding principles that "tobacco-control measures should not constitute a means of arbitrary or unjustifiable discrimination in international trade." Although this principle could have little bite, tobacco control advocates are up in arms that a provision such as this will be used to put free trade values ahead of public health values and will block efforts of individual nations from imposing additional tobacco control measures of their own. This flag has been raised notwithstanding the further guiding principle of the chair's draft that "the provisions of this Convention should be recognized as minimum standards, and Parties are encouraged to implement measured beyond those required by the Convention."

How the Treaty Approach Might Get Countries to Adopt Stronger and More Effective Tobacco Controls than They Would Without the Treaty

Whether the framework convention and protocols are a sweeping attempt to change domestic tobacco controls or a more limited attempt to address cross-border problems and domestic capacity building, the question remains: why might countries agree to measures they have not already either imposed on themselves or voluntarily adopted for the benefit of others?

The answer lies in the nature of international law making and the envisioned dynamic process that accompanies a framework convention and protocols approach. We can understand the distinctive ways an international process of this sort could result in progress on tobacco control if we consider the wide range of reasons why nations might agree to sign a tobacco control treaty.

First, consider the countries (several of which were noted earlier) that already have adopted comprehensive tobacco control regimes. They are probably most likely to sign the convention and all its protocols early on. After all, these nations (1) won't have to make many, if any, changes in national policy in order to comply, (2) will have "bragging" rights to say they have stepped up to do the "right thing" for public health, and (3) may genuinely benefit from the cross-border controls that are adopted. Indeed, it is perhaps not surprising that (despite some doubters within their own borders) the countries with strong tobacco control records have generally been among those urging the working group and the negotiating body to include tough requirements in the framework convention itself. Surely, treaty advocates have counted on countries like these all along to get something started, hoping that these pioneers would be willing to use some of their political and economic muscle to persuade others to join in.

A second type of country that would be drawn to sign the treaty early is a nation whose leaders would like to have tougher domestic tobacco control policies, but currently lack the capacity to impose and enforce such controls. As already noted, many advocates of the framework convention believe that it will help build that capacity, and several specific provisions suggested by the working group and the negotiating body that are targeted at that goal have already been were described. To repeat, the hope is that, over time, the convention's provisions will provide the needed training, expertise, and cash to support strong domestic tobacco control efforts—especially in developing nations (although whether richer nations will in fact provide cash remains to be seen). Support for the treaty along these lines is suggested by a declaration issued in March 2001 on behalf of 21 African nations following a meeting in Johannesburg of health officials.

Another way to think of the framework convention is as a political device for encouraging a group of nations to act in concert against the tobacco companies. The vision here is that, without the treaty, the industry is now able to immobilize weak governments one by one. But the solidarity of the treaty process (amplified by convention provisions relating to regular meetings, information exchange, and the like) may be a means of increasing the collective strength of these countries to resist the tobacco giants. Ironically, some counties in this group may be those with national tobacco industries who, their governments fear, are losing out in market competition with the international giants. These nations may now be afraid to impose tobacco controls that would harm the international companies because this could subject the country to free trade and other sanctions. But the framework convention may provide a more secure basis in international law for adopting those controls. Cooperative action along this dimension is suggested by an April 2001 agreement reached at meeting in Jakarta among health officials from eight Asian nations to support a total ban on cigarette advertising.

Third, from a "public choice" perspective, the internal politics of some countries might be influenced by the creation of the framework convention. That is, the political leverage of existing tobacco control supporters within a country (political entrepreneurs, leaders in key nongovernmental organizations, and important public health officials) may be enhanced by the process leading up to the adoption of the framework convention. The debate over the convention and its later adoption can help fairly powerful tobacco control advocates inside a country finally gain the upper hand, thereby facilitating the adoption of protocol requirements calling for additional domestic controls that would not be possible without the convention. Several aspects of the treaty might work in this direction. First, the convention and protocol process may establish international norms of "proper" regulation. This may give such norms more weight inside a country than they might have as mere WHO recommendations or policy positions of tobacco control advocates. In addition the visibility of the framework convention, the negotiations surrounding it, and the worldwide facts it brings to light through the convention-adoption process may help bring and keep tobacco control on the "front burner" as a domestic political matter in ways that would not happen without the treaty creation process. This too might tilt domestic politics in favor of committing to broader tobacco control than would otherwise be possible.

Fourth, countries facing specific tobacco control problems may be drawn to signing the treaty because of advantageous trade-offs within the terms of the tobacco control convention itself. That is, they would foresee more gain than loss from signing up. For example, Italy and Spain might agree to adopt new internal controls if they could get international help to fight their smuggling problems.

Fifth, once the framework convention is in place, even recalcitrant nations might be influenced to change their domestic policies over time. If there is a worldwide commitment to the tobacco problem, some nations can effectively be embarrassed into doing more domestically to control tobacco. The regular reporting requirements of the framework convention are intended to work in this direction by forcing the do-little signatories to lay bare both the extent of their tobacco problem and their failure to make progress in solving it. (This, of course, assumes that nations currently unwilling to embrace binding protocols will at least sign a framework convention that imposes reporting and meeting obligations.)

Easiest to influence in this way, perhaps, are nations that like to have a "good guy" international reputation. Many nations included in this group may have internal legal norms such that signing a treaty, even with binding promises included, yields few if any genuine legal consequences internally. For example, these countries may readily agree to adopt measures limiting youths' access to smoking but then not rigorously enforce them. Nonetheless, from the multinational perspective, even getting these "paper tigers" to sign the treaty (and perhaps some protocols) could be valuable. Eventually the treaty would allow these foot-dragger countries to be identified and isolated and thereby subject to further international pressures to fall in line.

One should not have great optimism about the United States ratifying the framework convention and its protocols. After all, the United States has not signed a number of other important treaties that have gained the support of most other nations—such as the treaties covering land mines or the rights of children. However, because of the ways the treaty-making process can shift internal political balances, as already discussed, even without formal ratification, the terms of a tobacco control convention and its protocols could have a positive influence upon internal U.S. policy.

Finally, some nations may embrace the convention and protocols because they are enticed or pressured into doing so. This happens all the time in the international law–making field. Sometimes, international organizations have some leverage points that can be used against recalcitrant member countries. Indeed, because of the leverage of the United Nations (UN), some initially favored having the UN rather than WHO take the lead on this effort. But it can be dicey, and perhaps illegal, for international organizations (whether the UN or WHA/WHO) openly and strongly to pressure countries into giving support to a new treaty. Think, for example, about a suggestion that the WHA should direct WHO to limit its support for the control of internal malaria problems or the cross-border spread of contagious diseases to nations that support the tobacco convention. Even if this were legal (which it might not be), this step is highly unlikely for the WHA to take. First, it is morally questionable, given who would be harmed if the threat is carried out; and second, it could create a logistical nightmare because it would invite a practice of reopening for renegotiation every international agreement each time a new one is put on the table.

It is one thing for avid tobacco control countries to campaign with words for others to follow their lead. It is another for them to make threats in other arenas, or offer sufficient bribes, to gain adherents. Nevertheless, in reality such efforts are probably necessary to gain certain nations' support. Indeed, some nations might secretly be welcoming the framework convention on tobacco control just because they will knowingly use it as an occasion to solicit and accept bribes.

In other world trade negotiations, for example, the United States was able to pressure China into adopting a domestic intellectual property law that would benefit U.S. companies because China did not want to lose access to the U.S. market. But, of course, it is by no means clear that the United States will be willing to exert any of its political or economic might in support of the WHO treaty. At the national level (as contrasted with the state and local levels), the United States has weak tobacco control laws—low taxes, few clean indoor air controls, limited advertising controls, and so on. Hence, the U.S. government hardly has a history of crusading for tobacco control. Moreover (or perhaps as an explanation of the former), Philip Morris and other U.S. tobacco companies have historically had considerable political power at the national level, and though that power may be eroding, the industry is still a strong presence in Washington.

Furthermore, American political entrepreneurs wanting to make a name for themselves in tobacco control are perhaps more likely to want to take on domestic issues (like giving the FDA control over tobacco products) than the WHO treaty. And because Japan's tobacco control record is even weaker than that of the United States, it looks as though the political muscle and economic grease for the treaty will come primarily from a combination of the European Union (which has adopted a strong European position on tobacco control) and former British colonies, such as Canada and Australia. What precisely these national groups will be willing and able to do to garner support from other countries remains to be seen.

The most talked-about "bribe" strategy so far concerns paying off poorer nations that are now large tobacco exporters by getting them to shift their agricultural investment to other crops. Zimbabwe and Malawi, especially, and Turkey and Brazil, secondarily, are significant exporters of unmanufactured tobacco that might be enticed into crop shifting. How much this would actually influence the worldwide supply of tobacco is another matter, however. The United States, China, India, and Italy, to give but some examples, are all also significant tobacco leaf exporters, many of which could readily increase production capacity if competitor nations dropped out of the business. Nonetheless, if the treaty deals with the plight of farmers in those poorer nations currently economically most dependent on tobacco growing, then at least one bothersome economic argument could be removed. In the end, however, other pressures and bribes may well be necessary.

If all (or even most) of these favorable possibilities fall into place, a strong tobacco control treaty could become a global reality in the next few years.

Risks

On the other hand, the framework convention on tobacco control could come to nothing, apart from the expenditure of WHO time and money. Now that the negotiating body has begun its work, it may well achieve consensus about the framework convention within the scheduled time period. But obtaining a consensus within the negotiating body is just a preliminary step. Whether the treaty will gain widespread ratification and actually result in substantial changes is still a question. And the risks of failure are significant.

It seems clear that the advocates for the convention are particularly concerned about the growth of tobacco-related health problems in developing nations. Many of the richer countries already have fairly strong tobacco controls in place, and many more will probably adopt such controls before too long even without the treaty; besides, tobacco consumption seems headed downward in most such countries (albeit at a much slower pace than tobacco control advocates would like). By contrast, developing countries have a much greater need for controls. Yet many of those countries have yet to experience the mounting number of tobacco-related deaths now common in richer nations. Moreover, many of them have other critical and immediate public health problems to worry about. Furthermore, in nations with short life expectancies and widespread poverty, measures that primarily prolong the lives of older people are not likely to have the highest priority. And, of course, the tobacco industry and its friends will do their best to prevent the adoption of a treaty, at least a treaty with any teeth at all (British American Tobacco 2000b; Scruton 2000).

From a numbers perspective, as with many international issues, high population nations such as China, India, Russia, and Indonesia are the key group on which to focus efforts at change, for by 2020 they are likely as a group to account for more than half of the death toll from tobacco outside the richer countries. Yet, as suggested before, these nations have many pressing problems in addition to the tobacco epidemic. Besides, when more than half of the men in a country smoke (as is now true in China, Russia, and Indonesia), the internal politics of tobacco control has tended to be much less promising. In countries with much stronger tobacco control programs today, men tend to smoke much less—such as Sweden, New Zealand, Australia, and Canada. Indeed, some have suggested that the causal direction of national tobacco control policy works primarily in this direction: that is, smoking reduction causes more tobacco control to be adopted than tobacco control causes smoking reduction. So far at least, leaders from China, India, Russia, and Indonesia have not made public their response to the WHO treaty effort (although China has joined the United States and Japan in asking for a sharp division between an aspirational framework convention and binding protocols).

Although the framework convention approach is designed to try to prevent the watering down problem that can plague comprehensive, fully binding treaties, obviously it will amount to much the same thing if, for example, most of the exporting countries refuse to sign the protocol regulating exports, or most of the countries responsible for smuggling problems refuse to sign that protocol.

A different problem is that a strong treaty would be signed by many nations that would then not comply (Chayes and Chayes 1995; Weiss and Jacobson 1998). For several other treaties, developing countries do not have splendid compliance records, even with reporting requirements. Often these countries do not have effective internal NGOs to pressure the government to meet its obligations, the press is weak or not interested, and, despite good intentions, the government is unable to deliver meaningful information about the state of its problem. Because this sort of noncompliance, based on the lack of an adequate infrastructure, could well plague the proposed tobacco control convention, its advocates are putting substantial emphasis on capacity building in developing countries.

Willful noncompliance is also a risk. Many nations could do a much better job, say, of reporting on their own internal human rights problems—but choose not to do so. Noncompliance could also happen with tobacco control for nations that weren't really keen to join in the first place but did so because of their wider agenda in the international community—or because the pro-tobacco forces regained political power that was temporarily lost around the ratifying of the treaty. All of this applies as well to countries that ratify protocols, but don't follow them in a meaningful way, either by adopting regulations with loopholes, by adopting regulations without sanctions, or by not enforcing their laws on the books. Tobacco control is especially problematic from this perspective because it requires changing the behavior of masses of ordinary citizens, and in many cases of large numbers of local businesses (e.g., around youths' access, advertising, and clear indoor air issues). This is very different from treaties with which the government can comply simply by getting government officials to go about their own business in new ways. Again, the working group and the negotiating body envision that these problems could be addressed through regular meetings of the signatories, in which these concerns may be aired and pressures brought to bear on nations to improve their compliance record; however, the long-term effect of these precautions is unclear.

Nevertheless, important progress could be achieved even if the WHO treaty suffered because many important countries refused to sign or signatories did not comply. After all, every country that imposes on itself stronger internal tobacco controls than it would have otherwise (or would have adopted only later on) would mean a public health plus. Some reduction in smuggling and cross-border ad leakage is better than none. And any gain in internal tobacco control infrastructure holds promise for the embrace of effective policies in the future.

Potential Implications for Tobacco-Related Disease Worldwide

Despite the concerns raised in the prior section, let us assume now that a strong framework convention and binding protocols were adopted and enforced by every nation in the world. What would be the impact on the worldwide toll of death and disease? That is, how much and how rapidly would such a treaty actually curtail the prevalence of smoking?

Controls that have a specific cross-border focus are likely to have relatively little direct impact. That is not to say they are unimportant, only that these measures need to be put in context. Suppose, for example, there was no more tobacco smuggling and no more leakage of outside advertising inside countries. By itself, this would surely reduce smoking only by a little in most places. If, as in a typical country, 5% of the cigarettes are now smuggled in and sell for a somewhat lower price on the street, the elimination of that supply could be readily replaced with legitimate sources, and the price effect on consumption would surely be modest. This would also be true even where a much higher share of the retail market is dominated by smuggled products (e.g., 20%), unless the price discount for those products is extremely large. In fact, the most important consequence of wiping out smuggling could well be to enhance the political will to stick with high domestic tobacco taxes; that indirect impact could, of course, be quite significant. A similar point applies to advertising from outside that evades internal bans. By themselves, these ads can have but a small impact on smoking levels, so, in turn, the direct consequence of their elimination cannot be great. But, again, if these ads are successfully kept out, a nation might be more willing to impose and enforce stronger internal ad bans that could have a greater impact.

Nevertheless, international experience to date also makes me cautious about how optimistic tobacco control advocates should be about the effectiveness of the domestic controls envisioned by the treaty. This caution derives from the fact that most of the nations that currently have strong comprehensive tobacco control programs still have significant smoking rates. I do not mean to say that tobacco control programs don't work or aren't well worth it from a cost-benefit perspective (National Academy of Sciences 2000). After all, a 10% reduction in deaths from smoking-related diseases by the year 2020 would mean more than 800,000 fewer deaths—a very large number indeed. And reducing the adult smoking rate worldwide below 20% would have an even greater positive long-run impact on public health. Nonetheless, my point is that one must be realistic about how far domestic tobacco control policies can directly bring about change. It is hard to find any nation with a strong tobacco control regime that by the year 2001 has moved its smoking prevalence rate below 20% (it appears that Sweden has finally achieve this goal [AP 1999]).

Moreover, one must face the fact that some countries with relatively weaker tobacco control regimes—such as the United States—have smoking rates that are generally no higher, or at times even lower, than similar nations with strong controls. Of course, the United States might have an even lower smoking rate were its controls tougher. After all, California, which has adopted significantly stronger controls than the United States on average, also has a substantially lower smoking rate among its citizens than among the nation as a whole. Still, it is unclear how much of this difference is due to tobacco control policies and how much is due to the state's "healthy lifestyle" culture.

From the international cultural perspective, it would be a mistake to draw many conclusions from the tobacco control experience of the rich Western countries. As noted at the outset of this chapter, in many developing countries, the greatest challenge from the tobacco control perspective may be keeping women from starting to smoke. But whatever the cultural norms are that create these vast gender differences, it is by no means clear that they can be directly and dramatically influenced by the levers available through tobacco control policy. Indeed, to the extent that other ongoing international efforts are aimed at creating greater wealth and equality in today's developing nations, substantial tobacco control efforts may be required to prevent the overall adult smoking prevalence rate from escalating.

That having been said, the proposed WHO treaty should be seen in the context of the wider cultural perspective. What is really needed is a global sea change in the social norms around smoking. This has in fact happened in many upper-middle-class and professional-class communities in the United States and elsewhere. In these circles, smoking is basically unacceptable; smokers are thought to be foolish and perhaps pitied; smoking is decidedly not cool; and as the social norms have changed, smoking rates have dropped dramatically, down to below 10% in such groups. Can these norms be embraced worldwide? It is by no means clear. But, over time, the proposed WHO treaty, both directly and indirectly, could indeed help promote changed social norms about tobacco, and perhaps therein lies its greatest hope.

NOTE

1. In India today, unlike most other high-consumption nations, tobacco is significantly consumed as bidis and as smokeless tobacco, and not as manufactured cigarettes. Bidis are made from a small amount of tobacco wrapped in a tembruni leaf. In 1992, for example, 20% of the tobacco (by weight) consumed in India was in the form of manufactured cigarettes as compared with 40% in the form of bidis. Despite their small size compared to cigarettes, bidis are thought to deliver at least the same levels of tar and carbon monoxide to their smokers.

REFERENCES

Abedian, I., R. van der Merwe, N. Wilkins, and P. Jha, eds. 1998. *The Economics of Tobacco Control: Towards an Optimal Policy Mix.* Cape Town, South Africa: Applied Fiscal Research Centre.

Ad Hoc Inter-Agency Task Force on Tobacco Control. 2000. *Report of the Secretary-General.* UNESCO Substantive Session of 2000, May 1.

Action on Smoking and Health (ASH). 2000. Online. Available: http://www.ash.org.uk.

———. 2001. Overview of the chair's text. March Online: Available: http://www. ash.org.uk/?international

American Lung Association Action Alert. Online. Available: *http://www.lungusa.org*

Associated Press (AP). 1999. *Sweden tobacco use declines.* Sept. 17.

British American Tobacco. 2000a. *Smuggling: Our view.* Online. Available: http:// www.bat.com.

———. 2000b. *The WHO Framework Convention on Tobacco Control: Our view.* Online. Available: http://www.bat.com.

Bettcher, D. 1998. WHO Framework Convention on Tobacco Control (FCTC): An accelerated workplan. Background document for presentation to the WHO Framework Convention on Tobacco Control: Meeting of Public Health Experts, 2 December.

Bloom, J. L. 1998. *International interests in U.S. tobacco legislation.* Health Science Analysis Project, Policy Analysis No. 3. Washington, DC: Advocacy Institute. Available: http://scarcnet.org/hsap/international.htm

Bodansky, D. 1998. *The framework convention/protocol approach: The experience of international environmental regimes.* Background paper for the proposed International Framework Convention on Tobacco Control, November.

Campaign Center for Tobacco-Free Kids. 2000. Online. Available: http://www. tobaccofreekids.org.

Chaloupka, F., and A. Laixuthai. 1996. *U.S. trade policy and cigarette smoking in Asia.* National Bureau of Economic Research, Working Paper 5543.

Chayes, A., and A. H. Chayes. 1995. *The New Sovereignty: Compliance with International Regulatory Agreements.* Cambridge, MA: Harvard University Press.

Chollat-Traquet, C. 1996. *Evaluating Tobacco Control Activities: Experiences and Guiding Principles.* Geneva: World Health Organization.

Council on Scientific Affairs. 1990. The worldwide smoking epidemic: Tobacco trade, use, and control. *JAMA* 263:3312–18.

Filder, D. P. 1998. The future of the World Health Organization: What role for international law? *Vanderbilt Journal of Transnational Law* 31:1079–1126.

Framework Convention Alliance. 2001. Briefing paper for the 2nd meeting of the intergovernmental negotiating body of the Framework Convention on Tobacco Control, comments on the chair's draft. March. Online. Available: http:// www.fctc.org

Galbraith, J. W., and M. Kaiserman. 1997. Taxation, smuggling and demand for cigarettes in Canada. *Journal of Health Economics* 16:287–301.

Hammond, R. 1998. *Addicted to Profit: Big Tobacco's Expanding Global Reach.* Washington, DC: Essential Action.

Holzman, D. 1997. Tobacco abroad: Infiltrating foreign markets. *Environmental Health Perspectives* 103:178–83.

INFACT. 1998. *Mobilizing NGOs and the media behind the International Framework Convention on Tobacco Control: Experiences from breast-milk substitutes, landmines, environmental codes and conventions.* Background paper, Tobacco Free Initiative, World Health Organization.

International Consortium of Investigative Journalists. 2001.Tobacco companies linked to criminal organizations in lucrative cigarette smuggling. Online Available: http://www.publici.org

International Union Against Cancer (UICC). 2000. *Tobacco and cancer programme.* Online. Available: http://uicc.ch/toba.

Joossens, L. 1998. *Improving public health through an International Framework Convention for Tobacco Control.* Background Paper, Tobacco Free Initiative, World Health Organization.

Joossens, L., and M. Raw. 1995. Smuggling and cross border shopping of tobacco in Europe. *British Medical Journal* 310:1393–97.

Levin, M. A. 1997. Smoke around the rising sun: An American look at tobacco regulation in Japan. *Stanford Law & Policy Rev* 8:99–123.

Levy, R., and R. Marimont. 1998. Lies, damned lies, and 400,000 smoking-related deaths. *Regulation* 21:24–9.

Lukachko, A. M., and E. M. Whelan. 1999. A critical assessment of "Lies, damned lies, & 400,000 smoking-related deaths." Online. Available: http://www.acsh.org/ publications/reports/cato99.html.

National Academy of Sciences. 2000. *State Programs Can Reduce Tobacco Use.* National Cancer Policy Board and Board on Health Promotion and Disease Prevention. Online. Available: http://books.nap.edu/catalog/9762.html.

Osaki, Y., K. Kawaminami, and M. Minowa. Forthcoming. Estimating adolescent cigarette consumption in Japan. *Journal of Epidemiology.*

Peto, R., A. D. Lopez, J. Boreham, M. Thun, and C. Heath, Jr. 1992. Mortality from tobacco in developed countries: Indirect estimation from national vital statistics. *Lancet* 339:1268–78.

———. 1996. Mortality from smoking worldwide. *British Medical Bulletin* 52:12–21.

Roemer, R. 1993. *Legislative Action to Combat the World Tobacco Epidemic.* 2d ed. Geneva: World Health Organization.

Sasamoto, T. n.d. *National policy on tobacco control in Japan.* Health Promotion and Nutrition Division, Ministry of Health and Welfare, Japan.

Scruton, R. 2000. *WHO, what and why? Trans-national government, legitimacy and the World Health Organisation.* Occasional Paper 113. London: Institute of Economic Affairs.

Smoking and Health Action Foundation and Non-Smokers' Right Association. 2000. Comments on draft elements of the WHO Framework Convention on Tobacco Control. Submission to *Health Canada.* Available: http://www.nsra-andf/ca/english/FCTC-NSRA.html. March 16.

Taylor, A. L. 1996. An international regulatory strategy for global tobacco control. *Yale Journal of International Law.* 21:257–304.

Taylor, A. L., and D. Bodansky. 1998. *The development of the WHO Framework Convention on Tobacco Control: Legal and policy considerations.* Background Paper, Tobacco Free Initiative, World Health Organization.

Taylor, A., F. J. Chaloupka, E. Guindon, and M. Corbett. 2000. The impact of trade liberalization on tobacco consumption. In *Tobacco Control in Developing Countries.* Edited by P. Jha and F. Chaloupka. Oxford: Oxford University Press. 343–64.

Tobacco Free Initiative. 1998. *Rationale, Update and Progress.* Online. Available: http://www.who.int/toh/. World Health Organization, December.

Tren, R., and H. High. 2000. *Smoked Out: Anti-Tobacco Activism at the World Bank.* Online. Available: http://www.iea.org.uk/wpapers/smokeout.htm. London: Institute of Economic Affairs.

Watanabe, B. 1997. *Smoking in Japan—1997 Profile.* Tokyo: Tobacco Problems Information Center.

Weiss, E. B., and H. K. Jacobson, eds. 1998. *Engaging Countries: Strengthening Compliance with International Environmental Accords.* Cambridge, MA.: MIT Press.

Weissman, R., and R. Hammond. 1998. In focus: International tobacco sales. 3 *U.S. Foreign Policy in Focus* 3, no. 17. Available: http://www.foreignpolicy-infocus.org.

World Health Assembly (WHA). 1998. *World Health Assembly paves way for Framework Convention on Tobacco Control.* Press Release, May 24. Online. Available: http://www.who.int/inf-pr-1999/en/pr99-wha14.html.

World Bank. 1999. *Curbing the Epidemic: Governments and the Economics of Tobacco Control.* Washington, DC: World Bank.

World Health Organization (WHO). 1997. *Tobacco or Health: A global Status Report.* Geneva: World Health Organization.

———. 1998. *Guidelines for Controlling and Monitoring the Tobacco Epidemic.* Geneva: World Health Organization.

———. 1999a. First meeting of the Working Group on the WHO Framework Convention on Tobacco Control, subjects of possible protocols and their relation to the Framework Convention on Tobacco Control. Provisional Agenda Item 8. World Health Organization, September 3.

———. 1999b. Report of the first meeting of the Working Group on the WHO Framework Convention on Tobacco Control. World Health Organization, October 28.

———. 2000a. Second meeting of the Working Group on the WHO Framework Convention on Tobacco Control. Annotated Provisional Agenda. World Health Organization, February 14.

———. 2000b. Second meeting of the Working Group on the WHO Framework Convention on Tobacco Control. Provisional texts of proposed draft elements for a WHO Framework Convention on Tobacco Control. Provisional Agenda Item 5. World Health Organization, February 29.

———. 2000c. Second meeting of the Working Group on the WHO Framework Convention on Tobacco Control. Secretariat update on progress since the first meeting of the Working Group. Provisional Agenda Item 4. World Health Organization. March 3.

———. 2000d. Second meeting of the Working Group on the WHO Framework Convention on Tobacco Control. Brief overview of discussion on 27th and 28th March. World Health Organization, March 28.

———. 2000e. Working Group on the WHO Framework Convention on Tobacco Control. Report of the second meeting of the Working Group. World Health Organization, April 26.

———. 2000f. Fifth-Third World Health Assembly, WHO Framework Convention on Tobacco Control, Report of the Working Group, WHO (Provisional Agenda Item 12.10, April 26, 2000 and with Corrigendum May 11, 2000).

———. 2001. Chair's text of a framework convention on tobacco control. January 9.

WHO Fact Sheets. 1996. *The Tobacco Epidemic: A Global Public Health Emergency.* N188. Online. Available: http://www.who.int/inf-fs/en/fact.html. May.

———. 1998a. *Governments for a Tobacco-Free World.* N159. Online. Available: http://www.who.int/inf-fs/en/fact.html. May.

———. 1998b. *Tobacco Epidemic: Health Dimensions.* N154. Online. Available: http://www.who.int/inf-fs/en/fact.html. May.

———. 1998c. *Tobacco Epidemic: Much More Than a Health Issue.* N155. Online. Available: http://www.who.int/inf-fs/en/fact.html. May.

World's best practice in tobacco control. 2000. *Tobacco Control* 9:228. Available: http://www.bmjpg.com/data/tob.htm.

Yach, D. 1995. Progress in achieving international tobacco control: Output of the 48th World Health Assembly, Geneva, May 1995. *Tobacco Control* 4:278–301.

Yach, D., and D. Bettcher. 2000. Globalisation of tobacco industry influence and new global responses. *Tobacco Control* 9:206–16.

Index